The Archaeology of
Disease

Dedicated to
Ann Manchester and
Ann Hunter

The Archaeology of Disease

THIRD EDITION

CHARLOTTE ROBERTS AND
KEITH MANCHESTER

CORNELL UNIVERSITY PRESS
ITHACA, NEW YORK

Third edition copyright © Charlotte Roberts and Keith Manchester, 2005

The authors have asserted the moral right to be identified as the authors of this work.

First published in this third edition in the United States of America in 2005 by Cornell University Press.

First printing, Cornell Paperbacks, 2007

Second edition first published in the United States of America in 1995 by Cornell University Press.

ISBN-13: 978-0-8014-7388-3 (pbk.)

Librarians: A CIP catalog record for this book is available from the Library of Congress.

Contents

7 Infectious Disease   164

8 Metabolic and Endocrine Disease   221

9 Neoplastic Disease   252

Acknowledgements

The authors would like to thank the following for their help in the production of this edition of *The Archaeology of Disease*: Ann Manchester and Stewart Gardner, for their understanding and tolerance; and the University of Durham, for allowing the first author the time fully to revise this edition. Many of the illustrations that are not credited to specific people were produced by Jean Brown (formerly of the University of Bradford, Department of Archaeological Sciences) or the first author; Jean's enthusiasm, understanding and dedication to the photography of human remains are gratefully acknowledged. The authors would also like to thank Johs Andersen, Arnold Aspinall, Cecil Hackett, William Jopling, Don Ortner and Freddie Wells for their guidance and encouragement for previous editions of this book, and Don for his continued help.

The illustrations were further enhanced by many colleagues providing us with permission to use some of their photographs. Particular thanks go to Art Aufderheide (University of Minnesota-Duluth), Pia Bennike (University of Copenhagen) (including on behalf of the Museum of Medical History, Copenhagen), Wilbert Bouts, Patricia Bridges (Queen's College, City University of New York), Domingo Campillo (University Autonoma de Barcelona), Peter Davies (Cardiothoracic Centre, Liverpool), Ian Dewhirst, Diane France (France Castings, Colorado), Anne Grauer (Loyola University of Chicago), Diane Hawkey (Arizona State University), Robert Jurmain (San Jose State University), Lynn Kilgore (University of Colorado, Boulder), George Maat (Leiden University), Charles Merbs (Arizona State University), Northumberland Health Authority and the Secretary of State for Health, England, Don Ortner (Smithsonian Institution), the late Juliet Rogers (Rheumatology Unit, Bristol Royal Infirmary, Bristol), Tony Waldron (Institute of Archaeology, London), and the late Calvin Wells for his tremendous slide collection, curated at the University of Bradford. Other institutions that have allowed the use of illustrations are: Reading Museum, Berkshire, England, the Royal College of Surgeons, London, the Science Museum, Science and Society Picture Library, London, and York Archaeological Trust.

The authors are grateful to a number of archaeological organizations for the provision of skeletal material, curated at the University of Bradford and the University of Durham. This material has provided invaluable data and illustrations for this book. Particular thanks are due to Malcolm Watkins (Gloucester City Museum; Gloucester cemeteries), Malcolm Atkin (formerly of

Gloucester Archaeology Unit, now Hereford and Worcester Archaeology Unit; Gloucester cemeteries), Northamptonshire Heritage (Raunds, Northamptonshire), Alec Detsicas (Eccles, Kent), John Magilton (Southern Archaeology and Chichester District Council; Chichester cemetery), Gil Burleigh (Letchworth Museum, Baldock; Baldock cemeteries), York Archaeological Trust (Ripon Cathedral) and Rosemary Cramp (Jarrow cemetery).

Finally, the authors would like to thank the numerous people at Sutton Publishing who have brought this third edition to fruition. Any mistakes in this book are the responsibility of the authors alone.

The Archaeology of
Disease

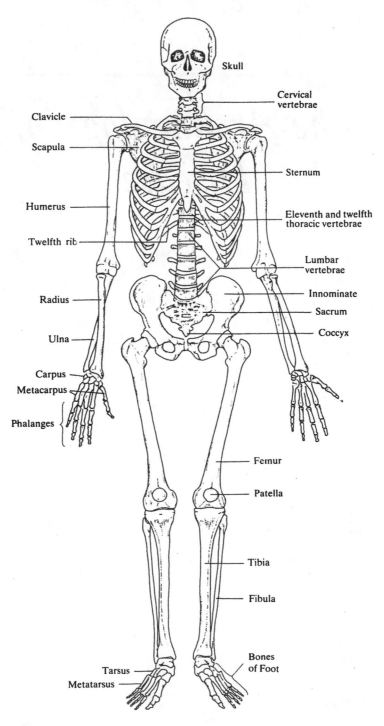

Skull

Cervical
vertebrae

Clavicle

Scapula

Sternum

Humerus

Eleventh and twelfth
thoracic vertebrae

Twelfth rib

Lumbar
vertebrae

Radius

Innominate

Sacrum

Ulna

Coccyx

Carpus

Metacarpus

Phalanges

Femur

Patella

Tibia

Fibula

Bones
of Foot

Tarsus

Metatarsus

The human skeleton.

CHAPTER 1

The Study of Palaeopathology

Disease is an inevitable part of life, and coping with disease is a universal aspect of the human experience . . . the experience of disease . . . is as inescapable as death itself. (Brown *et al.*, 1996: 183)

INTRODUCTION AND DEFINITIONS

The study of palaeopathology examines the evolution and progress of disease through long periods of time and looks at how humans adapted to changes in their environment. It provides primary evidence for the state of health of our ancestors and, combining biological and cultural data (the 'biocultural approach'), palaeopathology has become a wide-ranging holistic discipline. Current developments, and the future of palaeopathology, are exciting and are discussed further in the final chapter of this book.

Pathology is the study (*logos*) of suffering (*pathos*). In practice, pathology is defined as the scientific study of disease processes. Palaeopathology was defined in 1910 by Sir Marc Armand Ruffer (Aufderheide and Rodríguez-Martín, 1998) as the science of diseases whose existence can be demonstrated on the basis of human and animal remains from ancient times. Palaeopathology can be considered a subdiscipline of biological anthropology and focuses on abnormal variation in human remains from archaeological sites. The study of palaeopathology is multidisciplinary in approach and concentrates on primary and secondary sources of evidence. Primary evidence derives from skeletons or mummified remains. This type of evidence is the only reliable indication that a once-living person suffered from a health problem; whether a specific diagnosis can be made is more of a challenge. However, as Horden (2000: 208) indicates, palaeopathology 'would seem to provide our . . . hardest evidence for past afflictions'. Secondary forms of evidence include documentary and iconographic (art form) data contemporary with the time period under investigation. Unfortunately, artists and authors in the past have tended to illustrate and describe the more visual and dramatic diseases and ignored those which may have been more commonplace; the mundane, common illnesses and injuries are lost to the palaeopathologist if this type of evidence is considered alone. For example, the mutilating deformities of the infection leprosy, the devastating effects of the Black Death, and the curiosity factor in dwarfism have led to abundant representations of these conditions in art, but coughs, colds, influenza and gastrointestinal upsets, along with cuts, bruises, burns and sprains, would probably have been so common that they would have been 'irrelevant' in the eyes of the writer or artist. In antiquity, those diseases with the greatest impact in terms of mortality, personal disfigurement or social and economic disruption probably evoked the greatest response from society (and its authors and artists). In the past, attitudes towards illness have often been due to the failure in understanding the nature of the disease itself. However, when interpreting disease in the past from secondary sources care must be taken – opinions and preferences about what should be described and drawn will affect what is read and seen. Imprecise and incomplete representation may transmit incorrect information. All literary works must be studied carefully within the traditional framework in which their facts are presented (Roberts, 1971). Those aspects of an illness which we consider to be of vital importance in the understanding of a disease may have been considered of no consequence to the observer in the past and may not therefore have been given due prominence in the record. There are also circumstances where a disease description does not correspond with any known disease in the modern world. This may be because it actually does not exist or the disease is just not recognized because of the inaccuracy of its representation. Relevant too is the need to appreciate that different diseases may produce similar signs and symptoms. For example, how does one differentiate between the skin rash of chickenpox, leprosy and measles? It is true to say that specific areas of the body may be affected by the different conditions, and the nature of the 'lesion' may differ, but to be able to determine what disease is being displayed in writing or art necessitates a very detailed representation. Another example is the clinical picture associated with respiratory disease. Cancer, chronic bronchitis and tuberculosis can all result in coughing up blood (haemoptysis) and shortness of breath (dyspnoea), but how would they be distinguished from one another in the written record if only haemoptysis and dyspnoea were being described? However, the diseases which are not displayed in the skeletal record, i.e. those affecting only the soft tissue (e.g. malaria, childhood diseases such as whooping cough and mumps, cholera and typhoid), may be recorded only in art and documentary sources, and therefore, in these cases, this type of evidence is especially invaluable. We do recognize that solely considering skeletal remains for the evidence of disease allows us to deal with only a very small percentage of the disease load in a population. However, as Horden (2000: 208) states: 'the greater the number and variety of perspectives on the pathological past with which we can engage, the greater the chance that our analysis will not be completely disabled by problems of retrospective diagnosis.'

The study of human remains within their cultural context, i.e. the period of time, geographic area and material culture, aids enormously in the interpretation of the history of disease. For example, precise dating of skeletons with bone changes consistent with venereal syphilis is important for the discussion of the pre- or post-Columbian nature and origin for this disease (Baker and Armelagos, 1988; Dutour *et al.*, 1994). Some researchers also study populations in geographic areas which sustain contemporary traditional societies (e.g. Merbs, 1983; see McElroy and Townsend, 1996 on medical anthropology). Medical anthropology has been likened to palaeopathology because it considers disease within the population's context of living environment, diet, economy, work, etc. For palaeopathologists it is useful to interpret the archaeological (dead) population in the context of the living group if it is accepted that the latter bears close resemblances, in terms of culture, to the dead population. Of course, there are many limitations to this type of study, not least the vast differences in time and space between the living and dead populations in many cases. However, these societies are often unaffected by change (in the modern western sense) and their health and the effect of disease on their bodies is 'natural' and not influenced or changed by drug therapy. They can be, thus, useful analogues although very few societies today are immune to 'alien influences'. Nevertheless, appreciating how 'traditional' groups of people today perceive an illness, its causes and how it may be prevented undoubtedly broadens our horizons when we try to understand the impact of disease on past populations (for example, see Roberts and Buikstra, 2003).

HISTORY OF STUDY

Aufderheide and Rodríguez-Martín (1998) categorize the history of the development of palaeopathology into four phases: Antecedent (Renaissance to mid-nineteenth century), Genesis (mid-nineteenth century to First World War), Interbellum Consolidation Phase (1913–45) and New Palaeopathology (1946 to present). In the first phase work concentrated mainly on prehistoric animals (e.g. by the German naturalist Johann Friederich Esper), but there was a recognition that studying human disease would be beneficial to exploring the history of past human populations. At the end of this period the first application of the microscope to examining Egyptian mummified tissue is noted, but there was 'little scientific precision and . . . specimens (were viewed) as curiosities, not as sources of medical, pathological or historical knowledge' (Aufderheide and Rodríguez-Martín, 1998: 3). The second phase had much more of an anthropological focus, and large skeletal collections were available for study. As Aufderheide and Rodríguez-Martín (1998) point out, although 'racial' studies were the norm, pathological conditions in these collections were noted, especially by the German physician Rudolf Virchow (1821–1902). Again, it was mainly case studies that were reported and there was little consideration of what the occurrence of disease meant in epidemiological terms. Although cases provide information on, for example, the first occurrence of a disease, they are limited in providing broader views on the history of disease. Jarcho (1966: 5) also notes that researchers were so obsessed with crania they assumed 'that some diseases ended in the foramen magnum'. Happily, the study of palaeopathology today is such that students do now know that the whole of the skeleton (or as complete as possible) needs to be considered in disease diagnosis. However, as Buikstra and Cook note (1980: 435): 'we learn[t] little about population dynamics or disease evolution' from case studies. Focusing on individual experience of disease in both modern and ancient contexts can quickly lead to biased and 'patient'-centred data that may not represent the population experience from which that person derived. The French were instrumental from the late nineteenth century in developing the discipline of palaeopathology (e.g. Paul Broca, 1824–80, who published work particularly on the evidence for Peruvian trepanation (Buikstra and Cook, 1980)). At this time, too, the first palaeopathology manual was published in America in 1886 by William Whitney.

In the third phase palaeopathology expanded and methods beyond visual (macroscopic) examination were used more often to investigate pathological lesions and improve diagnosis, in addition to statistical analysis (Buikstra and Cook, 1980). This is described as the evolution of palaeopathology as a scientific discipline. Sir Marc Armand Ruffer (1858–1917) promoted the term 'palaeopathology' as defining the scientific study of disease observed in human and animal remains. A trained physician and Professor of Medicine in Cairo, Egypt, he made detailed records of his observations particularly on mummified remains (e.g. Ruffer, 1913 in Aufderheide and Rodríguez-Martín, 1998), although, as Aufderheide and Rodríguez-Martín (1998) note, the interest in mummies then waned. Other work in Egypt came from the enormous efforts of Grafton Elliot-Smith and Frederic Wood Jones (1910; Waldron, 2000), both trained physicians, and in the early twentieth century Roy Lee Moodie in North America published two very influential books on palaeopathology (Moodie, 1923a and b, cited in Aufderheide and Rodríguez-Martín, 1998). Aleš Hrdlička was also instrumental in the development of palaeopathological studies in the Americas (1941). Located at the Smithsonian Institution (National Museum of Natural History), he created a Division of Anthropology there and accumulated large skeletal collections from North and South America for study. In tandem, Earnest Hooton of Harvard University introduced a demographic perspective to palaeopathology and used an ecological and cultural approach (and statistical analysis) to understand the disease load in the Pecos Pueblo population (1930, in Aufderheide and Rodríguez-Martín, 1998). He also advocated the accumulation of pathological specimens with known histories as a tool for comparison with the past. Aufderheide and Rodríguez-Martín (1998: 7) note that this third phase is characterized by the 'introduction and gradual standardization both of new methods and of new interpretive concepts, resulting in the emergence of palaeopathology as a scientific discipline'.

The final phase is marked by an increased recognition of the link between palaeopathology and epidemiology and demography (Aufderheide and Rodríguez-Martín, 1998), with much more of a focus on raising hypotheses and testing them with skeletal data from large numbers of individuals. Wood et al. (1992: 344) also note that in the 1980s and early 1990s there was a move away from 'a particularistic concern with individual lesions or skeletons to a population-based perspective on disease processes'. Notable figures in the exploration of specific diseases early in the second half of the twentieth century included Møller-Christensen (1967) on leprosy and Hackett (1963) on the treponematoses. There has also been a focus on developing standardised methods for collecting palaeopathological data (Ortner, 1991, 1994; Lovell, 2000). Additionally, the use of biomolecular methods of analysis to identify diseases, primarily the extraction, amplification and analysis of ancient DNA specific to pathogens, has seen a considerable increase in use since the early 1990s.

The Paleopathology Club, later the Paleopathology Association, was formed in 1973 and the first meeting was held in 1974 (and the first European meeting a year later in London). This still thriving Association of several hundred members worldwide brings together people interested in, and studying, palaeopathology from a wide range of disciplines including anthropology, archaeology, medical history, medicine, pathology, genetics, biology and many more. Additionally, the World Committee on Mummy Studies, formed in 1992 after the first World Mummy Congress, 'looks after' the interests of people researching mummies, although the Paleopathology Association encompasses many of the same members. A survey of the membership of the American Association of Physical Anthropologists shows that palaeopathology as a field of physical (or biological) anthropology remains a prominent area for Ph.D. study, although not as popular as human evolution and human biological variation. It also showed that the majority of people practising palaeopathology were female, a feature that increased from the 1970s into the 1990s (Turner, 2002).

In Britain some key people in the development of palaeopathology as a discipline have included Calvin Wells (1964a), Don Brothwell and Andrew Sandison (1967), Juliet Rogers (Rogers and Waldron, 1995), Simon Hillson (1986, 1996), Theya Molleson (Molleson and Cox, 1993) and Tony Waldron (1994). However, as Mays (1997) notes, when comparing the publication content of US and UK researchers in palaeopathology, the emphasis in the UK is on 'case studies of health', whereas in the United States it is on 'population' health. In order that palaeopathology advances as a recognized discipline, the UK needs to turn more to this population approach to palaeopathology. North America, being a larger country with more research in palaeopathology being undertaken, has also seen a much longer history of study. Notable researchers here include: J. Lawrence Angel (1966a), George Armelagos (1990), Arthur Aufderheide (Aufderheide and Rodríguez-Martín, 1998), Jane Buikstra (1981), Della Cook (1994), Alan Goodman (Goodman et al., 1988), Anne Grauer (1993), Robert Jurmain (1999), Clark Larsen (1997), John Lukacs (1989), Charles Merbs (1983), Don Ortner (Ortner, 2003), Doug Owsley (1994), Mary Powell (1988), Doug Ubelaker (1989) and Phil Walker (1997). This list is of course not all-inclusive but is meant to show the main publishers of work in the field.

WORKING FROM A CLINICAL BASE

The study of palaeopathology naturally starts with understanding how disease affects the body in the modern clinical sense and, more specifically, the skeleton, since most of the human-derived material palaeopathologists work with is skeletonized. It is only after this stage that this knowledge can be applied to an archaeological context. However, this process is not quite so straightforward as we might hope. For example, the classic appearance and distribution of rheumatoid arthritis in the skeleton, described in clinical texts, may not always 'fit' what we may see in an archaeologically derived skeleton. Some features may be the same, but there may be differences; however, this does not mean 'our skeleton' did not have rheumatoid arthritis. There is certainly an assumption (not necessarily correct) that the bone changes have not altered during the evolution of the disease, but we cannot be certain. Additionally, there may be skeletal changes associated with a disease in the past that are not described clinically. We must also be aware that there may have been less virulent forms of a disease in the past compared to the present (or vice versa) that would have affected the eventual impact on the skeleton. Finally, while very subtle bone changes may be associated with disease in a living person, radiographic techniques may not identify these changes, and therefore they would not be described; in an archaeologically derived skeleton we see the bone changes but some may be puzzling when we do not see them described clinically. There are certainly some advantages to studying dry bones. But why should palaeopathology be studied?

The discipline provides a tool for investigating how people interacted with their environment and adapted to it over many thousands of years. Conversely, in modern studies of disease in living people, a doctor may only be considering a patient's progress over a few weeks, months or years. Thus, very detailed knowledge may be gained of a patient's (or group of patients') experience of a disease and the underlying reasons for its appearance. However, by considering longer periods of time we might explore major alterations in disease patterning which could have been influenced by climate and environmental change, or by significant changes in economy, housing and occupation. The disease processes studied in palaeopathology reflect the condition as seen on the skeleton or soft tissues without any influence from drug therapy, or the chronic form of the disease. What is observed is the record of a person's dental and skeletal health at the time of death. While some disease manifestations may be recognized as 'active' at death (and possibly an indicator of cause of death), most represent health insults over the period of the person's life. However, rarely can age at first occurrence of a disease be identified, because the changes observed are usually chronic, healed and long-standing. It is also possible that some disease processes today may not have been present in the past and, likewise, some pathological processes may have been present in the past but not seen today. For example, rheumatoid arthritis is a common condition today but in the archaeological record there are few convincing examples (Kilgore, 1989; Waldron and Rogers, 1994). There may be several reasons for its absence: non-diagnosis due to non-recognition, confusion with another joint disease or the fact that it really was rare in the past. It is a disease whose aetiology (cause) is ill understood. Climate, diet and environment may all have their part to play but may not, because they were different in the past, have predisposed populations to the disease.

Palaeopathology may also contribute to knowledge in modern medicine. For example, Møller-Christensen's work in the 1950s and 1960s on the skeletons buried in Medieval Danish leprosy hospital cemeteries highlighted a number of bone lesions characteristic of leprosy which had not been recognized by clinical leprologists at that time (Møller-Christensen, 1953); this work helped to identify skeletal changes of leprosy in living leprosy sufferers. A second example can be illustrated in a study by Rogers *et al.* (1990) where a palaeopathologist's and a radiologist's observations were compared. The bone changes of joint disease were recorded for twenty-four knee joints macroscopically by the palaeopathologist and radiographically by the radiologist. The results showed that subtle bone changes were not observed by the radiologist but the palaeopathologist could, on the basis of her findings, diagnose the early stages of osteoarthritis. This study was instructive in that it may explain why people today who suffer joint pain do not show radiographic osteoarthritic changes.

METHODS OF STUDY AND TISSUE CHANGE

The methods of study in palaeopathology range quite widely but usually, primarily, rely on macroscopic or visual observation and description of abnormal changes seen in skeletal remains. A description of these changes and their distribution in the skeleton or soft tissues is a prerequisite to attempting a diagnosis of the disease process being observed although, as Waldron (1994: Table 3.2) points out, diagnosis in modern contexts is difficult even with the array of diagnostic tests available. Some attempts at developing new methods of diagnosis are being explored currently (Byers and Roberts, 2003). In our description it is important to use unambiguous terminology so that readers and future workers who may wish to use these data understand its meaning, especially if they are to reinterpret the data, which may lead to a different disease diagnosis. Unfortunately, the clinical and palaeopathological literature abounds with terms describing different changes in disease, and, unless a common set of terms is used and agreed upon, there can be little hope of comparative studies of palaeopathological data on a global perspective. Buikstra and Ubelaker (1994) have gone some way towards addressing methodological standardization in palaeopathology, the British Association of Biological Anthropologists also has a similar document for use on British-derived skeletal material (Brickley and McKinley, 2004), and the 'Health in Europe Project' overseen by Richard Steckel, Clark Larsen and Philip Walker also aims to standardize the recording of thousands of skeletons so that comparative research can be undertaken.

The bone changes seen in palaeopathology usually represent chronicity, i.e. the individual adapted to the problem and the body reacted to it by forming and/or destroying bone. These people survived the acute phase of the disease and progressed into the chronic stage. An individual with skeletal abnormalities may therefore represent a healthier constitution than one without, although lack of any bone abnormality could either mean a healthy individual who died as a result of an accident, for example, or somebody who was unhealthy but died before bone change occurred; absence of evidence does not mean evidence of absence in all cases! In addition, Wood et al. (1992: 357) suggest that 'different disease processes interact with each other and also with an individual's constitutional susceptibility to stress in determining frailty', and hence what is observed on the skeleton. However, the degree of frailty in a population is not known for the past, nor is its association with the development of abnormal lesions, and knowledge of the amount and length of exposure a person had to a disease-causing organism is limited.

The bone changes of disease may be proliferative, i.e. bone forming and initiated by osteoblasts (bone-forming cells), or destructive, i.e. bone destroying and initiated by osteoclasts (bone-destroying cells). There may also be a mixture of the two activities. In the normal physiological state there is a balance between osteoblast and osteoclast activity which allows continuous remodelling and turnover of bone throughout life. However, as a person ages, bone loss overtakes bone formation and there is net loss of bone. Pathological stimuli may induce an imbalance, producing changes of atrophy, hypertrophy, hyperplasia or metaplasia. The cellular changes in bone are stimulated by a change in oxygen supply to the tissues – high blood oxygen tension stimulates osteoclast activity and low blood oxygen tension stimulates osteoblasts. Hypertrophy involves increase in cellular size and may be induced physiologically, e.g. the person has a heavy manual occupation and the muscles used become increased in size. Atrophy means that there is a decrease in cell size, e.g. when a limb is not being used in, say, paralysis of whatever cause. Hyperplasia indicates cellular division and an increase in cellular content of the tissue, and metaplasia involves the change in differentiation of cell type, i.e. a cell assumes the morphological and functional characteristics of another cell under pathological stimulus, e.g. in a tumour.

The bone formed in a disease process may be woven (or fibre), immature or primary bone (porous, disorganized; Fig. 1.1), or more mature, older, organized, lamellar bone (Fig. 1.2). The former indicates that the disease process was active at the time of death, and the latter indicates that the process was quiescent or had been overcome. However, the presence of active lesions may not indicate the process was the cause of death but that, with other factors, it contributed. It is also of importance to study whether an abnormal lesion appears healed (smooth bone with rounded edges) or unhealed (sharp unremodelled edges) because this gives an indication of the disease state at the time of death and perhaps whether this abnormality had contributed to the demise of the individual. However, determining the ante- or post-mortem nature of unhealed lesions can prove problematic.

It is essential to have a complete skeleton to study since observation of distribution patterns of abnormalities is necessary to attempt a diagnosis based on modern clinical criteria. Unfortunately, in archaeological contexts complete skeletons are not usually the normal occurrence and the palaeopathologist is often working with incomplete data. It should also be remembered that several diseases may induce similar lesions on bone and can occur on the skeleton at the same time, because bone can only react to a pathological stimulus in a limited number of ways, as we have seen. For example, new bone formation on the lower leg bones (tibia and fibula) may represent leprosy, treponemal disease, tuberculosis, trauma,

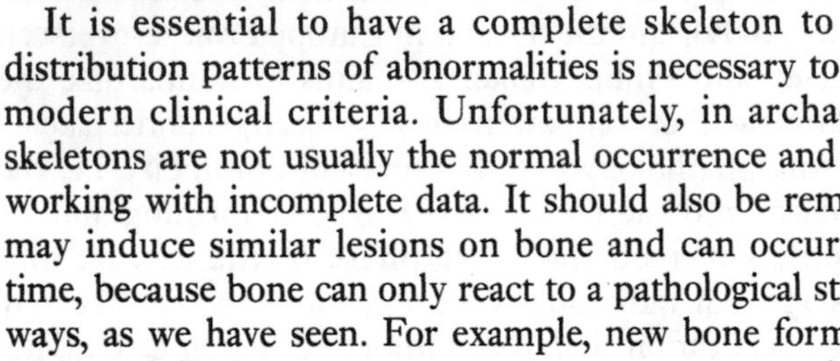

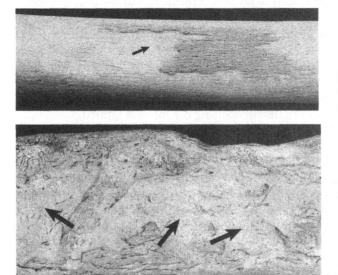

Fig. 1.1. Long bone with woven bone formation on top of the original cortex.

Fig. 1.2. Long bone with lamellar bone formation.

non-specific infection and scurvy. Of course, one would never diagnose any of these conditions solely on the basis of this change, because we would be considering the fuller picture (distribution pattern) of all the changes. Consideration of possible differential diagnoses for the abnormalities described is essential because of the potential for several disease processes to cause the same bony changes. This means recording the bone abnormalities and their distribution and considering all potential disease processes which could have caused the patterning; by a process of gradual elimination on the basis of known patterning in modern clinical circumstances a most likely diagnosis may be made. However, it may not be possible to make a definite diagnosis. Some workers in the field also like to attach some degree of 'severity' to lesions observed, but their appearance may not necessarily reflect a gradation in the disease. If grades are to be included, a definition of the grades (including photographs) should be given so that future researchers understand the meaning of the definitions. Recording detailed descriptions of abnormal changes, although accepted as essential, does take up space in a skeletal report but may be solved using CDs, microfiche or web archives. However, it is advocated that an archive is kept for all reports. Advances in the storage of both visual and textual data since the 1990s, may help this problem to be solved in the future. The use of zip and compact disks for the recording of large amounts of data has allowed the transmission of these data to other readers. Additionally, electronic transmission of images captured by digital cameras, and of scanned photographs, has enabled researchers to gain opinions on pathological specimens and their diagnosis much more quickly than previously. We also have wide access to the worldwide web, where web pages record type specimens of specific diseases, and the information can be accessed by anybody with the technology to do so.

Of especial interest to the palaeopathologist is the study of disease prevalence through time but basic data must be collected before meaningful prevalence rates can be obtained (see Waldron, 1994 for a discussion of the definitions of prevalence and incidence and their relevance to past human skeletal populations). For example, if the prevalence of left hip joint disease is to be studied, then the observers need to know how many left femurs and acetabulae they have observed in order to determine the prevalence of joint disease of the component parts of the hip – inventories of bones and teeth observed are essential data which should be included in all reports (Table 1.1).

Table 1.1 Prevalence of left hip joint disease in three hypothetical skeletal populations

No. of acetabulae	No. affected (%)	No. of femur heads	No. affected (%)
20	10 (50)	30	10 (33.3)
55	20 (36.4)	75	15 (20)
130	60 (46.2)	115	33 (28.7)

Note: One often does assume that if one bone of the joint is affected then the apposing element will similarly be affected, but this is not always the case. However, in the above example the frequency of joint disease in both acetabulae and femur heads in individuals with both elements surviving should also be examined.

The nature of the (often) fragmentary state of human skeletal material means that one cannot assume all bones are represented in all skeletons and, if prevalence rates for disease are presented according to individuals, e.g. five out of ten people had leprosy, the assumption has to be that all bones (facial, hand, foot and lower legs) were present for observation (even though five of the unaffected skeletons may have had no foot bones to observe).

In addition to macroscopic examination of the skeleton, radiography (Fig. 1.3) plays a large part in the diagnosis of disease and trauma (Roberts, 1989; Blondiaux *et al.*, 1994; Hughes *et al.*, 1996), especially in the case of unwrapped mummies (Zimmerman, 2000). Light, transmission and scanning electron microscopy (Martin, 1991; Bell and Piper, 2000; Pfeiffer, 2000) add an extra dimension and can increase accuracy for diagnosing disease (Fig. 1.4) and also pseudopathological changes, i.e. those post-mortem changes which appear to be pathological but are not. Physical and chemical techniques of analysis have been used increasingly over time to diagnose disease (e.g. lead poisoning, Vuorinen *et al.*, 1990; Klepinger, 1992) and also to examine dietary status (Katzenberg *et al.*, 1996; Wright and Schwarcz, 1998; Katzenberg, 2000; Lillie and Richards, 2000; Sealy, 2000; Cox *et al.*, 2001; Dupras *et al.*, 2001); of course, the latter has a bearing on a person's likelihood of acquiring a disease. More recently, work has focused on identifying disease at the molecular level, and there have been considerable advances in this area since the second edition of this book (e.g. Salo *et al.*, 1994; Brown, 2000; Gernaey and Minnikin 2000; Stone 2000; Taylor *et al.*, 2000).

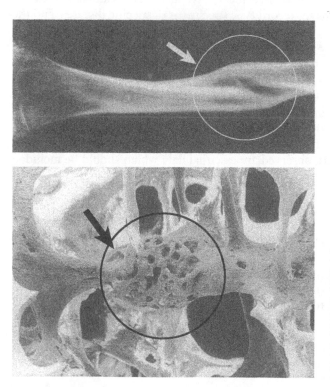

Fig. 1.3. Radiograph of tibia showing healed fracture.

Fig. 1.4. Scanning electron microscopy of section of a lumbar vertebral body showing a healed microfracture (early Medieval, eighth–tenth centuries AD, Raunds, Northamptonshire, England).

Since the 1990s attempts have been made to suggest how abnormalities should be recorded and to specify the minimum set of data which should be generated for skeletal population studies (Rose *et al.*, 1991; Buikstra and Ubelaker, 1994; Brickley and McKinley, 2004). Additionally, experimental studies have shown that there can be quite marked discrepancies in how data are recorded (Waldron and Rogers 1991; Miller *et al.*, 1996). To be able to compare data between different cemetery groups, methods of recording and the data generated must be comparable if palaeopathology is to be recognized as a scientific discipline.

TERMINOLOGY

There are several terms that the reader should become familiar with. **Aetiology** refers to the cause of the disease, **pathogen** is the foreign life-form which is capable of stimulating disease (e.g. *Mycobacterium tuberculosis* causes tuberculosis), and **pathogenesis** refers to the mechanism and development of tissue change in a disease. An affected individual's physical **signs** and **symptoms** are **clinical features** (e.g. the swelling and pain of joint disease respectively), and a **lesion** refers to the individual tissue manifestations in a specific disease. **Epidemiology** studies the incidence (or prevalence), distribution and determinants of diseases in populations. For example, pollution in an environment may determine the prevalence of upper respiratory tract infections. **Mortality** refers to death and **morbidity** describes the occurrence of illness. Clearly, there may be many factors contributing to the occurrence of disease – genetic predisposition, age, sex, ethnic group, physiological state and social status, prior exposure to the micro-organism, intercurrent or pre-existing disease and human behaviour, e.g. occupation, diet, hygiene (e.g. see Polednak, 1989 on racial and ethnic differences in disease, McElroy and Townsend, 1996 on ecological factors). A person may also have natural (i.e. inherited) **immunity** to a disease independent of any previous exposure to specific pathogenic micro-organisms. In addition, an acquired adaptive immunity may be stimulated by exposure to foreign proteins of invading pathogenic micro-organisms and the immune system will be dependent upon the properties of specific circulating white blood cells called lymphocytes. Adaptive immunity is characterized by the retention of a specific memory for the invading pathogen so that a 'tailor-made' defence mechanism for future invasion by the specific pathogen is in place. The problem with immunity in past human groups is that the levels of natural and acquired immunity cannot be ascertained. However, chronic evidence for disease does indicate that a person's immunity was effective enough to prevent death in the acute phase. A child who died with no bone changes of disease may also indicate that his or her immune status was not developed enough to prevent disease. Another example would be that a person with bone changes of leprosy usually has the lepromatous (or low-resistant) form of the disease, indicating a less-developed immune system (Fig. 1.5). As time goes by people may 'move' their immunity to the other end of the spectrum and develop tuberculoid leprosy, because of increased exposure (and adaptation) to the infection. Clearly, building up one's immune system by being exposed to pathogens in the environment is key to a healthy life (Hamilton, 1998).

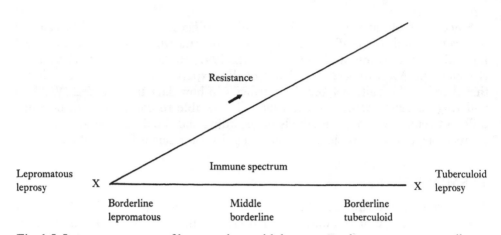

Fig. 1.5. Immune spectrum of leprosy; those with lepromatous leprosy are more easily identifiable in the skeletal record. *(After Ridley and Jopling, 1966)*

LIMITATIONS OF PALAEOPATHOLOGICAL STUDY

There are several limitations to the study of palaeopathology, as Wood *et al.* (1992) stated. In any discipline there are limitations, but some can be overcome. The hazards of selective mortality, individual variation in a person's risk of disease and death (i.e. there is an unknown mix of individuals who varied in susceptibility to death and disease, depending on biocultural factors), and the non-stationary nature of populations were highlighted by Wood *et al.* (1992) as major problems which it may not be possible to solve in palaeopathology. The following summarizes other limitations that should be considered.

The 'populations' being studied in palaeopathology are dead and therefore may not be representative of the living group; biological anthropologists are dealing with a sample of a sample of a sample . . . of the original living population, and total excavation of a cemetery is unusual. Partial excavation of a cemetery is the most common occurrence in archaeology and therefore only a portion of the original buried population will be examined (Fig. 1.6); the differential disposal of males, females, children and people with particular diseases, and their subsequent excavation, means biases in the produced data are inevitable. For example, in some cultures children were not always buried in the cemetery serving the general population – for example, in the Roman period in Britain (Philpott, 1991). In addition, skeletal material is often fragmentary and poorly preserved, with non-adult skeletons commonly suffering post-mortem damage (see Guy *et al.*, 1997), and therefore observation of the distribution pattern of abnormal changes is not possible; hence an attempt at a diagnosis often cannot be made. Researchers in biological anthropology often deal with small numbers of individuals and therefore cannot say much about disease prevalence at the population level because the group of skeletons being examined can only be a small sample of the original living population; sample representivity is often difficult to assess.

Acute infective disease is likely to have killed people very quickly in antiquity, especially if the individual had had no previous exposure or experience of the

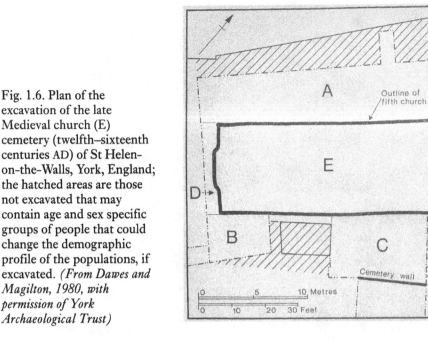

Fig. 1.6. Plan of the excavation of the late Medieval church (E) cemetery (twelfth–sixteenth centuries AD) of St Helen-on-the-Walls, York, England; the hatched areas are those not excavated that may contain age and sex specific groups of people that could change the demographic profile of the populations, if excavated. *(From Dawes and Magilton, 1980, with permission of York Archaeological Trust)*

invading organism. Therefore, no evidence of abnormal bone change would be visible (or expected) because the person died before the bone change developed. Many diseases also only affect the soft tissues and therefore would not be visible on the skeleton. It is therefore quite possible that skeletons from the younger (non-adult) members of a cemetery population were victims of an acute, or soft tissue, disease because frequently they do not have any signs of abnormal bone change. Additionally, their immune systems may not have been fully developed to defend against disease. Furthermore, pathological bones are inherently fragile structures and may, in some circumstances, become damaged while buried and not survive to be excavated, which precludes examination and recording; thus their frequency may be under-represented.

A further factor to consider is the inability, in most circumstances, to ascribe a cause of death to an individual. Without, for example, a weapon embedded in the skeleton in the grave, or an unhealed injury (Fiorato *et al.*, 2001), it is often guesswork determining a cause of death, although the observation of the posture of a skeleton within its grave may be an indication of cause of death. For example, the 'live' burials recorded from Kingsworthy, Dalton Parlours and elsewhere in Britain (Hawkes and Wells, 1975; Manchester, 1978a) were dependent for interpretation upon the observed posture. Beheadings, seen as cut marks to the neck vertebrae (Boylston *et al.*, 2000), or hanging, strangulation or trauma to the neck, seen in fractures to the hyoid bone or ossified neck cartilages, may also be clues. However, complete bodies such as those from north-west European bogs (Brothwell, 1986) may indicate a more obvious cause of death because of the survival of soft tissue. What can be indicated are the disease processes an individual may have been suffering from in life and whether the disease was active or not at the time of

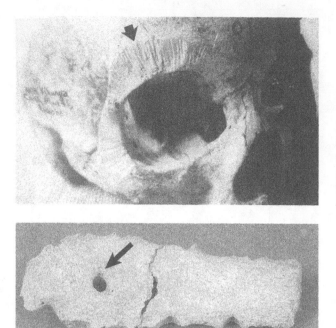

Fig. 1.7. Post-mortem (pseudopathological?) lesions around the eye socket due to gnawing from a rodent in the grave. *(Calvin Wells Photographic Collection)*

Fig. 1.8. Sternal foramen, a non-metric trait.

death. However, we should not dwell too much on our inability to assign a specific cause of death to skeletal remains. There is ample evidence from clinical research and historical data that assigning the correct cause of death was not, and is not, easy (see Hardy, 1994 on eighteenth- and nineteenth-century Cause of Death Statistics for England and Wales, and Alter and Carmichael, 1999 and Hanzlick, 1997 on the history of registration of causes of death). For example, a study of Irish general practitioners by Payne (2000) found that up to 50 per cent of cause of death data on death certificates could be based on guesswork. Likewise, Ermene and Dolene (1999), after correlating cause of death data on death certificates and autopsy reports in 444 individuals, found in 49 per cent of cases there was complete agreement, and in 19 per cent complete disagreement.

Apart from determining cause of death, there is also the problem of deciding whether abnormal bone change is the result of a disease or due to the post-mortem effects of deposition, burial and excavation of the body, or pseudopathology (Fig. 1.7 and Wells, 1967; Hackett, 1976; Bell, 1990). Finally, one should be careful of ascribing disease to an individual on the basis of normal variation in the skeleton, or non-metric trait presence (Fig. 1.8; e.g. see Saunders, 1989 regarding non-metric traits of bone and Scott and Turner, 1997 for teeth).

BIOCULTURAL PERSPECTIVES OF DISEASE FREQUENCY

Despite these limitations, a striking feature in the study of the history of disease is the constant nature and the different distribution of disease with the passage of time. Many diseases which have been recognized in skeletons from distant antiquity present the same physical characteristics as those diseases today. Diagnoses in palaeopathology are made with reference to the knowledge of modern pathology as we have seen. The agents of disease stimulate bone reactions which we assume were the same for the palaeolithic hunter as they are for the twenty-first-century office worker. However, with the development of ancient DNA analysis very recent work has started to explore whether strains of specific diseases were the same today as they were thousands of years ago (Buikstra, pers. comm.; Zink *et al.*, 2003). Nevertheless, it is the overall world frequency of disease and the differing geographical patterns of disease which have changed during the history of human populations. The following sections consider a number of themes and their impact on health.

Movement of people

Travel, trade and contact with people have spread disease, sometimes with devastating effect, and this is still seen today.

The human infectious diseases have achieved worldwide status through the migrations of humans and the animals associated with them (Wilson, 1995). For several thousands of years armies have crossed frontiers and seas and travelled on campaign to distant lands. Crowded together, poorly nourished and usually exhausted by the stress of battle, soldiers on active service are notorious for their spread of infectious disease, often of the enteric types. Today, refugees from war-torn areas of the world often endure similar living conditions in their new environment. They hope for a better life, but this is not always achieved immediately, and they take their diseases with them as they travel, while experiencing new health insults on weakened bodies (see Roberts and Buikstra, 2003, on the effect of travel and migration on the frequency of tuberculosis).

Unlike the immunity of indigenous populations as, for example, in the tropical diseases, people transporting infectious disease from one region to another were probably overtly infected themselves. With the notable exception of typhoid fever, there are very few asymptomatic carriers of human infectious disease. The population into which the disease was introduced was also no more and no less susceptible than the people actually transporting the disease.

When one population moves from the region to which it has become adjusted, to another, it shows increased susceptibility to the diseases of the area into which it moves (Mascie-Taylor and Lasker, 1988; Roberts *et al.*, 1992). This fact was noted with cynical effect in Kent in the nineteenth century. At that time, and for many years before, the north coast of Kent was an important focus of endemic malaria. The area was marshy and the frequent hot, dry summers resulted in outbreaks of the disease (Dobson, 1994). However, indigenous males appeared to be immune to a strain of the malaria parasite and so did not readily succumb to the disease. Another example is the effect of explorers from the Old World on the native population health of the Americas: new diseases were introduced to which they had no resistance (Larsen, 1994; Larsen and Milner, 1994).

Climate and weather

The latitude, longitude and associated climate and weather have a profound effect upon the incidence of certain diseases (Brimblecombe, 1982; Patz *et al.*, 1996; and see Lukacs and Walimbe (1998) for a palaeopathological example), and the constant relationship between respiratory disease and more recently seasonal affected disorder (SAD) and the winter climate is well known to all living in northern Europe. What may not be quite so well known is the seasonal and climatic variance of such diseases as meningitis, poliomyelitis, glaucoma and mental disease. It is possible that a knowledge of the geographical prevalence of specific diseases will provide clues to their causes (Learmonth, 1988). However, the ability of people to adapt to a totally new environment, climate and weather, and the associated diseases, is perhaps one of our most valuable characteristics.

Diet and economy

Until the advent of agriculture in all parts of the world, many people lived in reasonable harmony with their environment. The equilibrium was destroyed with deforestation and the development of farming. This still continues to be a problem (Morse, 1995). Ploughing, crop-rearing and tending flocks also increase exposure to new organisms. For example, cultivated soil containing organic refuse, particularly animal dung, is a good medium for survival of the spores of the tetanus bacillus. People cultivating land were liable to develop tetanus, which in antiquity must have been almost invariably fatal. In common with most of the acute infectious diseases, tetanus is not recognizable in the human skeletal record. We also know that some bacteria may survive for considerable amounts of time and be still viable (e.g. tuberculosis – Cosivi et al., 1995). The use of dung for fuel (Fig. 1.9), building and manuring could potentially introduce health hazards.

Environmental change has been a feature of all periods of time. In association with the change in environment, be it deforestation, land cultivation or urbanization, people have come to live in closer relationship with a variety of animals. Cattle, horses, sheep and pigs were accumulated and people lived life in close proximity to them, often sharing their houses. Only later were the dog, cat and a multitude of other animals seen as companions and pets. These animals are all subject to their own parasites which may or may not cause disease within them. Cattle are subject to tuberculosis, the pig to *Taenia solium* (tapeworm) and the dog and sheep to hydatid disease, to name but a few. In fact, many of our human diseases may have originated from animals (Waldron, 1989: table 3). Increasing domestication of animals brings people closer not only to animals but also to their parasites, be they worms, bacteria or viruses, and it may have been during this time of increasing contact with animals that people first became infected with the parasites of animal origin (zoonoses – see Brothwell, 1991). Close contact with

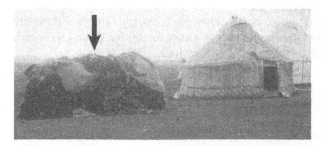

Fig. 1.9. North-west China: large pile of animal dung used for fuel for this nomadic population.

dogs and canine distemper may have been responsible for the introduction of measles to humans. The measles virus, which at present appears to have no primate ancestral parallel, is similar to the virus causing canine distemper. This transfer may have been the stepping-stone for the recurrent endemic and at times life-threatening disease of measles with which modern populations are so familiar. However, the community size at the introduction of the measles virus must have been large enough to sustain it as an endemic infection.

In the Americas, the introduction of agriculture, particularly maize, allowed the development of a more settled community with permanent housing to enable people to care for crops and animals. However, as population numbers increased, the local living environment became less healthy, diet became less varied and people's health suffered. Studies from the Americas consistently indicate a decline in health with the advent of agriculture (Cohen and Armelagos, 1984; Cohen, 1989; Larsen, 1995; see table 1.2 for an example) and note that hunter-gatherers were probably healthier because of higher mobility, less fat intake, a varied (and more reliable) diet and temporary housing. However, this does not mean that they did not suffer. For example, disease could be transmitted from hunting, butchery and consumption of wild animals, and water sources could become polluted.

Living environment

The rise of urban communities, which gathered momentum towards the later Medieval period in Europe certainly, pushed increased numbers of people into closer contact, often in poorly ventilated, un-hygienic houses, creating a situation that allowed transmission of infectious diseases more readily (Keene, 1983; Woods and Woodward, 1984; Cohen, 1989; Dyer, 1989; Rosen, 1993; Howe, 1997).

In the early and somewhat haphazard stages of village and town development, little thought was given to waste disposal (Keene, 1983). The health hazard of the open sewer and its attendant flies was not realized. The inadequacy of communal water supply was unrecognized (see Fig. 1.10 for a contemporary example). It is within this framework of public health ignorance that the largely water-borne infections of cholera, typhoid and infantile gastroenteritis flourished. These are the debilitating, sometimes fatal, illnesses of adulthood and the almost invariably fatal illnesses of infancy and childhood. The almost careless, at least unwitting, proximity of water supply and effluent discharge in the narrow Medieval

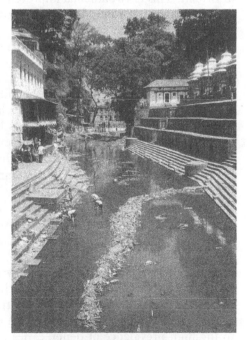

Fig. 1.10. Kathmandu, Nepal: children playing in a highly polluted river full of rubbish.

town streets of Europe allowed the easy transference of bacteria and viruses from one public service to the other. Later in time, a specific example in London reveals the problem of having a water supply which may not be beneficial to health. In 1854 the Soho area of London was subject to an epidemic of cholera and its source was centred on a pump in Broad Street (now Broadwick Street). Once the pump was removed from use, the infection declined. This suggested that the water supply had been infected, a common method of transmitting the disease (Learmonth, 1988).

In the twentieth century the health hazards of the large conurbations of industrial development have become apparent, albeit poorly understood. Lung cancer and chronic bronchitis showed a high incidence in the large centres of population in Britain (Howe, 1997). The coal-miner's pneumoconiosis and anthracosis, also seen in past humans (Munizaga *et al.*, 1975; Walker *et al.*, 1987), the business executive's coronary thrombosis due to stress, the ubiquitous mental illness, the gut and lung cancer of the developing world due to changes in diet, the adoption of smoking and the increases in health problems due to environmental pollution (Hassan *et al.*, 2003) are but a few of the many penalties of human adaptation to changing circumstances. The phenomenon is not new but is better documented today. Nevertheless, not all environmental change has favoured the parasite. Sometimes, quite unintentionally, people have altered the environment and destroyed the natural habitat of the vectors of some diseases and so, effectively, eliminated the particular disease. Drainage of marshlands and maintenance of adequate dykes were responsible for the eradication of malaria in the late nineteenth century in some parts of Britain. This environmental improvement, carried out by the farming community for reasons of economy, led unwittingly to the elimination of the mosquito by destroying the habitat favourable to it.

It is not only the change in landscape which results in disease variance; we must also consider the differences the range of environments could have on disease frequency. Coastal and inland, island and mainland, river, lake and estuary, highland and lowland, hot and cold, dry and humid; all these environments affect the range of diseases experienced. Occupation of unchanged land itself may also encourage the development of certain diseases. It has been suggested, for example, that people living in districts with a high soil content of copper, zinc and lead have a higher than average incidence of multiple sclerosis (Warren *et al.*, 1967), and copper mining in the past could lead to poisoning (Oakberg *et al.*, 2000). In Jordan, high levels of copper today affect populations' health (Pyatt and Grattan, 2001), and in the south-west of England granite-walled houses emit radon that could cause cancer. The causal relationship between the development of goitre and a nutritional deficiency of iodine is well known. This deficiency, due to a low iodine content of water, is most common in inland mountainous areas of the world, especially in parts of America and Switzerland (Drury and Howlett, 2002). In Britain the deficiency gave rise to the now classic 'Derbyshire neck'. The significance of fluorine as a nutritional trace element is a recent concept, although as early as 1892 it was suggested that a dietary deficiency of fluorine was related to the high prevalence of dental caries in Britain. Fluoridation of drinking water in Britain has caused great controversy over the years but studies do show that it reduces the frequency of caries in children (Thomas *et al.*, 1995). The properties of fluorine at the correct levels in the prevention of dental caries are now well known. It is also known, however, that excessive levels of fluorine in water can cause fluorosis (Blau *et al.*, 2002). However, differentiating between a disease caused by a deficiency or lack of a dietary element noted in skeletal and dental remains, and the infiltration of soil elements into the bone or teeth, needs great care in interpretation (Price *et al.*, 1992). Such problems of the relationship between disease and environment are ill-understood today. Their significance for the diseases of antiquity may remain unknown. The difference today is that an association between disease incidence and 'geographical' characteristics can be assessed and checked in contemporary societies; for the past this is more difficult.

There is also a factor in the causation of disease which is beyond the influence of the environment and which may have a bearing upon the differing geographical prevalence of certain diseases of antiquity. In 1953 it was reported that there was a significant association between cancer of the stomach and individuals of blood group A (Aird and Bentall, 1953). Since that time investigation has extended to many diseases and blood group associations (Vogel, 1970; Polednak, 1989), including the relationship of disease to certain proteins of the blood (Cattaneo, 1991). The results of these investigations are not without their critics (Weiner, 1970), but, as is observed, blood group frequencies do separate geographically, even in the present days of widespread travel.

Occupation

The health hazards of the type of work people have done, and do, are clear. You may be a hunter-gatherer and live in a healthy environment with a good well-balanced diet, but the dangers of trauma from hunting wild animals may compromise your health considerably! Working in the pottery, textile and mining industries creates particles in the environment that, when inhaled, can induce inflammation and infection in the respiratory tract (e.g. Lancaster, 1990). The trades of tanning, butchery and farming create an environment conducive to contracting zoonoses (e.g. see Reber, 1999 on tuberculosis in nineteenth- and twentieth-century Argentina), and spending long hours cooking over a smoky fire (Fig. 1.11) may lead to infection and cancer of the respiratory tract (Larson and Koenig, 1994; Dietz *et*

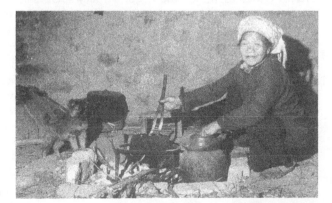

Fig. 1.11. China: woman
cooking over a smoky fire.

al., 1995). In the latter part of the twentieth century and now in the twenty-first century, certainly in westernized societies, health and safety measures have been introduced to prevent disease and injury, such as putting guards over dangerous machinery, and ensuring that people working in noisy or polluted environments wear ear-muffs and masks, respectively. However, in the past these regulations (in a less developed form) may or may not have been instigated. It is, nevertheless, likely that preventive measures were inconsistently exercised.

Treatment

The commonplace infections which killed or debilitated humans in antiquity are rapidly treated with antibiotics in modern western societies. Unfortunately, the use, and misuse, of the earlier antibiotics has led to the development of resistant strains of bacteria, for example in tuberculosis today (Grange, 1999), and in some instances the parasite has regained the upper hand. The manufacture of more and varied antibiotics has, however, once more mastered some diseases. Infectious diseases due to viruses are in a different class, since at present no universal and totally effective antiviral agent exists. The common cold, influenza, measles and smallpox, for example, are incurable once established. Success against them depends upon preventing their establishment. With very few exceptions, however, these viral diseases are not manifest in skeletal material and for this reason will not be discussed further.

More important for western populations is the increasing significance that circulatory, degenerative and neoplastic disease has in modern society. By their adaptability and knowledge, humans have exchanged one group of diseases for another. The conquest of cancer, AIDS (acquired immune deficiency syndrome) and circulatory disease remains a goal for the present. The increase in incidence of these diseases may be more apparent than real and due in part to the increased longevity of modern western populations. They are also due to environmental change and the industrialization of the past two hundred years. Of course, in the past sophisticated methods of treating illlnesses, e.g. using drugs, did not exist and would not have affected the course of the disease. However, what we would now call 'alternative therapies' were clearly exploited, as seen in documentary and artistic representation. They include blood-letting, including cupping (Fig. 1.12), to rebalance the humours, cautery (the application of hot irons to the affected part), herbal remedies, minor and major surgery such as setting fractures, amputation and trepanation, wound care, bathing and more unconventional remedies (Rawcliffe, 1997). We also have records for the founding of hospitals for specific diseases such as leprosy (Roberts, 1986a) and tuberculosis (see summary of sanatoria development in Roberts and Buikstra, 2003), although whether particular treatment regimes were used are debated. In Medieval Europe hospitals were often founded by a benefactor who was usually more interested in 'getting to heaven' than in treating the sick effectively. We know too that 'medical' practitioners existed, and ranged from village elders to barber-surgeons and bone-setters. Despite this long list of 'available' care and treatment, we do not know what proportion of people through time had access to therapy, whether only higher social status (older/younger?) males or females were favoured, and whether urban or rural populations were more likely to be treated. We know today that certain parts of populations are advantaged for various reasons (e.g.

see Roberts and Buikstra, 2003 on the problems of access to treatment for tuberculosis) and it is highly likely that this was the case in the past.

The problems of disease today in relation to environmental change, to advances in medical treatment and to the very nature of humans themselves are complex and the subject of continuous change. The understanding of disease in antiquity and the analysis of the changing patterns of disease throughout history are equally complex, but may be of paramount importance in the inter-pretation of medical problems today. While we may not detect all our ancestors' health history, we may start to understand what the presence of some diseases meant in terms of absolute impact.

In the following chapters diseases that potentially affect bones and teeth are discussed. Both congenital and acquired diseases are considered. Congenital disease is present at birth, and acquired disease is developed during life. This latter classification encompasses:

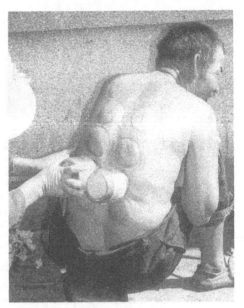

Fig. 1.12. China: treatment by cupping (a heated glass vessel is placed on the skin; this creates a vacuum and draws the blood to the surface).

1. Dental disease: those diseases or conditions affecting the teeth and associated tissues.
2. Traumatic lesions: due to injury or malformation of the skeleton and associated soft tissues.
3. Joint disease: diseases that affect the joints of the body and associated tissues.
4. Infectious disease: caused by invading living organisms (viruses, bacteria, parasites or fungi).
5. Metabolic disease: caused by a disturbance in the normal processes of cell metabolism.
6. Endocrine disease: caused by over- or underactivity of the endocrine glands which secrete hormones.
7. Neoplastic disease: 'new growths' which may be benign (localized to the site of growth) or malignant (progressive growth which invades and destroys surrounding tissues and spreads to more distant sites in the body).

In a book such as this it is not possible to consider all the possible skeletal and dental diseases that occur in past human remains; it is the intention to deal with those disease processes that are more commonly seen, with the aim of providing guidelines for scholars in the discipline and informing other interested readers about commonly occurring palaeopathological lesions and their interpretation within a cultural (archaeological) context.

CHAPTER 2

Back to Basics

The world's population is primed to start diminishing for probably the first time since the Black Death in the fourteenth century. (Pearce, 2002: 38)

INTRODUCTION

This chapter considers some of the most important information necessary to interpret the evidence for health and disease in skeletal remains: the age and sex of the individual, the demographic profile of the population under study, the person's height (stature), and his or her ancestry. Without knowledge about these key variables, it is simply not possible to make any meaningful interpretations and conclusions about individual skeletons showing disease, or about a population's health status. For example, population figures and their patterns are of immense value to the palaeopathologist because a circular feedback of data operates to calculate population size and growth and then this may be explained in terms of socio-economic development. Furthermore, the changing population pattern may have a bearing on modern disease and its possible causation. Important factors are the rate and pattern of growth of the population, the relationship of these to epidemic disease, famine and technological innovations, and the whole complex interrelationship of these to changing birth and death rates. Of course, not all parts of the world have contributed to the growth of the population uniformly (as we see today). For example, the initial upsurge, which may have been coincident with the development of tools, occurred on the African continent, and growth in the Fertile Crescent with the advent of agriculture may have contributed disproportionately to population increase. Nevertheless, population increases and declines are very much related to culture and the environment in which that culture operates, all producing opportunities for advance but also threats to survival.

POPULATION GROWTH THROUGH TIME

Population growth occurs when birth rates exceed death rates (McElroy and Townsend, 1996: 124), but Thomas Malthus (1798) stated that if a population increases faster than its means of subsistence it will be subject to the checks of war, famine and disease. The world's population has grown through time and has had surges with the invention of tools, the introduction of farming and the Industrial Revolution, each followed by a period of stability; each 'surge' was the result of opportunities provided by the new developments. These stable periods have been characterized by localized fluctuations caused by factors such as famine, disease and war. Advances in medical and surgical care, and the ability to sustain more people by intensification of agriculture, have allowed recent increases, particularly throughout the twentieth century. The world's population throughout time has been the result of the changing balance of births, deaths and migration (McElroy and Townsend, 1996: 121). The first two periods of upsurge are associated with increased food and material prosperity, a decrease in death rates, and a consequent mastery of the environment by newly found technologies. For example, the advantage of a tool user compared to a non-tool user in the killing of animals and preparation of food, and some of the advantages of settled, controlled farming with its regular year-round supply of food, are the most obvious factors accounting for population increase (although not the entire explanation). The establishment of permanent habitations, and practising agriculture, allowed the accumulation of stored food for leaner times, and enabled people to develop immunity to parasites in a specific area and allowed for the care of sick and older people (Strassman and Dunbar, 1999: 96). Settled communities, however, also encounter many negative consequences as a result of producing their own food, such as allowing the population to increase and living in permanent housing. Particular problems include increases in droplet-spread infectious disease through populations living in close contact, malnutrition as a result of harvest failures (and a lack of variety in the diet), and sickly domesticated animals transmitting their diseases to humans (see Cohen and Armelagos, 1984; Cohen, 1989). For example, hunter-gatherers are known to eat over 100 different plant species today, but in traditional agricultural communities only 10–15 are eaten (Strassmann and Dunbar, 1999: 97). However, an improvement in the quality and quantity of protein consumption (which may or may not have been associated with settled communities – Cohen, 1989) can lead to a lowering of the age of female sexual maturity and an increase in female fecundity, thus increasing the reproductive life of females (Hassan, 1973). The more settled agricultural village could also have resulted in a narrowing of birth spacing, meaning that more children overall could potentially be borne and reared by any one fertile female (Sussman, 1973). Nevertheless, frequent childbirth can create maternal stress (in its broadest sense), and childbirth was probably hazardous in the past (Chadwick Hawkes and Wells, 1975; Wells, 1978; Gelis, 1991). These factors may obviously act adversely on population growth by increasing female mortality in the reproductive phase of life. It is possible, but unproven, that induced abortion and infanticide were practised in hunter-gatherer populations. Even today some societies do practise these population-control measures, either because of a traditional requirement for the numbers of females to be controlled, for general population control, or to rid a population of 'abnormal' individuals (Daly and Wilson, 1984). For similar reasons, birth control in the form of sexual taboo and prolonged post-partum sexual abstinence has been practised; in addition, prolonged lactation would have induced a contraceptive effect.

The earliest date for which the population of the world can be estimated even to within 20 per cent accuracy was the mid-eighteenth century (Coale, 1974). Even so, written estimates of population size and structure in historical data cannot be taken at face value and may be influenced by the author's objectives in making such data available. Tombstones, parish records, wills and taxes may all contribute some knowledge of past population size, but care must be taken with their interpretation. The earliest population census in world history was made in China around 2000 BC, with a further and perhaps more reliable one in AD 2 during the Han Dynasty, while in the sixth century BC a Roman census was taken (Hollingsworth, 1969). However, it is not known what part of society was included in these censuses (the rich?), and therefore their value must be seen as limited. In England, the Domesday Survey of the population was carried out in the eleventh century, largely for taxation purposes (Welch, 1992), and is therefore inaccurate for the country as a whole. For the remainder of the Medieval period in England population counts were made by the clergy, but it was not until 1848 that regular censuses were taken. However, in Sweden censuses had been introduced by 1749 (Eversley et al., 1966). Therefore, it is only for about 0.5 per cent of the time since the emergence of *Homo sapiens* that population statistics based on reliable census data exist.

In the case of populations where written records do not exist, the job of recreating population numbers becomes much harder because there is a reliance on variables such as how many skeletons have been excavated, the size and density of settlements, the structure of houses, the amount of pottery discarded, the number and capacity of storage pits, the amount of refuse, and the carrying capacity of a landscape (Bintliff and Sbonias, 1999). Sbonias (1999: 1) describes some of these variables as 'crude'. In terms of surveying landscapes for settlement sites, potential problems to consider include how intensive the survey was, how accurate estimations of the carrying capacity of the environment can be, and how missing sites can be evaluated (for example, for prehistory it is likely that there will be fewer sites detected than for later periods). Another issue to consider with respect to the identification and characterization of settlements from pottery discard rates is whether the rates differ for varying economic and social regimes. Furthermore, the extent of sites (and hence estimates of the size of the population) are usually determined by the surface distribution of pottery through field walking; how representative is the distribution of the original settlements? Pottery can be moved by natural and human intervention, and can fragment with time, and when we consider the use of particular identified structures we must be careful not to attribute occupation by people to a structure used for storage or industry (Sbonias, 1999: 8). The number of skeletons excavated and analysed from an area, and their relationship to the original living population, will be determined by who was buried where, how they were buried and whether they survived burial to be excavated; all these processes determine the final number, and it is inevitable that this number will be only a fraction of the original (Fig. 2.1; see Waldron, 1994 for a discussion of how representative a skeletal sample may be; also Henderson, 1987, and Waldron, 1987a for discussions on preservational factors). Furthermore, if only part of the cemetery has been excavated, specific parts of the buried population may not be present for analysis. Finally, the assessment of the numbers of people living in a house by analysing the layout of the houses in which they lived can also be fraught with problems. It is dangerous to assume a certain number of people lived in a particular house by imposing on the past our notions of how many people can live in a defined space today; this can change considerably through time or even as status changes. While the study of traditional living populations may provide a view

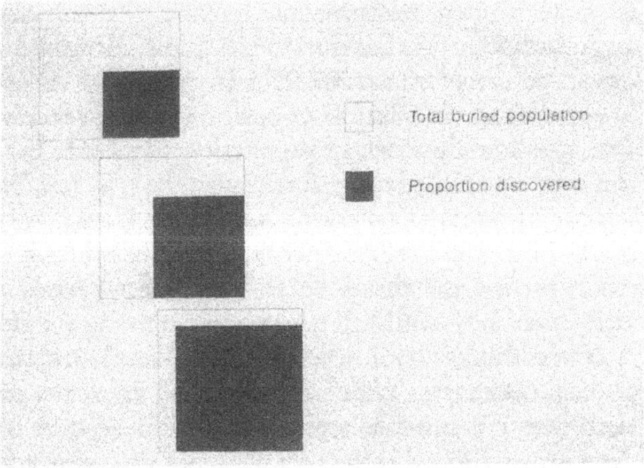

Fig. 2.1. Three possible scenarios for a cemetery excavation indicating the total buried population and the proportion discovered; this will affect the data analysis and interpretation. *(From Waldron, 1994 and with permission of Tony Waldron)*

of the numbers of people for a particular size of house, again we cannot assume an analogous situation for the past, both geographically and through time. While the use of historical data for population estimates has its problems, in prehistory our data can be a particular challenge to interpret.

However, today's population estimates, using the most sophisticated technology and calculations, may not necessarily be accurate, although there is now a better knowledge of the predicted impact of health problems on population mortality, and there is a good system of registering births and deaths, certainly in developed countries. For example, in England and Wales in 1999 the population was estimated to be 52.7 million, and predicted to be 57.1 million by 2023. The long-term decline in mortality rates continues for both males and females in most age groups, and by 2021 life expectancy for males is expected to be 78.8 years and for females 82.9 years (Anon., 2001); 1998 figures for the UK were 74.6 for males and 79.6 for females, with regional differences. Jurmain *et al.* (2003: 433) indicate that at the most recent United Nations International Conference on Population and Development the goal of containing the world's population to 7.3 billion by 2015 was set. If this did not happen, it was predicted that the population by 2050 would be approaching 10 billion. In developing countries the transfer of western technology to accelerate medical provision improvements and boost the economic base has allowed people to live longer and to have better nutrition and levels of hygiene (Pearce, 1998: 1). This has led to an increase in population growth rates per year for many countries (for example, 4 per cent in Africa), although in some areas of the world, such as Bangladesh, free contraception for fertile women has led to a decline in population growth rates (Pearce, 1999: 20). The consequence of having people live longer and also of low birth rates in developed countries is that the provision of medical care and state support in the form of pensions is very stretched.

However, the world's population may be set to decline in the future, in some parts of the world as a result of falling fertility (except in parts of the Middle East and sub-Saharan Africa – Pearce, 1998: 3), and in others as a result of increased mortality due to diseases such as HIV (human immune deficiency virus) and AIDS (as in Africa – Pearce, 1999: 20). Furthermore, with birth control being accessible to more women, many people moving to urban situations (and thus not needing large families to sustain agriculture), and decreased infant mortality due to medical care (and therefore the need for large families disappearing), the number of births is also falling. In some European countries, therefore, low birth rates will not be able to maintain existing population numbers. For example, in Italy the average number of children per fertile female is 1.2, a little more than half the figure needed to prevent excessive population decline (Pearce, 2002: 38). Of course, it could be argued that decreasing population numbers can only be good for the environment and that if there were fewer people in the world it would be more likely that they would all have better access to the necessities of life.

If one thinks about developing and developed countries as separate entities, the global economy as affecting developed countries and advances in technology are such that it is possible actually to sustain an ever-increasing number of people. In developing countries the picture is not the same and, until it is possible to provide an equivalent way of life for all people, rich and poor, a continuing increase in population cannot be sustained. As Buckley (1994) states, 95 per cent of population growth is in developing countries 'already struggling to provide a decent standard of living for their existing populations' (for example, a safe clean water supply). This does not by any means 'let off the hook' and 'allow' developed countries to increase their populations infinitely; it should, if nothing else, stimulate them to explore environmentally friendly ways of coping with too many people. The stark reality is that the gap between the rich (more often developed countries) and poor (developing countries) is widening as time goes by. Why is it that 61 per cent of Americans are classed as overweight and yet 14 million people in Africa face starvation and 1 billion people worldwide live in poverty (Edwards, 2002)? While there does seem to be some light at the end of the tunnel as estimates indicate that the world's population will stabilize at around 10 billion in the second half of the twenty-first century (Pearce, 1998: 3), it will be the developing countries that will continue to bear the burden of high populations.

POPULATION GROWTH, MORTALITY AND DISEASE

Important in the discussion of population size is disease load; while absolute population size will determine what diseases can appear and be maintained in a community, the occurrence of disease may limit the growth of a population and indeed eliminate it. In effect, people die because of ill health, and disease affects their ability to function normally; thus, the study of disease, both modern and ancient, sheds light on society as a whole. For example, the association between community size and infectious disease permanence has been studied in living isolated societies. Acute infections of short duration – for example, the viral infection of measles – are spread only by human-to-human contact and will not cause major periodic outbreaks unless the community is less than 250,000. Greater than this and the infection will either kill the person or infect and consequently immunize him or her. The virus, not having an intermediate animal host and not being carried dormant in a human, dies out (Black, 1975). Further outbreaks in the community will occur only if the virus is reintroduced from outside the community. The implication is that at the same time as one isolated group of people is free from and immune to such a disease, a neighbouring group is in the throes of an epidemic. It is only by inter-group contact in succeeding generations that the acute, infectious and totally human diseases will continue to thrive.

According to McElroy and Townsend (1996: 120), hunter-gatherers tend to suffer from chronic endemic infections until the development of larger permanent settlements (including the opportunity for more human contact) and the occurrence of acute infectious disease. These diseases therefore could not have made a lasting appearance in human populations until the size of these groups was large enough. The point in history at which population size reached the critical level is of course not known, and these acute infections do not leave their mark on the skeleton, except possibly in the rare case of smallpox (Jackes, 1983). However, with recent developments in the extraction and amplification of ancient DNA of specific disease-causing organisms, including those caused by viruses (Reid *et al.*, 1999) and other conditions that do not affect the skeleton (e.g. plague – Drancourt *et al.*, 1998, and malaria – Taylor *et al.*, 1997), the detection of acute infections as possible causes of death in skeletal remains from archaeological sites is now a possibility. Despite infectious disease being recorded in both living and ancient hunters and gatherers today (Cohen and Armelagos, 1984; Froment, 2001), our distant hunting and gathering ancestors were probably free from the common acute viral infections with which we are so familiar today.

While infectious disease was a significant cause of death after the development of agriculture up until the development of industrial nations, now it is the chronic degenerative diseases of old age such as heart disease that claim lives. These diseases are often termed 'diseases of affluence' because they are associated with lack of exercise, too much fat and sugar in the diet (and too little fibre), and obesity. For example, fibre in the diet initiates a quicker throughput of waste in the intestines; a lack of fibre slows the process and potentially allows longer exposure of the lining of the intestines to passing tumour-causing agents in the diet (Burkitt *et al.*, 1972, cited in Strassman and Dunbar, 1999). There are, of course, increased risks to health from environmental hazards, travel, migration and immigration, and extremes of poverty. Notable, however, are the disparities in mortality rates and causes of death around the world, and indeed even the differences seen regionally within particular countries. For example, Fitzpatrick *et al.* (2000) report that, in the United Kingdom, Wales, Scotland and Northern Ireland have the highest overall death rates for most age groups, that northern England has higher death rates than the south, and that the inequalities within regions of England are greater than between the four countries for all age groups. In Europe, the highland areas of Scotland, parts of Germany, Italy, Greece, Spain, Portugal and Corsica were also classed as areas of higher mortality (Shaw *et al.*, 2000). When it comes to causes of death in the United Kingdom, Pearce and Goldblatt (2001) record that for Scotland the highest death rates for all ages are those caused by heart disease, lung cancer, all tumours, 'strokes', alcohol, drugs, suicide and infectious disease. The latter is a particular cause of death for many developing (and developed) countries today, with new and re-emerging infections such as HIV and tuberculosis having developed as major threats to life. Between 1990 and 2000 diarrhoeal disease, tuberculosis and lower respiratory infections increased dramatically as causes of death worldwide (Edwards, 2002).

PALAEOPATHOLOGY AND THE QUESTION OF NUMBERS

The study of palaeopathology is not possible without understanding basic facts about the population being studied. Many factors determine a population's susceptibility to developing disease in modern contexts, as already discussed in Chapter 1; some of these factors may or may not be known for the past. Therefore, taking a multidisciplinary approach to the study of past health and disease is essential. Studying skeletal or mummified remains in isolation from their cultural context, although they provide the primary evidence for disease, cannot produce any meaningful interpretations about the origin, evolution and spread of disease through time. Likewise, the study of health and disease today cannot be undertaken without reference to factors determining the patterns we see.

It is important to know how many people were at risk of becoming ill as a first step to understanding why some diseases were more prevalent than others in the past. We have already considered the three major events in prehistory and history that contributed to increases in population, but how do we calculate how many people were present in a population? While discussion of the number of settlements, house size and arrangement, amount of pottery, and carrying capacity of the surrounding landscape have received attention, it is the skeletal remains that provide us with the direct evidence of numbers of people. However, it is extremely rare indeed for a complete cemetery to be excavated, exceptions perhaps including excavation in a rural area where there are no limits on the investigation. Even if a complete cemetery were to be excavated, the skeletons from that cemetery would be only a sample of the population that it served. We cannot assume, for example, that everybody living in the area was buried there; some of the people could have been migrants from another area (or even people who just wanted to be buried there but had not lived in the village/town). Neither do we know how many people had migrated from elsewhere into the community, or whether some parts of the population were buried in other places – for example, children, the disabled or diseased.

The determination of population numbers using just skeletal evidence relies on determining the number of individuals represented by the skeletal assemblage. However, often a number of graves are excavated, but some may contain more than one individual. Therefore, in cemetery reports the usual way of presenting the data is to describe the number of graves excavated and the number of skeletons recovered, and then to calculate the minimum number of individuals (MNI) as determined by counting the number of bone elements and teeth present. The calculation of the MNI starts with counting the number of left and right bones (as appropriate), and the bone element with the highest count becomes the MNI. For example, if there are 52 right femurs and 69 left femurs, then the MNI represented would be 69. The MNI is usually less than the number of skeletons excavated because many are fragmentary – that is, they do not contain all the bones they should. The importance of this calculation is particularly acute if a site contains not only discrete skeletons but also disarticulated bones. This bone (and tooth) count is also essential for determining the frequency of specific diseases in particular bone elements (and teeth). While reports on skeletons from archaeological sites often cite the frequencies of disease as the number affected as a percentage of the total skeletons excavated, this can be very misleading if most of the skeletons are fragmentary. For example, to ascertain how many people were *actually* affected by the more severe form of the infection leprosy, the facial bones need to be intact to allow examination. Often this area of the skeleton is damaged and not preserved, and if it is not preserved, we cannot know whether the person had leprosy or not. Therefore, the correct way to produce data on leprosy of the facial bones is to count the number of skeletons with facial bones existing, determine how many have leprous changes to the bones, and then work out the percentage rate compared to the number of facial bones preserved for observation. The same situation holds true for recording dental disease. Many skeletons lose teeth while buried, and, therefore, if the dental caries rate is being calculated, it really is important to state how many teeth have been observed and how many were affected; any further data such as how many people had dental caries can also be given but, if only those data were provided, one would have to assume that all skeletons had all teeth preserved to observe. This latter example is, of course, complicated by the fact that teeth can be lost generally because of dental disease, and dental caries can be one of the causes. When calculating the frequency of disease through the time period of a cemetery, the calculation becomes even more difficult. Some cemeteries span several hundreds of years, and stratification detail is usually not available to allow the division of burials into subperiods within the cemetery, although there are exceptions (Stroud and Kemp, 1993). In reality, a palaeopathologist may be dealing with 500 skeletons over 500 years, but archaeological data do not usually allow subdivision into smaller units of time. Therefore, examining the prevalence of disease through time for a population may be possible only in a very general sense. As Waldron (1994: 22) suggests, if there are no temporal subunits available for the population being analysed, then a mean prevalence rate for specific diseases is produced. This is all well and good, but it does not pick out the peaks in disease prevalence that may have occurred throughout the time span of the cemetery, and these peaks may have increased the mean disease rate when, for most of the time, the population was reasonably 'healthy'. This question of frequency rates in palaeopathology and how they are calculated is eloquently discussed by Waldron (1994), and to be able to compare population frequencies of disease temporally and geographically their correct assimilation is absolutely essential. However, it should be remembered that only around 15 per cent of burials in a typical archaeological skeletal sample will have evidence of disease (Ortner, 2003), and 80–90 per cent of those individuals will show evidence of trauma, infection or joint disease.

PALAEODEMOGRAPHIC STRUCTURE: AGE AND SEX

Not only are population numbers studied in the past but also the age and sex structure of those populations because these variables are instrumental in the contraction and maintenance of disease (e.g. see Reichs, 1986a; Grauer and Stuart-Macadam, 1998; Pollard and Hyatt, 1999). However, the age and sex structure of a population may be biased by a number of factors. Males, females, people with specific diseases and/or disabilities and different age groups may have been buried away from the main cemetery, thus eliminating certain sections of society. A possible sex bias in an excavated cemetery may be highlighted in the following examples. It may be expected that cemeteries associated with monasteries or battlefields would contain more males than females. This situation was found in the cemetery of St Andrew, Fishergate, York (Stroud and Kemp, 1993); here, in the monastic phase, of 228 adults 173 (73 per cent) were males. Likewise, the thirty-seven skeletons excavated from the Wars of the Roses battlefield at Towton, Yorkshire were all young males (Fiorato et al., 2001), as were the individuals from the Tudor battleship the Mary Rose that sank and was later excavated off the south coast of England (Stirland, 2000). With respect to the (frequent) absence of non-adult individuals from many cemetery sites, many factors could be responsible, including non-survival of the skeletal remains because of their size and fragility (Guy et al., 1997, although see Saunders, 1992), and burial away from the main cemetery in a context that is not excavated (Saunders, 2000). While some children's cemeteries have been excavated, such as the cremated remains of thousands of juveniles in the Punic cemetery at Carthage, Tunisia and on the island of Motya, off the west coast of Sicily (see Markoe, 2000), the numbers of non-adult skeletons compared to those of adults available for study from archaeological sites are generally much lower.

Methods of analysis for age and sex estimation

Determining the age and sex distribution of a cemetery population is the first step towards establishing a palaeodemographic profile for a group of skeletons. Methods used for age and sex determination have developed over many years mainly using skeletal remains of known sex and age (Bass, 1987). For example, the Terry Collection is a group of over 1,700 skeletons collected in the earlier twentieth century and curated in the Department of Anthropology in the National Museum of Natural History, Smithsonian Institution, Washington DC, and the Hamann–Todd collection comprises over 3,000 skeletons curated at the Cleveland Museum of Natural History, Ohio, both in the United States. Research on both groups has generated methods of analysis using specific parts of the skeleton that are then applied to archaeologically derived skeletal remains. However, it should be remembered that the methods are based on relatively modern populations with different diets, activities and living environments when compared to our distant ancestors, and thus the expression of sexual traits and age-related phenomena in the skeleton may be very different from what it was in the past. As Milner et al. (2000: 477) say, these documented collections 'are highly selected samples . . . [and] . . . age at death distributions of these two collections cannot be regarded as representative of any real community'.

Sex estimation

The sex of an individual is established at conception and indicates a chromosomal difference: XX is female and XY is male. Important to note also at this point is the definition of gender, because, in a modern context, gender is often (incorrectly) used instead of sex to describe biological sex. Sex refers to biological sex and gender refers to the socio-cultural differences placed on the biological differences between males and females – that is, cultural construction is linked to biological sex but not defined by it (Mays and Cox, 2000: 117). However, even though there is usually a correlation between sex and gender, it cannot always be

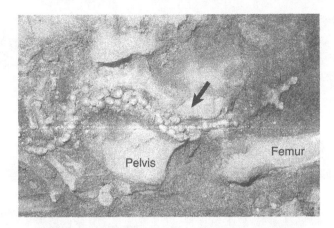

Fig. 2.2. Skeleton excavated in the Netherlands with buried grave-goods in the form of a rosary. *(With permission of Wilbert Bouts)*

assumed to be the case, and, as indicated by Walker and Cook (1998), these two descriptive terms should be kept separate. Unfortunately, the recent global introduction of the term 'gender' to refer to 'sex' has blurred the differences between the two. Furthermore, on many occasions the characteristics of grave-goods buried (Fig. 2.2) with a skeleton have been taken as indicating either male or female (weapons and jewellery, respectively) rather than the biological features of the skeleton being used to indicate sex; it is much more likely that grave-goods indicate gender rather than sex, and of course sex may be different from the gender indicated (for an example, see Effros, 2000). As Ucko (1969) points out, our assumptions about why and how people are buried in the past can be very much explained by ethnographic study. One should never substitute archaeological for biological data when sex is being determined.

Hormones produced in the bodies of males and females determine sexual dimorphism as seen in the skeleton. However, despite the presence of papers in the literature suggesting otherwise, the estimation of biological sex in the non-adult skeleton is not possible with any reliability because sexual dimorphism is not well expressed in the skeletons of people of such a young age; it is not until puberty that changes start to occur (see Saunders 2000; Scheuer and Black, 2000a). However, with the advance in ancient DNA analysis, it has now become possible to determine the sex of non-adult skeletons (and also fragmentary and cremated remains) based on the detection of X and Y chromosome-specific sequences within the amelogenin gene (Stone *et al.*, 1996; Brown, 2001). This development enables more probing questions to be asked of skeletal remains such as: what sex were these apparent infanticide victims (Mays and Faerman, 2001), or children buried at a convent (Cunha *et al.*, 2000)? Additionally, on the basis of this technological advance, it will now become possible to include non-adults, divided into males and females, in demographic profiles from cemetery populations, and explore mortality differences and reasons for patterns seen. Saunders (2000: 153) does note that there are 'still issues of consistency, control, false negatives and false positives . . . as well as current cost and expense of testing large samples from which substantial proportions may never yield amplifiable DNA'. However, developments in techniques are becoming rapid, as seen in a recent paper by Schmidt *et al.* (2003).

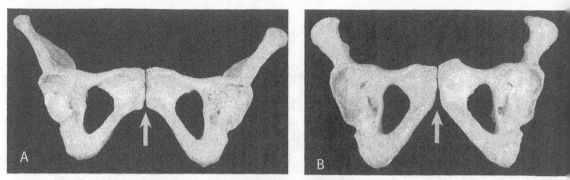

Fig. 2.3. Pelvis of female (A) and male (B) showing the wider subpubic angle of the female.

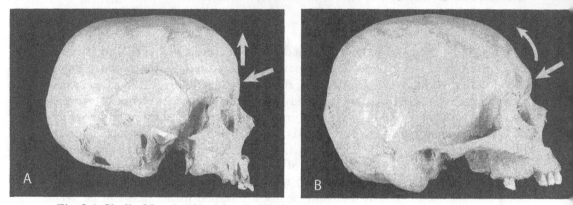

Fig. 2.4. Skull of female (A) and male (B) showing the more upright forehead and less prominent brow ridges of the female.

The estimation of sex of adult skeletons relies primarily on the pelvis, less so on the skull, and sometimes on measurements taken from certain parts of the skeleton (methods are described in Krogman and Iscan, 1986; Bass, 1987; Buikstra and Ubelaker, 1994; Mays and Cox, 2000; see Figs 2.3 and 2.4). The traits in the skull are observed, and metrical data generally tend to reflect the robusticity of the individual, with the assumption that larger measurements and more prominent features on the skull indicate maleness; this is, of course, not always necessarily the case. In some parts of the world even today very prominent cranial features can be seen in females, and they may also have very robust skeletons that may reflect an active lifestyle involving hard manual labour. Additionally, young males may appear more feminine and gracile in their skeletons while older females appear more masculine and robust (Walker, 1995). It should be noted that the expression of male- and female-related traits may vary within and between populations, and there may even be mixtures of male and female traits in the same skeleton. Therefore, sex estimation of different 'populations' can require some adjustments to the methodologies used. The final area to consider with regard to biological sex is that of 'parturition scars' (Cox, 2000a). These 'scars' on the pelvis were identified in the 1970s and 1980s as indicating evidence for childbirth (and the number of children a mother had borne). A number of different locations for the 'scars' were identified:

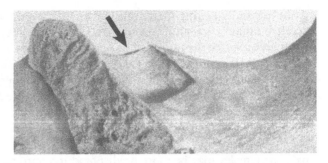

Fig. 2.5. Pre-auricular sulcus ('parturition scar') next to the joint surface of the ilium of the pelvis. *(Calvin Wells Photographic Collection)*

the pre-auricular sulcus next to the auricular surface of the ilium (Fig. 2.5), pitting on the posterior aspect of the pubic symphysis, and the pubic tubercle. These features are believed to be associated with stress (in the later stages of pregnancy) on the ligaments that attach to these sites. The most recent research by Cox on the eighteenth- and nineteenth-century skeletons from Christ Church, Spitalfields, London (summarized in Cox, 2000a: 135) indicates that, on the basis of observations of the 'scars' and an appraisal of the obstetric history of the individuals, there was 'no statistically significant association between absence, presence, severity, type or size of the pre-auricular sulcus with parity status; the same proved to be the case for pubic pitting'. However, she noted a statistically significant relationship between an extension of the pubic tubercle and the number of children a female had given birth to, although she also stressed that even 33 per cent of the women who had not had children had this feature. In summary, the use of these 'scars' cannot be reliably taken as indicating the biological sex of an individual because males may exhibit a pre-auricular sulcus or, indeed, whether a female has had children. Other methods that may help with the identification of sex (but ones that should never be relied on totally) are grave-goods (see discussion above), foetal bones in the pelvic area (Fig. 2.6), circumstances of burial, presence of sex-specific diseases and associated historical data. Obviously the sex estimation of complete bodies, for example, the 'Iceman' (Spindler, 1994) and 'Lindow Man' (Stead *et al.*, 1986), may be easier to identify because of the survival of soft tissue.

Estimating the biological sex of the skeleton is paramount to the interpretation

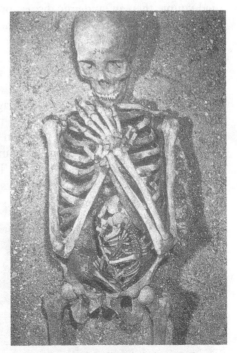

Fig. 2.6. Late Medieval skeleton of a woman who died with her baby unborn. *(Æbelholt cemetery, Denmark)*

of the person's health. It is well known that women have a stronger and more effective immune system (Stinson, 1985; Ortner, 1998, 2003) and therefore may be better able to resist the impact of disease. Additionally, research indicates that men (in this case, in the United States at the beginning of the twenty-first century) suffer more chronic conditions than women, and have a higher death rate for the top fifteen causes of death (Courtenay, 2000). They also increase their risks of poor health by following behaviour that indicates their masculinity, and do not seek health care as much as females; there are, of course, exceptions where women behave more like men and increase their risk of disease. However, there are many instances where either males or females may be more predisposed to contracting a certain disease, and this may be related to many variables in their life. This could include the diet they have access to, the work that they do and the environment in which they live. For example, in the early twenty-first century in some parts of the world women are more exposed than men to indoor air pollution produced by burning fuels such as wood and dung purely because they (and their children) are indoors for longer periods of time (Ozbay *et al.*, 2001). Thus it becomes vital to consider sex differences in health and behaviour, and estimating the sex of skeletons excavated from archaeological sites is the first step to exploring the reasons behind any differences seen.

Age at death estimation

Like sex, the age at death of individual skeletons, and of populations, helps us to understand and interpret their health status. For example, if a group of people have all died young, then an epidemic disease process must be considered as a cause of death. If it is a group of dead young males, then interpersonal violence may be a possibility (e.g. Fiorato *et al.*, 2001), and if a large group of infants is found in a strange burial context, then perhaps infanticide could be a likely explanation (e.g. Smith and Kahila, 1992). Furthermore, there are diseases that target certain age groups just as they do for the two sexes. The attribution of age at death in a non–adult or young adult skeleton (up to around 25–30 years of age) is relatively straightforward as long as the necessary parts of the skeleton are preserved. In the case of non–adults, the development, calcification and eruption of the deciduous (milk) and permanent teeth are key to estimating age, particularly up to the age of 12–13 years when the second permanent molar develops (Fig. 2.7). This is because they usually develop in a set sequence (in girls 1–2 years before boys) (Whittaker, 2000); the same can be said for

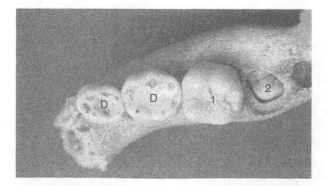

Fig. 2.7. Lower jaw showing that the two deciduous molars (D) and the first permanent molar (1) have erupted, but the second permanent molar (2) has yet to erupt; this individual was at least 6 years of age when he or she died.

the maturation of the bones. The growth of (and epiphyseal fusion in) the bones of the skeleton also provide a parameter on which to base age at death (Fig. 2.8), because there are certain ages at which the maturation of the individual bones of the skeleton occurs (see Scheuer and Black, 2000a (summary) and b for an excellent review of the juvenile skeleton; also Humphrey, 2000). As for all the age estimation methods, by necessity, data have been taken from relatively recent populations, and thus one has to question the validity of applying these data/methods to archaeologically derived skeletons. While there has been little specific palaeopathological research focused on juveniles (but see Lewis, 2002a), work is increasing and, as Lewis states (2000: 39), 'the health and survival of the offspring indicate the level to which a population has adapted to the environment in which it lives'. Therefore, the study of the demographic profile of juveniles in relation to their health status is an area of research that would benefit palaeopathology in the future.

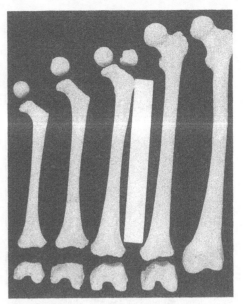

Fig. 2.8. Series of femurs showing youngest (left) to oldest (right) based on the fusion of the epiphyses; far right is the femur of an adult.

In the adult, as Maples (1989: 323) says, 'age determination is ultimately an art, not a precise science', and there has been much debate about the accuracy of ageing adult skeletons, with suggestions that people in the past were living longer than was once thought (e.g. see Molleson and Cox, 1993; Cox, 2000b). Molleson and Cox (1993) indicated that those aged over 70 years were being under-aged at the post-Medieval site of Christ Church, Spitalfields, London, and those less than 40 years over-aged. As Cox (2000b: 75) points out, the main problem is trying to correlate non-linear changes with passing linear time, because nowhere do we fully understand how and why the changes occur in the skeleton, and this makes it difficult to use the changes to assess accurate age. There is no reason to doubt that, once a person survived the hazardous years of infancy and childhood, he or she would live to a reasonable age. The problem we have today is that we do not have methods of age estimation that will age skeletons into the 70-, 80- and 90-year categories, and this is because the methods are based on documented skeletal material that often does not reflect those older age categories.

Following the development and eruption of the permanent teeth and the full development of the skeleton to its adult state – that is, when all epiphyses are fused – the body, including the skeleton, starts to degenerate, and people's skeletons will deteriorate at different rates, thus making a precise estimation of age using methods currently available very difficult (for overviews see Krogman and Iscan, 1986; Iscan, 1989; Buikstra and Ubelaker, 1994; Cox, 2000b; Jackes, 2000). There has been a

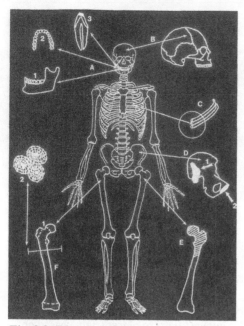

Fig. 2.9. Diagram of skeleton summarising the adult age estimation methods.
A: 1: Eruption of the third molars
   2: Dental attrition
   3: Dental root transparency
B: Cranial suture closure
C: Degeneration of the sternal ends of the ribs
D: 1: Degeneration of the auricular surface of the pelvis
   2: Degeneration of the pubic symphysis
E: Changes in the trabecular bone structure in the proximal end of the femur
F: 1: Late fusing epiphyses
   2: Changes in the histological structure of the cortical bone

tendency to utilize as many methods as possible with the hope that the majority will result in a similar age (e.g. see Bedford *et al.*, 1993; Fig. 2.9). However, it should be remembered that virtually all the methods (apart from dental wear analysis) have been developed and tested on known aged and sexed populations of different ancestries (see above) who have particular diets, diseases and lifeways that will affect how fast or slowly their skeletons age. Thus the methods used reflect the age structure (and rate of degeneration) of the skeletal population that the method has been developed on; this may or may not be appropriate for use on an archaeological skeletal population. The methods used include dental wear or attrition (e.g. Brothwell, 1989; Miles, 2001), closure of the cranial sutures (Masset, 1989), degeneration of the joint surfaces at the pubic symphysis (Meindl and Lovejoy, 1989) and auricular surfaces of the ilium (Lovejoy *et al.*, 1985), degeneration at the sternal ends of the ribs (Loth and Iscan, 1989), radiographic and histological analyses of bones (Sorg *et al.*, 1989 and Robling and Stout, 2000, respectively) and teeth (Whittaker, 2000), and the eruption of the third molar and fusion of the late fusing epiphyses such as the sternal end of the clavicle and vertebral end plates. Some of the methods require knowledge of the sex of the skeleton before they can be used, and often an age range is usually assigned to a skeleton or even a label such as 'young' or 'older' adult. Clearly, from the current literature, in order to counteract the inherent problems in ageing adult skeletons, sophisticated statistical methods of analysis are now being used (Aykroyd *et al.*, 1999; Jackes, 2000; Schmitt *et al.*, 2002); this has been extended to analysing perinatal skeletal material (Gowland and Chamberlain, 2002). However, it has been suggested that we should rather move away from trying to assign a specific age or age range to a skeleton and use developmental stages in relation to survival (Wiley and Pike, 1998). We do not know how important (or not) assigning an age to a person was in the past; it is highly probable that progression through life was related to specific events, and when the person reached that development stage such as crawling or walking then his or her status in their group changed. These achievements may also have affected their health. For example, walking increases the risk of having more accidents and weaning may lead to diarrhoea; both these experiences could ultimately lead to death.

Palaeodemography

Once age and sex have been estimated for each skeleton, it then becomes possible to build up a demographic profile. Palaeodemography considers the size, structure and dynamics of an ancient population (Chamberlain, 2001: 259), but 'there is no quick and easy route by which population size and structure can be inferred from archaeological data'. Pennington (2001: 170) is adamant that as everything that humans do ultimately depends on life and death then the study of demography is 'fundamental to understanding everything about our species'. A palaeodemographic profile reflects the age at death structure of a dead (not living) population, and its morbidity (the occurrence of disease), which is intrinsically related to age- and sex-specific diseases, genetic inheritance and fertility (Reichs, 1986a, b; Polednak, 1989). Diseases may be seen in skeletons from the site, but many will not because soft tissue (and acute) diseases do not leave any mark on the skeleton. However, a demographic study may be the only way to explore the impact of a soft tissue disease on a population, as has recently been undertaken for a Black Death cemetery in fourteenth-century England (Margerison and Knüsel, 2002). Palaeodemography is also related to extrinsic factors such as diet, social status, living conditions, climate, migration in and out of the group, and occupation (e.g. see Learmonth, 1988 for a discussion of ecological aspects of human disease), as we have seen. We might expect in the past that many people died in infancy because of acute infections and respiratory and diarrhoeal diseases, with few making it to older ages (as in many developing countries today). This is often the case, even though it is not possible to assign adults to older age categories and relatively few non-adult skeletons survive to be analysed. Additionally, the hazards of childbirth in the past may determine in some mortality profiles the higher frequency of deaths in young adult women compared to men (although this cannot be proved). Before the twentieth century and the advent of modern obstetric care, of course, childbirth was a very hazardous process indeed. Reproductive death is not merely a problem of parturition but is a hazard throughout pregnancy. In respect of complications, particularly haemorrhage, the greater the number of pregnancies, the greater is the likelihood of such complications. The number of pregnancies in antiquity may have been high by modern western standards and this could have influenced female mortality greatly. Of course, apart from young adult female mortality in demographic profiles, there are instances of foetal and newly born infant bones being found with buried females (e.g. Wells, 1978). However, the numbers are not large. For example, a recent survey of obstetric deaths in Britain revealed just 29 obstetric-related deaths out of nearly 35,000 individuals surveyed dating from between the Neolithic period (as early as 4000 BC) to the post-Medieval period (as late as the mid-nineteenth century AD) (Roberts and Cox, 2003).

The demographic profile may incorporate a mortality profile (Fig. 2.10), a survivorship curve and a life table. Mortality is the relative frequency of deaths in

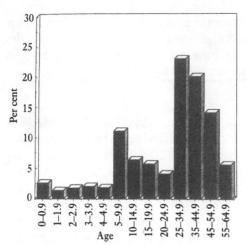

Fig. 2.10. Mortality rate for the late Medieval (twelfth–sixteenth centuries AD) population excavated at St Helen-on-the-Walls, York. *(From Grauer, 1991, and with permission of Anne Grauer)*

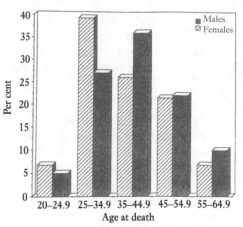

Fig. 2.11. Mortality rate by sex for the late Medieval adult population excavated at St Helen-on-the-Walls, York. *(From Grauer, 1991, and with permission of Anne Grauer)*

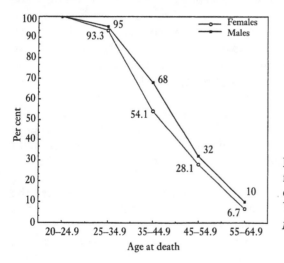

Fig. 2.12. Survivorship curve by sex for the late Medieval adult population excavated at St Helen-on-the-Walls, York. *(From Grauer, 1991, and with permission of Anne Grauer)*

relation to population numbers, and the mortality profile shows at what age people were dying and whether there are any differences between male and female adults (Fig. 2.11). Death affects all age groups but in differing frequencies depending on time period, geographic location and intrinsic and extrinsic factors referred to above. A survivorship curve (Fig. 2.12) is another way of presenting the data and shows the proportion of people in each age group, starting at 100 per cent for the youngest age group represented. Life tables provide a wide range of information on mortality and survivorship in a population, and this includes the probability of dying in an age category and the average number of years a person could expect to live when entering a particular age category (life expectancy). As

Chamberlain (2001: 260) points out, it is a mathematical device used to represent the mortality experience of a population. Each component is derived from the original raw data on age at death for the individuals. Inherent in all these calculations is the problem of lack of accurate age estimations for adult skeletons and lack of sex estimation for non-adults, and many have reiterated the need to address the problem particularly with respect to age estimation (e.g. Buikstra and Konigsberg, 1985; Chamberlain, 2000). Additionally, as for calculating frequencies of disease over the time span of a cemetery (see above), because of the (often) lack of stratigraphic data for many cemeteries, it is not possible to chart changes in mortality through time. This means mortality rates are calculated for the whole population. The study of palaeodemography has had, as Milner *et al.* (2000) point out, a long history that has been fraught with problems of accuracy of biological sex and age data, selective mortality, the presence of inherent frailty and unknown in- and out-migration. However, the integration of demographic profiles with data on health and disease for archaeologically derived populations is essential for us to understand the impact of disease on our ancestors. Fortunately for palaeopathology, Milner *et al.* (2000) are very optimistic about the future of palaeodemographic study as more researchers tackle and conquer problems with methodological advancements.

STATURE AND HEALTH

Of particular relevance to health is stature or attained height. Although 'genes are important determinants of individual height' (Steckel, 1995: 1903), any genetic differences 'approximately cancel out in comparisons of averages across most populations, and in these situations heights accurately reflect health status'. Steckel (1995: 1910) emphasizes this by describing studies of genetically similar and dis-similar populations in different environments and indicating that height differences are 'largely attributable to environmental factors' (especially during childhood and adolescence). There is also a very strong correlation between nutritional status and height, and susceptibility to disease may be enhanced by poor nutrition, a depressed immune status and poor absorption of nutrients. Additionally, work demands food to fuel the body, and excessive hard manual activity may deprive the body of nutrients necessary for growth (Steckel, 1995: 1910). A reduced stature may indicate less than adequate nutrition and poor health when the person was growing, although 'catch-up' growth can occur where there is an increase in the growth rate following suppression in older juveniles (Bogin, 1988). Measures of height have been used by many researchers to assess inequality, in the form of nutritional deprivation and level of income, especially in the twentieth century. This has revealed, not surprisingly, that higher-status people were taller, reflecting inequality in the biological standard of living (Steckel, 1995: 1922).

The assessment of juvenile growth is a more sensitive measure of changes in health and nutritional status than adult growth; variation in juveniles is usually because of immediate conditions, but for adults it is more likely to be the result of a chronic condition (Goodman and Martin, 2002). Unfortunately, because of the problem of sex estimation of non-adults, it is not usually possible to examine sex differences in growth. However, research on the growth of juveniles by measuring the length of the long bones and correlating them with dental age has allowed comparisons of growth to be made between archaeologically derived juvenile populations and also living populations in developing and developed countries (for a good overview of research and problems, see Humphrey, 2000). Additionally, there have been correlations made between growth, as seen in long bone length, and the presence of indicators of stress such as dental enamel defects (e.g. Ribot and Roberts, 1996), and Gunnell *et al.* (2001) found that individuals with shorter bones died younger; both these studies focused on Medieval English skeletal populations. Finally, Lewis (2002a) considered the impact of urbanization and industrialization on mortality and morbidity and found that the growth of juveniles was affected, particularly at post-Medieval Christ Church, at Spitalfields in London, as a result of industrialization, but the children's growth at St Helen-on-the-Walls in York, northern England, in the late Medieval period was not affected by urbanization.

Adult stature is calculated by measuring the maximum lengths of the long bones (preferably the femur and tibia) and, for most biological anthropologists, using the regression formulae of Trotter (1970) to produce a stature. Of course, these equations were developed on individuals with known age, sex and height from the early twentieth-century Americas, and must therefore be used with some caution in archaeological studies of stature. For adult stature, it is very difficult to determine the cause of reduced height, and, because of the loss of juveniles to death before adulthood and the process of 'catch-up' growth, adults tend not to be as sensitive to any changes in the 'environment', in its broadest sense (Goodman and Martin, 2002: 22). Nevertheless, a study of long bone growth and height in archaeological populations should always consider possible variables within the population's environment such as genetic make-up, nutritional status, environment and disease (see various studies in Steckel and Rose, 2002). An example of data from Britain shows stature in skeletal populations from the Mesolithic (as early as 10,500 BC) to the post-Medieval period, revealing interesting patterns (Table 2.1).

Table 2.1 Mean stature (cm) from the Mesolithic to the post-Medieval period in Britain

Period	Male	No.	Female	No.
Mesolithic	165	3	157	2
Neolithic	165	71	157	36
Bronze Age	172	61	161	20
Iron Age	168	113	162	72
Roman	169	1,296	159	1,042
Early Medieval	172	996	161	751
Late Medieval	171	8,494	159	7,929
Post-Medieval	171	558	160	540

Source: Roberts and Cox, 2003: 396.

While the increases and decreases in stature may be small, and the data are collated from many cemeteries from different geographic regions and contexts, the apparent *rise* in stature in the early Medieval period (mid-fifth to mid-eleventh centuries AD) may suggest better health for this essentially rural-based society. This can be compared to lower stature in the previous urban-based skeletal populations of the Roman period, and the subsequent late Medieval period characterized by increasing population density and poorer living conditions. However, higher early Medieval stature may be the result of the mixing of the British population with new influxes of people, if the 'migration theory' is believed (for a discussion, see Lucy, 2000). However, we do not know how many people came to Britain at that time from the Continent, and Tanner (1978 in Steckel, 1995) notes that 'outbreeding' has a minor effect on stature. Furthermore, Steckel (1995: 1922) has noted that it is only recently that urban populations have seen a height advantage over their rural counterparts. Perhaps the most dramatic *declines* in stature have been seen in studies of populations making the transition to agriculture, and several contributions to the volume edited by Cohen and Armelagos (1984) document this decline. However, some studies found the opposite, some document an increase in one sex but not the other, and there was much discussion about the validity of using attained height as an indicator of economic status (in its broadest sense). Less obvious, however, are those factors affecting stature that depend on the structure of society itself. It is well known that inbreeding may lead to smaller people. No doubt in the past in some societies where there was little movement, and contact with others was limited, inbreeding during many generations took place. However, any benefit from the reduction of inbreeding and increase in stature would probably be offset by the more rapid spread of disease (especially infections) that results from travel, trade and contact.

Of all the myths surrounding human populations in antiquity, perhaps the most widely believed and the most easily disproved is that concerning stature. The popular picture of the world inhabited by small people cannot be supported. Stature estimates for human skeletal remains demonstrate that both males and females were more or less of similar stature to modern groups at least until the mid-twentieth century in Western society. Over more recent time, certainly for developed countries, maximum stature has increased (and been attained earlier in life), and the most obvious reason must be improved childhood nutrition and medical care to prevent and treat disease. In 1950 in the United States and Britain mean stature of men was 175cm, but in other European countries such as the Netherlands height was 178cm. As Steckel (1995: 1920) notes: 'Although Americans were once the tallest people in the world . . . [they] now lag behind some Western European nations in international comparisons of stature.' Currently American males have a mean stature of 177cm while in the Netherlands it is 181cm. However, up until the end of the eighteenth century, when agricultural productivity increased in Europe, stature could not have reached that of American populations because diets were so inadequate for the majority and calorie intake was much lower (Steckel, 1995: 1925). Americans also had low population density, a low incidence of epidemic disease and lots of land to cultivate for food and on which to raise stock. Clearly, knowledge of stature and its relationship to causative variables is vital to our understanding of disease today, and the same can be said for the past. A correlation of stature data with indicators of disease stress, along with a consideration of 'environmental' factors for specific archaeological populations, is essential.

SOCIAL STATUS AND HEALTH

There have been many studies in clinical contexts where social status has been examined with respect to health (e.g. Krieger *et al.*, 1995; Fein, 1995). It makes sense that poorer people have more disease because they are often eating a less varied and nutritious diet, living in poor-quality housing, and often working in occupations that have a significant increase in health risks (e.g. see Schell and Czerwinski, 1998). However, in the archaeological record there have been relatively few studies of health and social status (e.g. Powell, 1988; Cohen, 1998), although inferences of higher social status individuals (monastic) having more diffuse idiopathic skeletal hyperostosis (DISH) have been made frequently (e.g. Rogers and Waldron, 2001). Nevertheless, Robb *et al.* (2001), in a recent study of grave goods and disease in an Iron Age population from Italy, found that some health indicators such as enamel hypoplasia and enamel defects had no relation to status, but that trauma, Schmorls nodes and periostitis seemed to relate to activity, and hence social status. Clearly, more studies of this nature are needed when one considers the amount of research conducted on living populations in this area, but to be able to carry this out effectively, sound archaeological data concerning the status (identity) of populations are needed at the outset.

ETHNICITY AND HEALTH

To complete this chapter, we must not forget that ethnic identity can be another factor in the occurrence of disease. Now also termed 'ancestry', as opposed to 'race', ethnicity refers to social identities and cultural differences. Ethnic groups are characterized by cultural distinctions such as those of history, heredity, religion and language (Brown, 1998: 259). However, the boundaries between different ethnic groups can be blurred, and the considerable amount of intermixing of people makes identifying a person to a particular 'group' much more difficult today. Of course, hereditary factors, or the presence of genes that can lead to traits in an individual that cause disease, can be influential in disease causation (Weiss, 1993). It should be noted that today the term 'race' is considered by many as an historic artefact, and the term has attracted (and still does attract) stigma, exploitation and injustice associated with certain groups throughout history (as does the term 'leper') (see the American Association of Physical Anthropologists' statement on biological aspects of 'race' (1996)). However, we should be aware that in forensic anthropology 'race' is an aspect of the identification process when a forensic anthropologist examines human remains from a crime scene (see chapter in Krogman and Iscan, 1986, and Sauer's 1992 discussion of the existence of 'races'). 'Race' is also a category defined on the police force's 'missing persons list', and 'Caucasoid', 'Mongoloid' and 'Negroid' are listed as the main 'racial' groups, with many subdivisions (Jurmain *et al.*, 2003). Forensic anthropologists tend to focus on the cranial and facial characteristics and measurements (and multivariate statistical analysis) of a skeleton to categorize 'race', and also on the characteristics of the teeth (Scott and Turner, 1997), but we do know that many factors can contribute to the shape of the skull, such as diet and climate. Nevertheless, identification of traits in a body or skeleton that are associated with particular ethnic or 'racial' groups shows that there can be a mixture of traits related to more than one 'group'.

In spite of these discussions about terminology, it is important to consider how ethnicity contributes to disease in any population, and authors have documented that some diseases are more common in some populations (e.g. Reichs, 1986b; Polednak, 1989). For example, sickle-cell anaemia occurs almost exclusively in 'Negroid' populations or in populations from the southern Mediterranean (Polednak, 1989). Due consideration should therefore be given to the geographic location of a skeletal population and the intrinsic and extrinsic factors that might be relevant to the patterns of disease seen. Added to this, it is obvious today that some ethnic groups treat males, females, children and particular age groups in different ways, which will affect what health problems they encounter. Important too is a consideration of health beliefs in different groups, which will, in turn, affect whether and how a disease might be treated (see Roberts and Buikstra, 2003 on tuberculosis in a variety of populations around the world today).

EPILOGUE

This chapter has discussed the inherent importance of considering the age, sex, stature, social status and ethnicity of individuals and populations, and their demographic profiles, in order to understand the patterns of disease seen; without these data a study of palaeopathology would be meaningless. The changing rates and patterns of disease throughout prehistory and history clearly (and obviously) reflect changes in disease prevalence through different times of life for populations. The further advent of new diseases, and re-emerging ones, brought about by modern complex industrial technologies, increased travel, warfare and refugee status, poverty, increased lack of access to medical care for the unfortunate, and more drug resistance, will cause further changes in mortality patterns in the future; differences will also be maintained (and increased) between the rich and poor in developing and developed countries. Clearly, though, mortality rates are influenced by many factors both past and present and, sadly, many such as poverty are much the same today as they were in the distant past.

CHAPTER 3

Congenital Disease

Detecting developmental defects within a prehistoric skeletal population permits interpretive projections for the occurrence of major defects, biological affinities, and both cultural and environmental influences. (Barnes, 1994: 5)

INTRODUCTION

If one considers the skeletal characteristics of the males and females of all nations, it is noted that there is a marked similarity of form between them. The number and size of the bones are fairly constant. The marks of muscular attachment on bones are the same for all humanity. The internal soft tissue organs are likewise uniform. In terms of skin colour and hair form, the ancestral groups exhibit wide differences. There is, however, quite marked normal variation in the shape and structure of some bones, in particular the skull, in different groups. Berry and Berry (1967) have observed many morphological deviations from normal in the cranium and correlated some with a genetic origin. Finnegan (1978) and Scott and Turner (1997) have also noted deviations from the normal appearance in the post–cranial skeleton and teeth, respectively. However, some work suggests that these traits may have other causes, for example, some may be occupationally related (Saunders, 1989; Tyrrell, 2000). These observations perhaps demonstrate that there is a remarkable degree of genetic constancy in the various ancestral groups. These facts are perhaps no more than evolutionary expectations.

And yet, at the individual level, problems in normal development do occur. Developmental abnormalities occur both in soft tissues and in the skeleton; these commence during foetal development and present themselves at birth or shortly thereafter. These developmental defects constitute the range of what can also be termed congenital disease. This range extends from the most minor anomaly of development which may never produce signs or symptoms in the individual, to the most severe abnormality which is incompatible with life itself. The full extent of abnormalities of foetal development is not, and may never be, known, since spontaneous abortion may, in some cases, be nature's way of eliminating the grossly abnormal. In contemporary societies these defects can, however, be documented, but in the less developed areas of the world even this may be an ideal not yet achieved. How much more difficult it is then to determine the range of congenital disease present in antiquity, and yet few population-based studies have been attempted (but see Barnes, 1994 on American south-west populations, Sture, 2002 on a comparison of urban and rural Northern English Medieval populations, and Masnicová and

Beñus, 2003 on Middle Age Slovakian populations). It is, without doubt, this class of abnormal variation in palaeopathology that dominates the published literature in the form of case studies. Perhaps we should also consider that children with congenital malformations may have been subject to infanticide, buried away from the main cemetery and/or stigmatized when alive. This will affect whether they survive in the archaeological record and therefore are available for study.

Soft tissue abnormality is, of course, recognizable only in preserved bodies, and these represent only a very small proportion of humanity in the archaeological record. In the context of biological anthropology only the skeletal abnormalities can be catalogued and it is only since the mid-1990s that minor abnormalities of skeletal development have been recorded. Developmental defects can occur in any body tissue, and some populations are more likely to have specific defects than others. For example, Barnes (1994: 9) notes that spina bifida and anencephaly occur more frequently in north-western Europeans, and that the Japanese have the highest frequencies of cleft lip. Recent figures for developmental/congenital malformations indicate that in 1998 in England and Wales malformations rose by 2 per cent on 1997 rates (Anon., 1999), and the rate was 87.8 per 10,000 live births. In 1999 rates for some conditions increased (Anon., 2000), and for Wales were the highest overall for all countries of Britain (171 per 10,000 total births compared to 105 for England – Pearce and Goldblatt, 2001: 39). The most common disorders for 1998 were those involving the musculo-skeletal system, which, of course, has implications for their recognition in the archaeological record. Numerically, therefore, skeletal malformations are more significant than individual system soft-tissue malformations in live births. It must not be forgotten, of course, that in archaeological terms it is mainly the live births which are preserved and examined, and only rarely are still births recognized; even then they are usually too fragmented or poorly preserved to be of palaeopathological interest. The numerical significance of these skeletal malformations is clear, but their survival significance is not great. Looking at the survival of malformed and of normal individuals, in a 1960s study (Table 3.1) it was noted that in the first year of life there is a great mortality difference between the two groups, and that this persists to the 5 year age group. Doubtless, the infant survival rate of antiquity was much less than today, so, bearing in mind the added disadvantage that malformation confers in terms of care, feeding and susceptibility to intercurrent infection, the discrepancy between the two groups in Table 3.1 would have been greater in antiquity than it is today. However, for the reasons of preservation just given, the recognition of such malformations in skeletal remains of these age groups is rarely possible.

In antiquity, the actual percentage of infant and childhood deaths attributable solely to developmental defects was probably low. Doubtless, many infantile deaths were due to the common infections of gastroenteritis and pneumonia, diseases that affect both normal and congenitally malformed infants. In the modern antibiotic era in which control of infantile infection is usually successful and commonplace (in developed countries), the percentage of deaths due directly to developmental defects has therefore increased. Numerically, though, the deaths attributable to the problem may have remained fairly stable; it is their significance relative to other infantile disease which has changed.

Table 3.1 Survival of malformed and of normal children to age 5 years (%)

Age	Malformed	Normal
28 weeks' gestation	100.0	100.0
Birth	83.5	98.2
1 day	76.5	97.5
1 week	69.6	96.9
1 month	63.0	96.8
1 year	53.8	96.0
5 years	51.3	95.7

Source: McKeown and Record, 1960.

In modern investigations it is noted that there is often an association between different malformations. An individual possessing one abnormality is likely also to possess a second and different abnormality (e.g. see Botting *et al.*, 1999). For example, an infant with a cleft palate or a club foot is more likely also to have an abnormality of the nervous system, and Down's syndrome is commonly associated with a malformation of the heart (McKeown and Record, 1960). It is as if nature deals a double blow. The occurrence of such different and seemingly unrelated abnormalities in a single individual is due, in fact, to a disruption of foetal development at a specific age. Any disturbing factor during the early life of the unborn child may affect several different areas of bodily development and so produce multiple abnormality. In many cases the association may be of skeletal and soft tissue malformation. In antiquity the latter is more often than not undetectable and such associations of malformation may be impossible to record. However, they are likely to have the same pattern and, for reasons of causation, more or less the same prevalence in antiquity as today (Turkel, 1989).

Because they are abnormalities of development, malformations (defects or anomalies) may be considered as the total failure of development (aplasia), the partial development (hypoplasia), the overdevelopment (hyperplasia), or the abnormal development of part of the body, which in terms of the skeleton means affecting one or more of the bones. Like most medical classifications, this is perhaps too simple, but it is nevertheless practical and convenient.

CAUSES OF DEVELOPMENTAL DEFECTS

Just as with other diseases, developmental abnormalities can rarely be ascribed to a single cause. The potential causes are many and can be grouped into genetic, or intrinsic (hereditary and affecting the constitution of the foetus), and environmental, or extrinsic, influences on the mother; their varying importance will of course differ in populations spread geographically and through time. Genetic influences cause 90 per cent of developmental defects (Patton, 1987 in Barnes, 1994). While identifying exactly what caused a particular condition in the past is impossible, it seems that the task may not even be easy today. Recent work has stressed the importance of linking developmental abnormalities and birth records in order to identify risk factors (Botting and Abrahams, 2000). The environmental influences include factors such as viral infection of the mother (e.g. rubella, measles, mumps, chickenpox and shingles), the effects of drug therapy (including alcohol) and exposure to chemicals and radiation; even in-vitro fertilization (IVF) has been suggested as being a cause of major birth defects, albeit in a small Western Australian population study (Brown, 2002). During pregnancy drugs can pass across the placenta to the unborn child, and between 2 weeks and 3 months of intrauterine development is when very serious foetal abnormalities can occur (Benjamin et al., 2002: 964). For example, phenytoin, used to treat epilepsy, can cause cleft lip and palate, and tetracycline, an antibiotic, can lead to damaged bones and teeth (Benjamin et al., 2002: 965). No doubt people in distant antiquity sought to remedy their physical ills with herbal remedies in many cases. By modern standards these crude, unrefined agents may not have been efficacious but they, too, may have had effects upon the development of the unborn. This is, of course, speculative, but these herbal remedies may have had a place in the aetiology of congenital disease in antiquity.

Exposure of the mother to radiation may also lead to birth defects developing in the unborn foetus. For example, in Iraq American weapons firing depleted uranium projectiles are believed by many to be behind the increases in birth defects in the population (Allen, 2003). The projectiles disintegrate into fine particles and contaminate the soil, water, air and people. Furthermore, in Vietnam, some thirty years after the war, there are still many people suffering birth defects and other conditions such as cancer probably because of contamination of the land by Agent Orange, a herbicide used to decimate the jungle, which contains one of the most virulent poisons known to humans (Scott-Clark and Levy, 2003).

With respect to genetic causes of these defects, many of the abnormalities can be attributed to single genes (a third – Barnes, 1994: 10), and their transference through generations should follow the patterns of Mendelian inheritance (Jurmain et al., 2003). However, some individuals are so malformed that even if they survive to adulthood, they are unable to reproduce and hence their genetic abnormality will not be passed on directly to new generations. These individual malformations arise either by the mutation of a gene, or by the maternal and paternal combination of recessive genes for the abnormality. Evidence for a genetic influence in many congenital diseases rests upon the recording of the repetition of the abnormality in siblings and other close blood relatives. Such evidence can only be obtained from contemporary and closely documented families. Its relevance to the abnormalities noted in skeletal material can only be inferred and must remain unproven. It is perhaps worthy of remark that the likelihood of congenital malformation is increased if parents are themselves close blood relatives. For example, marriage between first cousins is commonplace within certain religious groups today and it is found that there is an increase in the rate of congenital malformation in their offspring. Breeding between closely related males and females in the small isolated groups of antiquity may, of necessity, have been common and, if so, will have had a similar influence upon the malformation rate.

The majority of defects, however, are caused by multiple factors (Barnes, 1994: 10) that comprise an interaction between genetic and environmental variables.

These disorders occur when there is disturbance of development at a 'threshold level'. This level is genetically determined, and variant genes and non-genetic factors can upset this normal development, usually as a delay in timing of the threshold event as the embryo develops. The defect that results reflects disturbance in a particular developmental field in the body. Determining the causes of developmental defects in the past proves very difficult, first because the causes are usually multifactorial and secondly because there are often very few specific archaeological data to provide clues to a specific cause. However, we can hypothesize that poorly ventilated smoky housing, and the mining, metalworking and pottery industries both in prehistory and history, may have exposed parts of the population to contaminants that predisposed to these conditions.

Developmental defects are more often than not recorded as individual case studies in the literature and, as has already been noted, rarely appear as population frequencies. However, various conditions, some more common than others, have appeared in the literature throughout the history of palaeopathological study (e.g. for British contexts see Anderson, 2000 and Roberts and Cox, 2003), and what is most apparent is that they are fairly rare compared to other pathological conditions such as infectious disease. Furthermore, many of the conditions noted would be of no significance to the person concerned. Before we consider the more common, or dramatic, conditions, some discussion on the inference of disability based on the presence of a developmental defect should be given. While many authors describe what appear to be major crippling conditions in the skeletal record, the direct correlation between the condition and its significance to the afflicted person cannot be assumed (e.g. see Lebel *et al.*, 2001 and Lebel and Trinkaus, 2002 on Middle Pleistocene 'care of the disabled', and DeGusta, 2002 and 2003 for an alternative scenario).

However, there have been innovative studies on how disability may be reconstructed from the skeletal record. Clinical data, joint mobility measurements and musculo-skeletal markers were used to assess impairment and disability in an adult male from a New Mexico site in the United States, and Hawkey (1998: 337–8) concluded that, 'although severely impaired, Gran Quivara 391 was well cared for, permitting him to survive to middle age' (Fig. 3.1). Buckley and Tayles (2003) have also considered the effect of anterior humeral bowing, joint deformity and destruction, and enthesopathy development in treponematosis (yaws) on the function of individuals from a prehistoric Pacific Island. Nevertheless, we must remember that disabilities can be major or minor, temporary or permanent, visible or not, and, importantly, can be adapted to by both the individual and the society in which they live (Roberts, 2000a). Furthermore, people's experience of the same condition/disability may differ because of the nature of their personality, or even spiritual beliefs (King *et al.*, 1999), and their impact on how they view their condition, what pain they may or may not experience, and how those factors impact on their recovery. They may also be differentially stigmatized through time, by different populations and in different economic contexts. For example, a hunter-gatherer population almost continuously on the move would have more problems supporting a physically disabled person than a settled agricultural/horticultural community. In a recent study by Sugiyama (2004) of the Shiwiar forager-horticulturists in Ecuador, it was found that provision was made for people who became disabled by illnesses and injuries and this ultimately reduced mortality. This, of course, is much more difficult to assess in the past. However, an archaeological study by Murphy (2000) of developmental defects in two Iron Age semi-nomadic Siberian populations concluded that they were accepted by their peers and supported in life, because there appeared to be no differential disposal of the people affected compared to the rest of the cemetery population. It is important that due consideration of the burial context of an individual affected by a major developmental defect in the past should always be made, such as where the grave is located and whether it differs in structure from the rest of the cemetery graves.

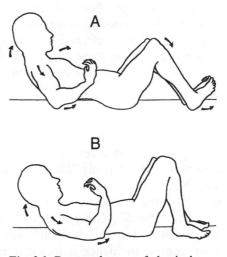

Fig. 3.1. Proposed types of physical movement possible for a diseased male skeleton (arrowed) at juvenile–subadult (A) and early adulthood (B) stages (New Mexico, United States). *(With permission of Diane Hawkey)*

The following discussion considers some of the developmental defects that have been observed in the archaeological record. For the purposes of this chapter the terms attributed to 'congenital disease' are used interchangeably and may include developmental defect, anomaly, abnormality or malformation. However, all these terms are taken to refer to conditions present at birth, or later in life, that are abnormal because of disturbances in development of a part or parts of the skeleton; they include minor and major variations. As Barnes (1994: 2) points out, most conditions seen at birth are usually severe, while those detected later on in life are not and are asymptomatic. She also argues that, if we use 'congenital disease' as the overarching term for these conditions, then we are referring only to those defects seen at birth. While this chapter is entitled 'Congenital Disease', these thoughts should be borne in mind. The identification of 'congenital disease' in non-adult skeletal remains is often fraught with problems including poor survival of immature bones for analysis due to various factors such as differential disposal of juveniles, soil conditions at burial and excavation techniques. Furthermore, incomplete development of these immature bones does not allow identification of many defects (Barnes, 1994: 5). However, Barnes indicates that, if those born with minor defects survived to adulthood, it is then that we as palaeopathologists would detect the defect.

There is, of course, great potential for the recording of developmental defects at the population level to examine family relationships and explore the causative factors behind these conditions. Barnes (1994) notes that similarities in patterns of defects represent a homogenous population but that different patterns suggest separate populations and gene pools. However, despite these attractions, there is a tendency for them to be ignored in palaeopathology for the more dramatic and more common conditions such as infectious disease.

We shall focus first on conditions affecting the skull and vertebrae (the axial skeleton), secondly on the lower limb bones (the appendicular skeleton), and finally on conditions where both axial and appendicular skeleton can be affected. Inevitably it has not been possible to consider all conditions that have been identified in past populations. Those defects that seem to be more commonly reported archaeologically in skeletal remains, those that would have been obviously visually deforming and conditions that may have led to disability and/or stigma are considered here.

AXIAL SKELETON

Anencephaly and microcephaly

Perhaps the most severe congenital abnormality known in palaeopathological contexts is anencephaly. The abnormality is incompatible with independent life after birth; only 25 per cent are born live and those die within seven days, and the condition has a modern incidence of 1 per 1,000 (Aufderheide and Rodríguez-Martín, 1998: 55). There seems to be a genetic factor in the causation of the abnormality, but this is clearly not the sole aetiology, since a difference in geographical incidence is found in modern societies. Quite possibly the same multifactorial causes operated with the same frequency in antiquity, but the failure of postnatal survival of the afflicted infants accounts for the extreme rarity of evidence from the past. The thin, fragile bones of neonates do not readily survive to allow for the recognition of skull vault abnormality.

The basic defect is the lack of development of the cranial vault and the associated failure of brain development (Fig. 3.2). A mummy from the Catacombs of Hermopolis demonstrates the abnormality; although considered at one time to be the mummy of an ape, it is in fact that of an anencephalic human (Brothwell and Powers, 1968). The failure of postnatal survival of the anencephalic child is a problem of equal significance today as it must have been in antiquity. Because of the very nature of the defect, medical management is powerless. Yet the personal grief of the new mother in the Neolithic village was probably as great as that of the mother of the twenty-first century. Notwithstanding the resigned acceptance of infant death in antiquity, pregnancy, then as now, held an expectation of success. The delivery of an anencephalic baby must have been psychologically very traumatic.

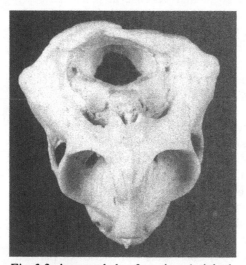

Fig. 3.2. Anencephaly of cranium (original modern example: Armed Forces Institute of Pathology 1001019, Anatomical Collections, National Museum of Health, Washington DC, United States; photograph of cast). *(Cast by France Castings, Colorado, United States)*

A less severe congenital abnormality, but one which is of profound significance in the social interpretation of antiquity, is microcephaly. This abnormality has genetic and environmental determinants and is characterized by a statistically significant subnormal skull circumference (Aufderheide and Rodríguez-Martín, 1998: 56) and general severe mental impairment (the brain weight is considerably reduced). The frontal and parietal bones recede, the occipital bone is flattened and the cranial capacity is reduced to less than 1000cc, with a circumference of less than 46cm. In addition, the cranial sutures fuse earlier than normal and the face is larger compared to the rest of the head (Aufderheide and Rodríguez-Martín, 1998: 56). Frequencies for microcephaly may be up to 1 in 2,000 births in isolated (inbred) populations (Barnes, 1994: 158). It is a rarity in skeletal remains, but a review of recorded cases has been undertaken (Richards, 1985).

Cleft palate

Although encouraged to do otherwise, many mothers in western society today choose to feed their offspring artificially with a bottle. In the past, breast-feeding must surely have been the norm (Stuart-Macadam and Dettwyler, 1995). A new-born baby needs to be able to suck in order to feed adequately at the breast. The normal infant does not find this a problem, but the infant with a cleft palate, in which there is an open connection between the mouth and nasal cavities, is unable to perform this simple function. The bony defect of cleft palate, which is due to a failure of bone union of the two halves of the palate during foetal development (Fig. 3.3), may be associated with a defect of the upper lip and bone beneath, called the cleft or hare lip. The modern incidence of the two conditions is 1 in 700 live births (Cohen, 2002: 16), but of cleft palate alone it is 1 per 1,000 live births (Aufderheide and Rodríguez-Martín, 1998: 58).

The two problems of cleft palate/lip and of cleft palate alone are in fact somewhat distinct entities with different causative factors. Cases of cleft palate are multifactorial in cause but have a strong family history and are therefore predominantly genetic in origin (Barnes, 1994: 175). The problem was probably as common in the past as it is today (and is seen more in females). Cleft lip frequency does not vary as much as cleft palate among populations (Barnes, 1994: 174) and may possibly be more related to environmental influences.

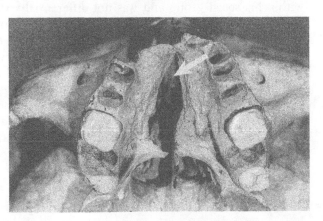

Fig. 3.3. Cleft palate (National Museum of Natural History, Washington DC, United States 316482, adult female, date unknown, south-west Colorado, United States). *(With permission of Don Ortner)*

Neonates with cleft palate require very time-consuming and laborious spoon-feeding of maternally expressed milk, or specialized artificial teat adaptation. Such care is accepted and can be provided in western societies today, but may have been unacceptable or impossible in earlier people, for example, in hunter-gatherer populations. Neonatal death of babies with cleft palate may therefore have been common in the distant past. In fact in many developing societies today, and in the past, deformed neonates, including those with manifest cleft palate and hare lip, were probably killed (or, at least, no effort was made to ensure their survival). Such actions may have been motivated by socio-economic attitudes. People with a cleft palate can suffer respiratory, speech and breathing problems (Barnes, 1994: 174) in addition to not being able to feed properly, and people with cleft lip will appear outwardly disfigured. Some of these characteristics may attach stigma to, and indeed ostracism of, people affected, especially in past communities where the conditions were not understood as they are today. However, there are instances such as those recorded in early Medieval Britain and ancient China where surgical correction of a cleft lip was undertaken (Vrebos, 1986 and Ma, 2000 respectively). Nevertheless, this depth of attention must surely have been extremely rare in the annals of congenital abnormality.

The preservation of fragile neonatal skulls is rarely good enough to allow a diagnosis of cleft palate to be made. Even diagnosing the condition in adult skeletons is fraught with difficulty because of the fragility of the palate bones, and the problem of distinguishing post-mortem breakage from ante-mortem cleft palate. There are, however, some examples in older individuals from archaeological contexts and Barnes (1994) discusses the various skeletal manifestations of cleft palate and lip. A child from sixth- to seventh-century AD Britain has been illustrated (Brothwell, 1981), but in this case the palatal defect is incomplete and may not have been associated with a deficiency of the soft tissue of the palate. Crania exhibiting both cleft palate and deformities of the maxilla indicative of hare lip have been excavated in California and dated to 2,000–4,000 years BP (Brooks and Hohenthal, 1963). These native American individuals were between the ages of 25 and 35 years at death. Another example of both palatal and lip deformities comes from Britain (Anderson, 1994a) in an eleventh- or twelfth-century 40–50-year-old male. The cleft lip made his face asymmetrical, but his age suggests he was accepted within his social group and was not differentially treated after death. The child from Britain may have been able to breast-feed, but quite probably these other examples were not. Feeding by spoon, or by some other modification lost to us through time, would have been employed, although evidence for feeding bottles has been found in the archaeological record (Drinkall and Foreman, 1998). These examples show that, perhaps contrary to the general practice in many communities, parental devotion to infant rearing is not just a phenomenon of our times but was also an ethic of distant antiquity; the use of palaeopathology to show evidence for 'care in the community' has of course been discussed (Dettwyler, 1991).

Hydrocephalus

Of all the multitude of abnormalities of development affecting people, few are more dramatic in their presentation than hydrocephalus. Literally, hydrocephalus means water on the brain, but, in strict terms, it is applied to the condition in which there is an enlargement of the normal fluid-containing spaces within the brain substance, associated with increased pressure due to accumulation of fluid. If untreated, 50 per cent of children today with the condition will die within five years of birth (Aufderheide and Rodríguez-Martín, 1998: 57). The usual clinical presentation is of a rapidly enlarging head in infancy or childhood, and this can be recognized in skeletons from the past. The condition can arise as a congenital abnormality (25 per cent of cases – Aufderheide and Rodríguez-Martín, 1998: 57), in which case the unborn foetus itself has a large head. Because of the enlargement of the unborn child's head, congenital hydro-cephalus was probably not compatible with foetal or maternal survival in antiquity. Such a case would result in obstructed labour, which, notwithstanding the documented classics of Caesarean section operations, was a fatal problem of childbirth of the past. Safe Caesarean section is a relatively modern concept. The condition may also arise due to acquired disease, and it is found that in modern populations most cases are due to the latter and arise in the first six months of life (Laurence, 1958). Infection of the brain substance by the viruses of mumps and measles is a known cause of hydrocephalus today (Aufderheide and Rodríguez-Martín, 1998: 57). Notwithstanding the limitations of these infections imposed by the group population sizes of antiquity, these viruses may also have been a cause in the distant past. However, bacterial infections, which today are cured by antibiotics but which, nevertheless, may still result in hydrocephalus, were probably fatal in antiquity before creating hydrocephalus. The possibility of a slowly growing tumour within the skull causing hydrocephalus must also be remembered, but this, too, is speculative.

The diagnosis of hydrocephalus from archaeological contexts rests upon the recognition of skull enlargement (Fig. 3.4) and upon the anatomical configuration of the facial and cranial skeleton (Richards and Anton, 1991), but hydrocephalus developing in later childhood may not result in appreciable enlargement of the head (Vaughan and MacKay, 1975). Therefore, the examples of palaeopathological interest probably had their origin within the first six months of life. Survival of such children, many of whom must surely have had physical disabilities, possibly indicates a caring attitude in the society of antiquity. If, in addition, the child was mentally subnormal, the care and

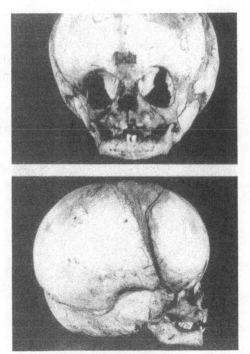

Fig. 3.4. Hydrocephalus of cranium (modern example: Pathology Museum of Barcelona University School of Medicine, Spain). *(With permission of Dr D. Campillo)*

attention given must have been considerable and would have been a particular burden to a small, intensive social group. In these same individuals the progress of the disease may have become arrested and not ended in death. Laurence (1958) noted that 46 per cent of cases become arrested between the ages of 9 months and 2 years, and a similar state may have existed in antiquity.

In palaeopathological records hydrocephalus is rare, but Richards and Anton (1991) indicate that about thirty possible cases have been identified, mainly from the Old World and dating from 10,000 BC onwards (Gejvall, 1960; Brothwell, 1967a; Manchester, 1980a; Richards and Anton, 1991). The earliest case hitherto recorded in Britain is of Romano-British date, and is of an adult with a cranial capacity of 2,600cm^3 compared with the normal capacity of about 1,500cm^3 (Trevor, 1950). The condition in both an early Medieval child of the sixth century AD, aged 14–16 years of age at death (Manchester, 1980a), and a Medieval child of 16–18 years from Westerhus, Sweden (Gejvall, 1960), was probably caused by an intracranial tumour. A young adult Egyptian male of the Roman period has asymmetry of the limbs suggestive of paralysis associated with his hydrocephalus (Derry, 1913). More recent cases include a possible example observed in a thirteenth-century 6–7-year-old child from Northern Ireland (Murphy, 1996), a 4–5-year-old child from Iron Age Aymyrlyg, southern Siberia (Murphy, 2000), and a 3-year-old child from Middle Palaeolithic Qafzeh, Israel (Tillier et al., 2001). Studies have shown that most hydrocephalic individuals have been found to be of normal intelligence and the same considerations probably applied in the past. The cases recorded from archaeological contexts, albeit rarely, probably fulfilled a useful role in society if mental capability is the yardstick. However, if affected individuals had significant physical handicaps in an early work-centred society, this may have been a limiting factor in determining the role of the individual.

Abnormalities in cranial suture development

The cranial sutures may also be subject to problems in normal development: this might include lack of a suture or premature closure of sutures (Fig. 3.5).

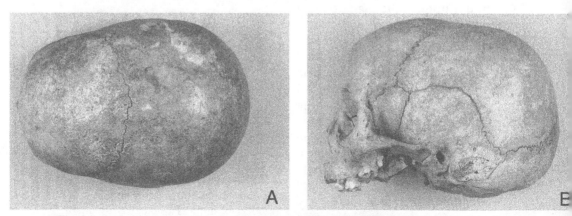

Fig. 3.5. A: superior view of skull with premature closure of the sagittal suture; B: lateral view of same skull. (Photographs by Jeff Veitch, Department of Archaeology, University of Durham)

The former is usually termed sutural agenesis and a genetic basis is indicated for its occurrence (Cohen *et al.*, 1971 in Barnes, 1994). The latter is called craniosynostosis, and several factors are believed to be behind its development, including birth trauma and intrauterine infection. Females more than males are affected. Agenesis, most often of the sagittal suture, leads to changes in the shape of the skull (the resulting shape depends on what sutures are affected), and the brain becomes displaced (Barnes, 1994: 152). Mental and neurological problems may result as increased intracranial pressure may be a sequel, although the relationship is not clearly understood (Aufderheide and Rodríguez-Martín, 1998: 52). A number of reports of agenesis/premature fusion of sutures have appeared in the palaeopathological literature and are well summarized in Barnes (1994).

Spina bifida

Spina bifida is probably the most common developmental defect to be reported archaeologically, and this 'neural tube defect' varies in frequency worldwide today. Barnes (1994: 41) indicates that the highest frequencies are in the British Isles (e.g. 62 of 5,607 babies for 1998 – Anon., 1999), the lowest in Japan, with North America in between. Males are more frequently affected than females generally, and genetic and environmental factors are potential causes – for example, deficiencies in maternal folic acid (vitamin B12), zinc and selenium while the foetus is developing (Barnes, 1994). However, it is the occulta type, rather than cystica, that is described most frequently. Spina bifida occulta defines incomplete fusion of the posterior neural arches of the sacral segments and/or lumbar vertebrae (Fig. 3.6). No structures such as the spinal cord protrude out through the space and, thus, no complications such as infection or paralysis occur. *Occulta* means hidden, and this condition is usually not detected in a living person because of the lack of associated signs or symptoms (unless radiography is undertaken), and the absence of any effect on the person's life. It should be noted that the 1st, 4th and 5th sacral vertebrae may be open as the norm for a particular person or population, and this must not be confused with spina bifida. To be able to compare population frequencies, an accepted standardized recording system must be used.

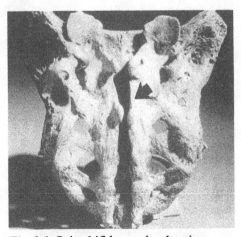

The more severe form is spina bifida cystica, which is often fatal. Aufderheide and Rodríguez-Martín (1998: 61) describe three forms of severity: meningocele, myelomeningocele and myelocele. The first involves protrusion of the nerve roots and meninges through the defect, with the spinal cord

Fig. 3.6. Spina bifida occulta showing open posterior sacrum (early Medieval, sixth–eighth centuries AD, England).

remaining in the vertebral canal, but a covering of skin is in place. The second (60 per cent of cases) involves the added protrusion of the spinal cord through the defect without normal skin covering, and in the third (the most severe) the skin and meninges fail to close at the defect and infection leads to death. Barnes (1994: 45) notes that myelomeningocele will produce a very wide defect in the sacrum/lumbar region because of the protrusion of the soft tissue structures described. However, it is very unlikely that a person in the past would have survived such a severe problem, which perhaps explains why there is so little evidence. However, if someone did survive, the complications of such a condition would include paralysis, incontinence and hydrocephalus. For example, Dickel and Doran (1989 in Barnes, 1994) describe a 14–16-year-old individual buried in Florida with spina bifida cystica from lumbar vertebra 3 to the 2nd sacral vertebra, with subsequent disuse atrophy of some of the bones; this may represent paralysis as a result of the condition. More data are available for spina bifida occulta. For example, for the early Medieval period in Britain (Roberts and Cox, 2003), of three sites reporting absolute frequencies (percentage of sacra affected), the frequency was 8.7 per cent (15 of 173), while Brothwell and Powers (1968) indicate an average rate of 2.7 per cent for some early British populations.

Lumbarization and sacralization

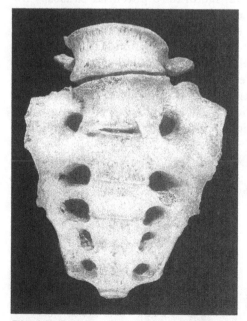

Fig. 3.7. Sacralisation of the sacrum (late Medieval, twelfth–sixteenth centuries AD, England).

Lumbarization and sacralization occur in the spine as a result of what is termed upwards or downwards 'border shifting' (Barnes, 1994: 79), and the affected vertebra takes on the features of the adjacent vertebra in the neighbouring region. If the shift is upwards, then it is called a cranial shift, or sacralization, and the 5th lumbar vertebra takes on the appearance of the 1st sacral vertebra. If the shift is downwards, it is caudal, or lumbarization, and the 1st sacral vertebra looks like a 5th lumbar vertebra, but identifying these conditions can be difficult if the complete spine is not preserved (often the case in archaeology). López-Durán, (1995 in Aufderheide and Rodríguez-Martín, 1998: 65) reports that 3–5 per cent of the population today may be affected by shifting at the lumbosacral border and that two-thirds are sacralizations (Fig. 3.7). Both conditions have been reported in the palaeopathological literature (e.g. for British populations, see Roberts and Cox, 2003, and for North America, see Barnes, 1994).

Spondylolysis

The lower parts of the spine are also the site of another, probably developmentally related, abnormality. This, too, is insignificant but may, as a complication, become symptomatically serious. The defect to some extent bridges the gap between congenital and acquired abnormalities. In the bony union of parts of a vertebra early in life, the bone development may be disorganized and, due to the continual stresses and strains of the upright bipedal posture, may fracture early in adult life. This defect is known as spondylolysis and is recognized in skeletal material as a separate and seemingly ununited posterior part of a vertebra. In most instances the defect does not create symptoms. Occasionally, however, the defect creates sufficient instability of the spine to allow one vertebra to move in anatomical alignment upon its neighbour, compressing the spinal cord and the nerves issuing from it, so creating symptoms of pain in the legs and back. This dislocation, known as spondylolisthesis, is sometimes recognized in skeletal material. Spondylolysis is further discussed in Chapter 5.

APPENDICULAR SKELETON

Congenital dislocation of the hip

In modern medical practice the congenital diseases of anencephaly and spina bifida cystica are readily apparent. In the former case the lesion is totally untreatable and in the latter case the lesion is sometimes treatable, allowing survival of the affected infant. In past societies, both lesions would have been obvious and both were probably universally fatal. There is also a congenital defect with genetic factors of causation which, with modern knowledge, is both diagnosable and curable shortly after birth. The neonate of antiquity was not so fortunate. The problem is that of congenital dislocation of the hip joint, perhaps more correctly termed congenital acetabular dysplasia, indicating that the defect is in the development of the acetabulum of the hip joint. In past societies the abnormality became apparent only when the child started to walk, by which time treatment, had it been available, would have been ineffective. The swaying gait due to the recurrent dislocation of the joint on weight-bearing is characteristic. The abnormality predisposes to the early development of degenerative arthritis in the hip joint. Fig. 3.8 shows the abnormality at a stage when it is recognizable in skeletal remains, i.e. when a new joint has been created. Note also the lack of development of the acetabulum, which may also be very shallow. The femoral head can also be flattened. The condition has a genetic predisposition, is more common in females, on the left side if only one hip is affected, and is associated with breech deliveries (Sartoris, 1995).

Clearly, with such an abnormal gait and with such severe arthritis, an individual would have been unable to perform efficiently any activity which involved walking. The individual may also have had constant incapacitating pain. His or her role in society in the past, particularly in those societies dependent for their existence upon hunting or agriculture, must have been restricted. The modern incidence of the condition is 10–20 in 1,000 live births (Sartoris, 1995), and, in more than half the individuals affected, the condition affects both hip joints. There is marked geographical variation in incidence and perhaps both

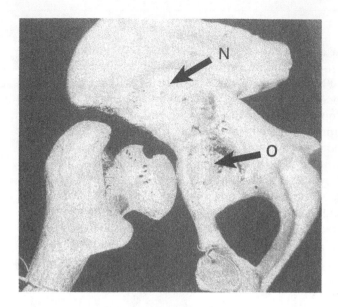

Fig. 3.8. Congenital dislocation of the hip showing 'new acetabulum' (N) that has formed above the original (O), which has not developed normally. *(Cleveland Museum of Natural History, Ohio, United States; with permission of Art Aufderheide)*

genetic and environmental factors are responsible for this. The abnormality has been recognized in skeletons from many periods from both the Old and New Worlds (e.g. see Roberts and Cox, 2003 for British examples, and Aufderheide and Rodríguez-Martín, 1998).

Club foot

A less common abnormality in palaeopathology is the individual with club foot, or talipes equinovarus. The most numerous and perhaps visually convincing evidence is in pictorial sources from Egypt. The classically inverted feet of this abnormality is admirably demonstrated in drawings. The modern incidence is 1 in 800–1,000 births, is more common in males and has been shown to have a familial predisposition (Aufderheide and Rodríguez-Martín, 1998: 75). Recognition of the abnormality in skeletons is difficult and perhaps it was more common in the past than the reported evidence suggests. Brothwell (1967a) details the skeletal changes that may be expected, by reconstruction of the foot and ankle, comparison with a normal foot (or the opposite unaffected side), and consideration of the consequences of such a condition (e.g. lack of use of the leg and disuse atrophy, and even the use of crutches to move around). Because of the difficulties in skeletal diagnosis, palaeopathological examples of talipes equinovarus are rare. Perhaps the earliest recorded specimen is of Neolithic date from Nether Swell (Brothwell, 1967a) and from a fourth-century AD skeleton from Kingsholm, Gloucester (Roberts *et al.*, 2004), both British. The latter case revealed atrophy (wasting) of the affected lower limb bones, indicating the possible effect of the condition on the mobility of the individual (Fig. 3.9). Later examples have been identified and their anatomy admirably described and analysed (Mann and Owsley, 1989; Owsley and Mann, 1990). Careful examination of skeletal material and reappraisal of all evidence is just as necessary for the recognition of club foot as for many other

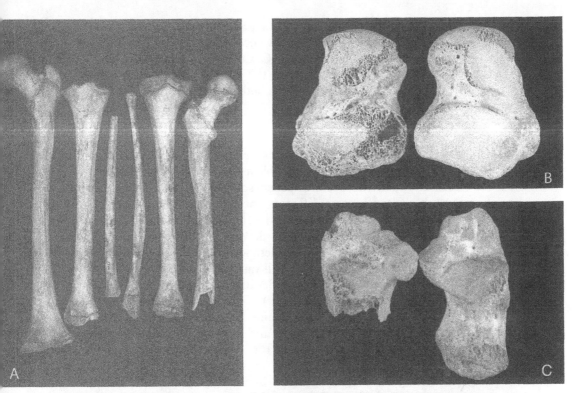

Fig. 3.9. Club foot evident in an individual from Kingsholm 131, Gloucester, England (Romano-British, fourth century AD). A: Affected (left) lower leg bones on the right side of figure; affected side shows medio-laterally flattened fibula, and more slender femur; B and C: talus and calcaneum, respectively, of the affected (left) and unaffected sides, showing changes in the articular surfaces.

abnormalities in palaeopathology. Just as with congenital dislocation of the hip, the main problem of club foot is in walking, and no doubt the same restriction of activity would have applied.

Other rarer developmental problems of the appendicular skeleton have also been reported in the palaeopathological literature – for example, polydactyly or the congenital duplication of one or more toes or fingers (Murphy, 1999), congenital absence of the patella (Patrick and Waldron, 2003), Madelung's deformity of the radius (Anderson and Carter, 1995) and arthrogryposis multiplex, where muscles are undifferentiated or absent (Anderson and Thomas, 1997).

AXIAL AND APPENDICULAR SKELETON
Achondroplasia

Skeletons representing people of short stature are rare in the palaeopathological record, although there are many types of dwarfism described in the clinical literature. For example, in Britain from the prehistoric to post-Medieval periods there are only about five skeletons that have been identified with proportionate or disproportionate dwarfism (Roberts and Cox, 2003), the former being a person who is short but in proportion and the latter being one who is short disproportionately (e.g. some parts of the body may be normal while the rest is short/stunted in growth).

An example of a genetically based abnormality is the most common form of dwarfism, termed achondroplasia. It is an abnormality of simple dominant inheritance but most commonly develops as a result of a gene mutation, and today affects males and females equally. The problem arises in the process of ossification, or bone formation, in the skeletal precursors of the foetus. Simply stated, ossification takes place by two different methods: in one, intramembranous ossification forms the bones of the skull vault, the face and the clavicle; the remaining bones of the skeleton develop by the other method, i.e. intracartilaginous ossification. In achondroplasia the first method progresses normally whereas the second method is defective. Hence the skull vault, face and clavicle are normal but the nasal area is depressed and the remainder of the skeleton is manifestly retarded in development ('short-limbed dwarfism'). The limbs are shortened and adult stature is usually not more than 140cm (Aufderheide and Rodríguez-Martín, 1998: 360). Consequently, the dwarf stature and short-limbed appearance of the achondroplastic are quite characteristic (Fig. 3.10) and recognizable even from artistic work of antiquity. The modern incidence of the condition is 1 per 10,000 live births (Aufderheide and Rodríguez-Martín, 1998: 358), and the incidence in antiquity was probably of the same order.

It is perhaps because of this distinctive appearance that the achondroplastic individual has drawn the attention of the artist in the past, and it is from pictorial sources that much of the evidence for the antiquity of achondroplasia comes (Enderle et al., 1994). More than any other developmental abnormality of the past, achondroplasia is portrayed in statuettes, tomb illustrations and even in the Bayeux Tapestry. The role of the achondroplastic individual in society seems also to have achieved undue prominence. The Egyptian god Phtha (and probably Bes) was given dwarf status. While achondroplasia is the most common disorder leading to dwarfism, not only this form but

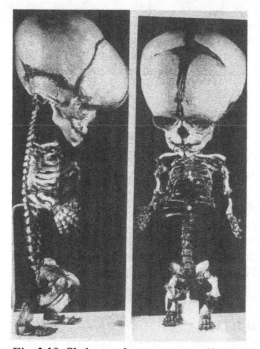

Fig. 3.10. Skeleton of person who suffered achondroplasia. *(With permission of the Royal College of Surgeons, London, England)*

several other dwarfism syndromes also achieved social and ritual significance in Egypt (Dasen, 1988). For example, the Roman emperors Tiberius and Alexander Severus (and also Mark Antony) retained achondroplastic dwarfs as counsellors (Johnston, 1963), and the little figure of Turold in the Bayeux Tapestry clearly held a position of importance in the entourage of Duke William of Normandy (Denny and Filmer-Sankey, 1966). Their role as 'objects of interest' in the Medieval period is shown by a record of a gift of nine dwarfs to Charles IX of France from the king of Poland. Precisely why honours such as Egyptian deification, and roles as Roman Imperial advisers, or Medieval court entertainers should be bestowed upon the congenitally malformed is impossible to say.

Although rare, and rather less emotive than the statuettes, there is skeletal evidence of achondroplasia from both the Old and New Worlds. In the Old World the earliest recorded skeletal example is from Italy and of late Upper Palaeolithic date (Frayer et al., 1987). What role in society such an individual played at this time can only be wondered at. Typical squat limb bones and characteristic skull shape have been described in remains from pre-Dynastic Egypt and from the Dynastic tombs of King Zer and King Mersekha (Brothwell and Powers, 1968). Two examples of achondroplastic adult skeletons have also been described from Poland (Gladykowska-Rzeczycka, 1980). In the New World fairly complete dwarf skeletons of an adult male and an adult female have been reported from a prehistoric Indian site at Moundville, Alabama, United States. The height of the female was estimated to be 125cm and the bones of the dwarfs were described as rugged and muscular (Snow, 1943). Other New World cases are described in Ortner (2003).

Since achondroplastic persons are not mentally retarded and, as is evident, performed useful and often prestigious functions into adult life, it is expected that their skeletons will be preserved and not suffer the fate of the bones of the young, dying in infancy from their congenital malformations.

Osteogenesis imperfecta

A similarly generalized, genetically determined abnormality of connective tissue is osteogenesis imperfecta or 'brittle bone disease'. It is an abnormality of great rarity today and the evidence from the past consists of two skeletons only. As its name suggests, the disease is the result of the inadequate formation of bone collagen (protein), but it also affects the dentine of the teeth, skin and ligaments (Goldman, 1995). The bones are, in consequence, brittle and distorted. Their fragility leads to frequent and multiple fractures. Aufderheide and Rodríguez-Martín (1998: 365) describe the different forms of severity of this condition, where in the mild form some people will be unaware of it until they break a bone. Type I is most common and is seen today in 1 in 30,000 births (Goldman, 1995). Although today the afflicted individual can be nurtured into adulthood, this may have been rare in the past. Death from fractures and their complications must have been the pattern in early childhood, as is indicated by the Egyptian 2-year-old infant of the XXI Dynasty, around 1000 BC (Gray, 1969). A single individual from Britain, dated to the early Medieval (seventh century AD) period, has been described, but the evidence rests only on the fractured and distorted femur (Wells, 1965).

Down's syndrome

Except in a very few instances, mental defect is not associated with gross skeletal manifestation. It is mainly upon skeletal manifestations that palaeopathological evidence rests, and that is clearly lacking in mental deficiency states. The evidence for this sort of problem must rest with historical documentation.

Down's syndrome (previously termed 'mongolism') is an abnormality resulting from an additional chromosome 21 (three rather than two), and is characterized by mental defect and by certain typical physical features. The skeletal features are principally of the skull and consist of a relative shortening of skull length associated with some flattening at the back and nose. These features, together with a retardation of growth of the base of the skull and the facial skeleton, give rise to an overall reduction in the capacity of the skull. Growth rates are slowed in adolescence, and the distal segments of long bones have growth deficiency. The individual may experience delay in walking and talking, and mental retardation (Cronk, 1993: 685). Individuals affected may also suffer infections, heart problems and acute leukaemia. Skeletally they are of short stature and can have hip dislocation.

The condition has been described in at least two cases from archaeological contexts. The first is of the tenth to eleventh century AD from Breedon-on-the-Hill in Leicestershire, England. This child was about 9 years of age at death. It is suggested that survival to this age was the result of care provided in the monastery at the site (Brothwell, 1960). A second case is described from the late Hallstatt period (350 BC) at Taubischofscheim, Germany, showing characteristics similar to the example from Breedon-on-the-Hill (Czarnetski, 1980). Although a child with Down's syndrome may be born to any mother, and the frequency today is 1 in 800 live births (Aufderheide and Rodríguez-Martín, 1998: 368), it is much more common in women who are over the age of 40 years at childbirth (up to 1 in 25 births). Exposure to drugs, tobacco, alcohol, coffee, contraceptives, fluoridated water and radiation have been investigated as potential causes but results are inconsistent (Cronk, 1993: 684). In early populations, the number of women surviving and subsequently bearing children at that age may have been small. Down's syndrome may therefore have been an extremely uncommon abnormality in antiquity and, for this reason, the extant evidence may also be rare. Of course, as with many other congenital abnormalities, those affected children dying in infancy will probably go unrecognized in archaeological material; it is only the survivors to late childhood or to adulthood that present the preserved bone manifestations of their misfortune.

In this outline of the palaeopathology of congenital disease, only the most common or dramatic and significant abnormalities have been discussed. The less significant abnormalities and the myriad of skeletal features, which may be counted as variations of normal, have been omitted. The diseases discussed were doubtless of grave significance to their possessors and to the community. They may illustrate also the care and tolerance shown by communities to those less fortunate men, women and children of past society.

CHAPTER 4

Dental Disease

No structures of the human body are more likely to disintegrate during life than teeth, yet after death none have greater tenacity against decay. (Wells, 1964a: 121)

INTRODUCTION

Teeth (the hardest and most chemically stable tissues in the body) are often the only part of the body that survives to be excavated from a cemetery, because of their hard and robust structure; this is fortunate, as they provide a wealth of information about, for example, diet, oral hygiene and dentistry, 'stress', occupation, cultural behaviour and subsistence economy. Furthermore, their use in documenting developments in human evolution testifies to their good preservation. The mouth functions primarily as a food processor (Lukacs, 1989: 261); food type determines the micro-organisms present in the mouth, and the condition of a person's teeth can reflect the composition of the food that has come into contact with those teeth. The oral cavity also produces sound, and is involved with respiration, and heat and fluid regulation, among other functions. Dental disease and anomalies are, with the joint diseases, the most commonly occurring abnormalities reported for ancient human remains and, when integrated with other forms of evidence from an archaeological site, are valuable sources of information about individuals and populations (Gilbert and Mielke, 1985). Their study may involve macroscopic and microscopic analysis, and the use of art, documentary, archaeological and ethnographic evidence to supplement the dental data. Normal variations in structure have also been used to explore relationships between populations (e.g. see Scott and Turner, 1997, Corruccini *et al.*, 2002), and isotope analysis of enamel has documented movements of people in the past (White *et al.*, 1998; Montgomery *et al.*, 2000; Price *et al.*, 2001; Budd *et al.*, 2004) and helped to reconstruct past diet (Lillie and Richards, 2000; Cox *et al.*, 2001; Privat *et al.*, 2002).

Infectious disease is one of the more common dental diseases in archaeological populations, e.g. caries, whereas the **degenerative diseases** of the jaws include ante-mortem tooth loss following periodontal disease and recession of the bone of the jaw, usually as the person ages; **developmental problems** include enamel hypoplasia and genetic anomalies, which incorporate, for example, lack of or more than the expected number of teeth. It has to be emphasized here that the dental diseases do not develop in isolation from one another; there is a complex relationship between them (see Lukacs, 1989: 265, fig. 1). For example, a person could develop plaque deposits on their teeth which irritate the soft tissues (gingivitis) and underlying bone (periodontal disease), which, in turn, may lead to reduction or loss of alveolar bone and ante-mortem tooth loss.

Today there is a great emphasis on caring for our teeth; use of toothpaste and dental floss, and visiting the dentist play a regular and consistent part of most people's lives. This will of course vary globally. In the past, access to dental surgery and dental cleaning implements and substances, although evidently available to some individuals in some populations (see below), is not seen consistently across all populations. In effect, it is likely that the dental problems observed in archaeological populations are not affected or influenced by significant oral hygiene or dentistry, and are more a pure reflection of particular dietary components eaten by the individuals being studied. However, it is clear from archaeological evidence that some dental diseases increase through time (e.g. caries) while others decline (e.g. dental plaque accumulation).

Although teeth survive well in archaeological contexts, care is needed in processing and cleaning them and the jaws that contain them, once excavated. The mandible, or lower jaw, is more robust than the maxilla, or upper jaw, and the latter does tend to suffer fragmentation during burial and/or excavation. Great care is needed with cleaning this area, where soil may become impacted in the nasal aperture and the integrity of this part of the facial skeleton may be affected. The reader is referred to Van Beek (1983: 5, 100) for the structure of a tooth and the number and types of teeth expected in the deciduous (milk) and permanent dentitions. Obviously, as the dentition develops there will be a mixture of the two types of teeth until all the deciduous teeth are lost and replaced by the permanent teeth. The single-rooted teeth often become separated from the jaws during burial and/or excavation or during processing, and care should be taken in their preservation; the multi-rooted teeth (e.g. the molars) are more stable in the jaws. Vigorous brushing of the teeth and jaws to clean them is inadvisable in an archaeological context; calcified plaque (calculus) deposits are easily dislodged and should be treated carefully, and the alveolar bone surrounding the teeth can be very fragile and become damaged. Loss of evidence is to be avoided.

There are several different dental diseases and anomalies which occur in the archaeological record, and some diseases of the human body may affect both bones and teeth (e.g. congenital syphilis). The dental diseases are now considered in terms of their aetiology (cause), appearance on the dentition, methods of recording (where appropriate), and examples of studies. In some respects the use of modern clinical observations as a base for interpretation is more appropriate for the dental diseases than for bone disease. Dentists today can observe the tooth surface (as in an archaeological situation), although they cannot visualize the surrounding bone, except by using radiographic analysis. The bones of a living person are usually only viewed through radiography, while the biological anthropologist can view skeletal elements directly.

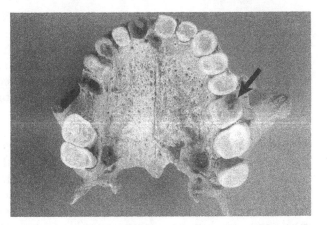

Fig. 4.1. Dental caries in a first upper molar tooth (late Iron Age/early Roman, first century BC–first century AD; Beckford 54104, Hereford and Worcester, England); note also the wear on all the teeth.

DENTAL CARIES

Dental caries (Latin: *caries*, or rottenness) is perhaps the most common of the dental diseases (Fig. 4.1) and is reported for archaeological populations more frequently than other dental diseases; it may occur as opaque spots on the tooth surface or as large cavities (Hillson, 1986: 287). An infectious and transmissable disease, it is the result of fermentation of food sugars, especially sucrose in the diet, by bacteria that occur on the teeth in plaque, e.g. *Lactobacillus acidophilus* and *Streptococcus mutans*. Starches in the diet may also cause caries but less frequently (Hillson, 2000: 260). Progressive destruction of the tooth structure is initiated by microbial action on the tooth surface (Pindborg, 1970: 256). If the correct combination of plaque bacteria and sucrose occurs, then the acids produced demineralize the teeth and leave cavities. Any part of the tooth structure that allows the accumulation of food debris and plaque could predispose to the development of caries. Therefore, two areas of the teeth may be affected: the crown of the tooth, where plaque can get trapped in fissures (molars and premolars, especially), and the roots of the teeth, including also the cemento-enamel junction, when exposed due to recession of the gums and bone surrounding the teeth (periodontal disease). Powell (1985: 317) usefully divides the causes of caries into several areas: environmental factors (e.g. trace elements in food and water), pathogenic agents (the bacteria causing the disease), exogenous factors (e.g. diet, oral hygiene) and endogenous factors (e.g. the shape and structure of the teeth). A recent cross-national study has also linked increased caries rates to urbanization (Miura *et al.*, 1997), and in British contexts this appears also the case in the past.

These factors should all be considered in an archaeological population study of caries because no one factor can necessarily be attributed to their development. For example, a relatively recent study of caries in 12-year-old children in ninety countries found no strong relationship between the amount of sugar consumed and the occurrence of caries in westernized countries (Woodward and Walker, 1994). Some trace elements may prevent caries or predispose the person to develop caries (Powell, 1985: 315). For example, certain levels of fluoride may protect a person's teeth, and Sibbison's study (1990) suggests that children in fluoridated areas in the US suffer 18 per cent less caries. Furthermore, Thomas *et al.* (1995) in their study of the dental health of children in Anglesey, North Wales, found that withdrawal of fluoride in the water reduced dental health and affected bones. However, levels that are too high may lead to fluorosis, which affects the integrity of the teeth and bones (Ortner, 2003: 406), and some parts of the world have naturally high levels in water (e.g. see the study by Littleton, 1999 in Bahrain). Other dental problems may weaken the teeth and allow caries to occur. For example, deciduous teeth with developmental defects in fifty-seven non-adults in the Libben population (Late Woodland, Ohio, United States) were found by Duray (1990) to show a moderate increase in caries when compared to normal teeth. The theory was that the normal structure of the teeth was already weakened and therefore more susceptible to carious attack. Severe wear on the surfaces of the teeth could also weaken the tooth structure, allowing the entry of bacteria into the pulp cavity through its exposure, with consequent abscess development at the root of the tooth – another infectious lesion.

Recording of caries should involve stating the tooth affected, the position of the caries on the tooth and the size of the lesion; all these variables help to explain underlying aetiological factors. Lukacs (1989: 267) describes a grading system incorporating four grades: no caries, less than half the tooth crown destroyed, more than half the tooth crown destroyed and all the crown destroyed. Care should be taken not to record caries when caries does not exist, i.e. discoloured, darkened areas of teeth, and soil in the occlusal surface fissures may be mistaken for caries. Obvious cavities should be recorded; recording any lesion which is not immediately obvious or convincing increases prevalence rates unnecessarily. To be able to indicate the prevalence of dental disease in a population the number of teeth observed needs to be known so that caries prevalence as a percentage of the numbers of teeth can be determined. These data should be available for all population studies. Hillson (2000, 2001) has recently produced a more detailed system. However, this is not without its problems (see Hillson, 2000 for a discussion). In addition, some authors present prevalence of caries per individual studied, but this assumes that all teeth were preserved or that the teeth lost post-mortem were not affected by caries. A recent survey of caries recording by Lukacs (1995) recommends that the method by which caries data are presented should be clear: is it caries rate in teeth observed, corrected caries rate in teeth observed using his correction factor, individuals affected by caries or mean caries per individual?

Of course, the determination of prevalence by sex has implications for differential access to diet for males and females, for example, and females today and in the past tend to have higher rates (Larsen, 1997: 72–6; Hillson, 2000: 261). While age prevalence for caries is always given for archaeological populations, the correlation of age with caries is not clear. For example, a person with caries, aged 40–50 years at death, may have developed the lesion two, five or even ten years before death. However, as age increases it is more likely that caries will develop. Consideration of caries prevalence in the very young can also obviously provide more information about its epidemiology than for somebody in adulthood (the speed of development of caries, for example). With regard to social status, one should expect to find differences in caries rates between higher and lower social statuses. One could also hypothesize that people of higher social status may have easier access to cariogenic foods, including exotic products with high levels of sucrose (as seen by Cucina and Tiesler, 2003). Alternatively, one could also argue that the higher classes would eat more protein in meat and therefore would suffer fewer carious lesions. However, did higher status people practise more oral hygiene and have better access to dental care? Larsen (1997: 76–7) summarizes studies of caries and social status in past human groups with the overall conclusion that people of higher social status have fewer caries because of increased protein consumption.

Many studies have been undertaken on the prevalence of caries in past human and non-human populations around the world, and the data interpreted in terms of factors operating within the living environment of individuals, particularly their subsistence base. At the transition to agriculture, fermentable carbohydrates become available and initiate the increase in caries, although not all crops (such as rice) will lead to a rise (e.g. see Tayles *et al.*, 2000). In the New World Larsen (1984) studied pre-agricultural (1000 BC–AD 1150) and agricultural (AD 1150–AD 1550) dentitions from thirty-one cemetery sites from the Georgia Coast in the United States. Caries appeared to increase by around 10 per cent with the shift to agriculture for both sexes and all tooth types. The increases were more pronounced in females than males. He attributed the increase to the adoption of maize agriculture, as maize has a high sucrose content. A number of other studies have also looked at specific population groups to determine caries prevalence with a change in subsistence. For example, Perzigian *et al.* (1984) found that caries prevalence increased through time in the Ohio River Valley in Late Archaic (hunter-gatherers), Middle Woodland (mixed economy) and Fort Ancient (agriculture) populations. Of 159 permanent teeth from the Late Archaic only 4 teeth (2.5 per cent) were carious. The Middle Woodland prevalence was five times that of the Late Archaic, and in the Fort Ancient population 24.8 per cent of the teeth were carious. Some studies have also concentrated on caries rate change with the intensification of agriculture (Hodges, 1989; Lukacs, 1992). Hodges examined skeletal material representing time periods from the Formative (1400 BC) through Classic to Postclassic (AD 950) periods in the Oaxaca Valley, Mexico, a time when agricultural intensification was being experienced. Here, a decline in caries rate from 17.9 per cent in the Formative to 16.9 per cent in the Classic to 11.1 per cent in the Postclassic was observed. The frequency of caries therefore did not increase with agricultural intensification except in male posterior teeth, which suggests a similar level of carbohydrate ingestion through all periods (Hodges, 1989: 68). A recent innovative study of a Mayan population dated to the Classic period in Mexico (AD 250–900) considered the frequency of caries related to social status (Cucina and Tiesler, 2003). Results showed that the lowest rate of caries and the highest rate of ante-mortem tooth loss occurred in the elite males; this correlated with poor oral hygiene and a softer and more refined diet. Finally, a study by Pietrusewsky and Douglas (2002) of a north-east Thailand population from Ban Chiang dating from as early as 2100 BC to as late as AD 200 found in sixty adult skeletons a caries rate of 7.3 per cent (74 of 1,016 teeth). Detailed analysis revealed more carious molar teeth, and more caries on the occlusal or biting surfaces, with males being affected more than females (2002: 57). The patterns revealed that the low rate of caries was consistent with a mixed economy and that males may have had differential access to caries-producing foods. The overall frequency was lower than at the Central Thailand site of Khok Phanom Di, where the skeletons studied by Tayles (1999) are dated to 2000–1500 BC. Here a frequency of 11 per cent caries of all intact teeth was noted, but females were more affected than males. Tayles (1999: 276) suggests, on the basis of Stephan (1966) and Wilson (1985), that the population's high rates may be related to ingestion of highly cariogenic sugars from bananas or from 'palm sugar' made from the coconut palm.

Interesting studies have also been made in the Old World. Meiklejohn *et al.* (1984) reported for Mesolithic populations (8300–4200 BC) a caries frequency of 1.9 per cent (33 of 1,780 permanent teeth). This low rate is seen in hunter-gatherers today (Hillson, 2000: 263), although there appears to be no consistency for low caries rates in Mesolithic populations (see Larsen, 1997: 70–1 for a discussion). For the Neolithic period (4200–1800 BC), when farming was being adopted, the caries rate was 4.2 per cent (69 of 1,654 teeth), with the difference between the Mesolithic and Neolithic samples being highly significant. In all, 80 Mesolithic and 51 Neolithic sites were examined. Bennike (1985) also produced similar figures for Denmark; no Mesolithic teeth of 423 available for examination had caries, whereas 160 of 7,062 Neolithic teeth (2.3 per cent) were affected. Interestingly, Bennike (1985) found much lower rates of caries for Danish Medieval populations (3.7 per cent) than are seen in British contexts.

Recent collated data for British populations from the Mesolithic to the post-Medieval period (as early as 8,000 BC to as late as the mid-nineteenth century AD) suggest a correlation between an increase in dental caries and sucrose and refined flour consumption through time, apart from the early Medieval period, where frequencies decline (Roberts and Cox, 2003). During all these periods agriculture was being practised to a greater or lesser extent, apart from in the Mesolithic. During the Roman period levels were relatively high compared to the preceding periods (7.5 per cent of teeth), whereas for the early Medieval period levels declined to 4.2 per cent, with an increase in the later and post-Medieval periods of 5.6 per cent and 11.2 per cent, respectively (Table 4.1). Moore and Corbett (1973) also noted this in their study. It was not until the twelfth century that cane sugar, containing high amounts of sucrose, was imported into Britain and it is 'unlikely that sucrose formed a significant part of the diet in Europe or in American aboriginal tribes before this date' (Moore and Corbett, 1971: 166). In both the Roman and the early Medieval periods honey was probably the main sweetening agent, with bread being the main source of carbohydrate. Cane and beet sugar were unknown, but small amounts of fructose were consumed in fruit. In the Roman period it is conceivable that some individuals had access to luxury imports such as figs and dates. Until the early sixteenth century cane sugar was generally unavailable to the majority of the population, and a study of seventeenth-century British teeth revealed an increase in caries rate (Moore and Corbett, 1975). At this time cane sugar industries became established in the New World and exports came mostly to northern Europe. In 1641 the first sugar factory was set up in the West Indies, and, as the price of sugar fell, consumption increased. By the end of the nineteenth century sugar consumption was rated at 20 pounds per person per year. By AD 1900 90 pounds of sugar per person per year were being consumed, including large amounts of chocolate, treacle and jam. The increased availability of sugar and fine white flour, with relaxation of import duties, contributed to caries increase from about the sixteenth century AD in Britain.

Table 4.1 Dental caries in Britain

Period	*% total teeth observed*
Neolithic	3.3
Bronze Age	4.8
Iron Age	2.9
Roman	7.5
Early Medieval	4.2
Late Medieval	5.6
Post-Medieval	11.2

While post-Medieval rates in Britain were 11.2 per cent of 12,993 teeth observed in 3,790 individuals from 15 cemetery sites, by contrast, in Ontario in Canada a nineteenth-century population showed rates of 41 per cent in females and 30.9 per cent in males (Saunders *et al.*, 1997). This probably indicates that the focus in this latter study was on a single population whereas the British data are pooled geographically. Molnar and Molnar (1985) also found a change in dental disease in dental remains from seven Hungarian populations covering 1,800 years (late Neolithic to late Bronze Age). However, the major difference was the caries rate, which ranged from 0 to 14.7 per cent over the seven cultural groups, increasing to 14.7 per cent for populations of the late Bronze Age. Studies such as these in one geographic area over a long period of time start to make possible a temporal correlation of dental disease and subsistence economy.

Clearly, the recording, analysis and interpretation of dental caries is complex, and the multifactorial aetiological nature of caries in populations both past and present warrants strong consideration when assessing results of studies. For example, dental caries and dental abscessing may lead to ante-mortem tooth loss, and Lukacs (1995) developed a 'caries correction factor' method for compensating for ante-mortem tooth loss due to caries based on rates of dental disease specific to individual skeletal samples. However, in palaeopathology, in order for valid comparisons of this most commonly recognized and recorded dental disease to be made between populations, agreement on the methods of recording the primary data is paramount.

DENTAL ABSCESS

Dental caries can predispose to the development of a dental abscess through exposure of the pulp cavity and infiltration of the cavity by bacteria; attrition or trauma may also expose the cavity. However, Dias and Tayles (1997) have emphasized that a cavity in the bone around the tooth root may not necessarily be an abscess and could be a more benign condition such as a cyst. Abscess formation can also occur if an individual develops periodontal disease and a peridontal pocket. This is initiated by the accumulation of plaque between the soft tissue of the gum and the teeth (Hillson, 1986: 306). When micro-organisms accumulate in the pulp cavity, inflammation begins and a body of pus (dead cells and bacteria) collects; this is termed an abscess. This can track to the apex or base of the tooth root and into the surrounding tissues (Hillson, 1986: 316). As the pus accumulates, pressure builds up, and eventually a hole, or sinus, develops on the surface of the jaw bone to allow the pus to escape (Fig. 4.2). The pain may be severe before this occurs. At this stage in the process the abscess can be identified archaeologically. Prior to this stage identification is not possible unless radiography is undertaken and shows a translucent destructive area at the tooth's apex. Potentially, the tooth can die and eventually be lost ante-mortem.

Because of the problems of identification it is likely that the estimate of dental abscess prevalence in the past is an underestimate of the true prevalence, especially when the high prevalence of caries, calculus deposits and periodontal disease in some populations is considered; these are all predisposing factors to dental abscess formation. One of the complications of an abscess might be maxillary sinusitis as a result of abscessing of an upper molar tooth. Recording of a dental abscess is variable between authors, but a sinus presence is often accepted as evidence. However, especially in the maxillary bone, pseudosinuses can be very convincing; the roots of the teeth, especially in the anterior area of the upper jaw, are very close to the surface of the bone and post-mortem damage can occur, exposing the tooth root through a hole. Identification of healed (rounded) edges to the sinus would be indicative of ante-mortem disease. Hillson (2000: 271) makes suggestions for more detailed recording of abscesses. Figures for dental abscess prevalence in Britain indicate that frequencies are indeed low, ranging from 3.8 per cent of total tooth sockets in the

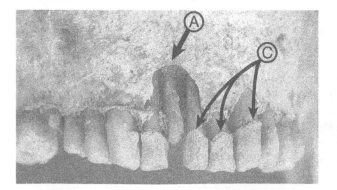

Fig. 4.2. Dental abscess (A) around the roots of the anterior teeth (late Medieval, twelfth–sixteenth centuries AD, France); note also the extensive calculus (C) deposits on the teeth.

Neolithic to 1.0 per cent in the Bronze Age (Roberts and Cox, 2003) (Table 4.2). By contrast, Pietrusewsky and Douglas (2002: 58) found at Ban Chiang in north-east Thailand that abscesses in adults had a frequency rate of 6.4 per cent of total tooth sockets, with a significant difference between male (7.6 per cent) and female (4.9 per cent) frequencies. This latter finding is concordant with the differences in rates for caries and antemortem tooth loss at the site, and the overall rate was similar to that observed by Tayles (1999) at another Thailand site.

Table 4.2 Dental abscesses in Britain

Period	% tooth sockets observed
Neolithic	3.8
Bronze Age	1.0
Iron Age	1.1
Roman	3.9
Early Medieval	2.8
Late Medieval	3.1
Post-Medieval	2.2

CALCULUS (CALCIFIED PLAQUE)

Other commonly observed dental diseases are calculus accumulation and periodontal disease. Dental plaque consists of micro-organisms which accumulate in the mouth, embedded in a matrix partly composed by the organisms themselves and partly derived from proteins in the saliva (Hillson, 1986: 284; Lieverse, 1999). It accumulates on the teeth faster when there is a high protein and/or carbohydrate diet favouring an alkaline oral environment. Plaque can

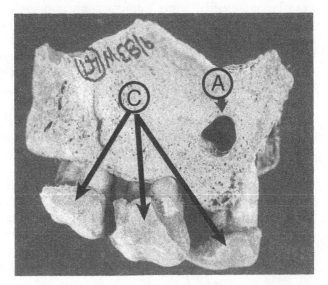

Fig. 4.3. Calculus (C) deposition on the upper and lower teeth (late Medieval, twelfth– sixteenth centuries AD, France); note also dental abscess sinus (A).

become mineralized into dental calculus (Fig. 4.3) where crystallites of mineral are deposited in the plaque. Two types of calculus are seen: supragingival calculus (above the gum) is more common and is usually thicker and grey or brown in colour, while subgingival (below the gum), often seen on exposed tooth roots, is harder and green or black in colour. Calculus develops most commonly on the teeth nearest the salivary glands (tongue side of the lower incisors and cheek side of the upper molars) and appears to be a common finding on archaeological teeth, which perhaps reflects a lack of attention to removing plaque (and thus calculus) from the teeth.

Methods of recording calculus have developed and vary from the basic (Brothwell, 1981) to the more detailed (Dobney and Brothwell, 1987), where thickness and extent of deposit are considered. Calculus has also been analysed to assess its composition; this has provided valuable insights into more specific information about, for example, the diet of an individual. Dobney and Brothwell (1988) used scanning electron microscopy to locate microscopic fragments of food debris in calculus on human and non-human teeth. Another study examined the presence and character of phytoliths in calculus from individuals from late Roman Spain (AD 300–550). Phytoliths are created as plants absorb silica dissolved in the soil with nutrients through their roots. This silica becomes solid in the plant tissue and adopts different sizes and shapes depending on the plant species and tissues (Piperno, 1988 in Fox *et al.*, 1996). Results of the analysis showed that, on the enamel surface where microwear had occurred, cereal plant phytoliths were present, and in the dental calculus itself *Poacae* family phytoliths were present. Results generally correlated with archaeological, ecological and historical data for a Mediterranean diet. A later study of Archaic hunter-gatherers in the lower Pecos region of West Texas, United States, found evidence for microwear on the teeth and interpreted this as being the result of phytoliths from the dietary staples prickly pear and agave, found in coprolites at the site (Danielson and Reinhard, 1998). Clearly, much more detailed information about calculus (and microwear) can be obtained by using a microscopic approach. Klepinger *et al.* (1977) also analysed calculus from skeletons from a population in Ecuador from 840 BC and later; the hypothesis in this study was that heavy calculus accumulation reflected habitual coca-chewing with lime. The site of calculus was different to its normal occurrence, i.e. the deposits were on the cheek side of all teeth. This was in accordance with the practice of holding the coca quid between the cheek and the teeth (1977: 506). Major and minor trace elements were analysed by X-ray diffraction. The magnesium concentration was higher than in modern calculus deposits, but magnesium is a constituent of chlorophyll (present in plants) and a co-factor of some enzymes (1977: 507). It was suggested that the results did support the hypothesis posed.

Dental reports from some archaeological human populations indicate that calculus was common in all periods, although comparison between different groups suffers because most authors report calculus on the basis of individuals affected, and not total teeth affected as a percentage of teeth observed. For example, of twenty-one Romano-British sites reporting calculus, only five provided rates calculated for the number of teeth observed; this rate was 43.4 per cent. However, when the number of individuals affected for all twenty-one sites was calculated, 26.8 per cent had calculus on their teeth (Roberts and Cox, 2003: 132). In contrast, nearly all the teeth from Ban Chiang, Thailand, had deposits on them (Pietrusewsky and Douglas, 2002).

PERIODONTAL DISEASE AND ANTE-MORTEM TOOTH LOSS

Calculus accumulates in crevices between the tooth and the soft tissue and bone of the jaw, forming periodontal pockets; it is a major predisposing factor in the development of periodontal disease. As the occurrence of calculus appears to have been so common in the past, it would be expected that the prevalence of periodontal disease would also have been high; this appears to be the case. Periodontal disease is also one of the most common dental diseases in modern populations and a major cause of tooth loss. It commences with inflammation of the soft tissues (gingivitis) of the jaw and subsequent (but not inevitable) transmission to the bone (periodontitis). Resorption of the bone and loss of the periodontal ligament holding the tooth take place, the distance between the bone and the cemento–enamel junction increases, and eventually loss of teeth occurs (Fig. 4.4). Details of the development of periodontal disease and its different types are described in Hillson (1986: 305–9).

Identification of this dental disease in archaeological material is problematic. The distance between the cemento–enamel junction and the alveolar crest may increase, but this may not be due to periodontal disease (Clarke and Hirsch, 1991); it may merely be a reflection of continuing eruption as a response to severe attrition (see above). Signs of inflammatory pitting, new bone formation on the jaw bones around the teeth, or 'periodontal pockets' around the teeth are more likely to secure a positive diagnosis for this dental disorder. Bone may be lost horizontally or irregularly, and increasing age, poor oral hygiene and diets rich in sucrose are major predisposing factors, although this condition is multifactorial in cause. The antiquity of this condition is illustrated by its presence in a 2.5–3 million years BP dentition from *Australopithecus africanus* (Ripamonti, 1988).

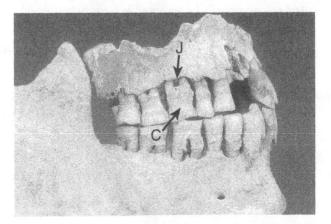

Fig. 4.4. Extensive calculus, periodontal disease and exposure of the tooth roots (late Medieval, twelfth–sixteenth centuries AD, France); note distance between cemento–enamel junction (C) and the bone of the jaw (J).

The current suggestion is that periodontal disease is overdiagnosed in skeletal material and may only be reflecting the body's compensatory mechanism for extreme attrition. The problem with assessing the prevalence of this disease is a general lack of standardized recording and knowledge of what actually constitutes periodontal disease. Davies *et al.* (1969), Brothwell (1981), Levers and Darling (1983), Karn *et al.* (1984) and Lukacs (1989) all describe different methods to record and classify this dental disease. Apart from the problems already outlined, the post-mortem damage that occurs to the jaws often mimics loss of bone around the roots of the teeth; care in diagnosing this disease is required. However, Larsen (1997: 79–80) indicates that in general there appears to be an increase in periodontal disease with a transition from traditional to western-style processed diets, that past populations eating a lot of plant carbohydrates or processed foods also have high rates, but that foragers with a lot of animal protein in their diets have lower rates.

Periodontal disease leads ultimately to tooth loss, and it is likely that it was a major factor in tooth loss in the past as it is today, although caries and abscess can lead to loss too. Ante-mortem tooth loss can only be recognized if there has been some healing of the edges of the tooth sockets and/or infilling of the affected sockets with new bone. Rates of tooth loss for British populations through time show similar patterns to caries, with increases and decreases occurring together. In Britain, as a percentage of total tooth sockets observed from pooled archaeological site data, the lowest frequencies are seen in the Iron Age at 3.1 per cent (800 BC–100 AD), with an increase in the Romano-British period to 14.1 per cent (third–fifth centuries AD), a decline in the early Medieval period to 8 per cent (mid-fifth–mid-eleventh centuries AD), with further rises to 19.4 per cent and 23.4 per cent in the late and post-Medieval periods respectively (from the mid-eleventh century to the mid-nineteeenth century AD) (Roberts and Cox, 2003). This may reflect the fact that caries was a major cause of tooth loss, but may also indicate periodontal disease was a factor. Unfortunately in Britain no systematic survey of periodontal disease has been undertaken, so comparisons between reliably collected, and standardized, population data are impossible. Increases in caries and tooth loss at the transition to agriculture were also noted for many of the studies in Cohen and Armelagos (1984), and in studies for the Western Hemisphere Health Project (Steckel and Rose, 2002), along with a general decline in health with increasing complexity, although some research indicated that it need not necessarily be accepted as a consistent trend.

Table 4.3 Ante-mortem tooth loss in Britain

Period	% tooth sockets observed
Neolithic	6.1
Bronze Age	13.2
Iron Age	3.1
Roman	14.1
Early Medieval	8.0
Late Medieval	19.4
Post-Medieval	23.4

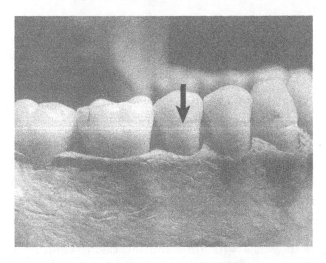

Fig. 4.5. Enamel hypoplastic defects on the buccal surfaces of the mandibular teeth (early Medieval, eighth–tenth centuries AD, Raunds, England).

ENAMEL HYPOPLASIA

Teeth can also indicate other events in a person's life, particularly during the growing years when the body is developing. In biological anthropology dental enamel defects, the most common being enamel hypoplasia, have attracted the attention of many researchers, in studies of both modern and ancient populations (Goodman and Capasso, 1992); they are often termed a non-specific 'indicator of stress' and are defined as 'deficiencies in enamel matrix composition' (Goodman, 1991: 281). Defects on teeth are, however, one of many 'stress indicators' (see Chapter 8). Defects in teeth are observed as lines, pits or grooves on the enamel surface, which are usually more easily seen on the cheek surfaces of the incisors and canines (Fig. 4.5). These defects can occur only while the teeth are developing, and remain as a permanent record into adulthood. Many factors are relevant to enamel defect aetiology (see table 2:1 in Hillson, 1986) but they can be categorized broadly into hereditary anomalies, localized trauma, and systemic metabolic stress such as a nutritional deficiency or a childhood illness such as measles (Goodman and Rose, 1991).

Much of the work in palaeopathology in this area has concentrated on examining rates of defect prevalence and changes in subsistence economy and the influence diet might have. For example, Goodman et al. (1984) studied the Dickson Mounds skeletal group from Illinois, dated AD 950–1300. Three groups of skeletons from different periods were considered: the Late Woodland (AD 950–1100), which consisted of a group practising hunting and gathering; the Acculturated Late Woodland (AD 1100–1200), representing a mixed hunter-gatherer/agricultural economy; and the Middle Mississippian (AD 1200–1300), representing an agricultural economy. Frequencies for enamel hypoplasia increased through time (1984: 285). Mean frequencies of defects per individual rose from 0.9 in the Late Woodland to 1.18 in the Acculturated Late Woodland and 1.61 in the Middle Mississippian. These findings were also supported by Larsen's work in prehistoric Georgia, looking at the change from hunting and gathering to agriculture (Larsen, 1984). In fact, many similiar studies have suggested that this change in economy led to increased stress. However, further agricultural intensification (as shown in an Oaxacan population; Hodges, 1989) may not increase the prevalence of enamel defects.

Data from Britain show low frequencies of enamel hypoplasia until the Romano-British period (9.1 per cent of teeth from six sites providing the requisite data, or 13.5 per cent of individuals from twenty-five sites). This rises in the late Medieval period to 35 per cent of individuals affected from twenty-eight sites, but this ranges from 4 per cent to 76 per cent (Roberts and Cox, 2003). Interestingly, in the intervening early Medieval period there is a decline to 7.4 per cent of total teeth from five sites, or 18.8 per cent of individuals from twenty-seven cemetery sites. This latter finding correlates with the figures for caries, ante-mortem tooth loss and dental abscesses (and also an increase in stature). The Western Hemisphere Project (Steckel and Rose, 2002) also found a general increase in hypoplasia with time and increasing complexity. A more innovative study explored the relationship between enamel hypoplasia, climatic deterioration (1100–700 BC) and change in subsistence in children at Inamgaon, in India. Contrary to expectations, health improved as a consequence of a climatic shift to aridity and a change to nomadism and hunting and foraging (Lukacs and Walimbe, 1998).

To explore the theme even further, not only have studies of ancient populations been undertaken, but populations from developing countries have been examined to determine a more specific cause for these defects. Groups of children were given either supplemented or normal unsupplemented diets, and their defect rates were compared. The results appear to support the hypothesis that diet may be one of the major causes of dental enamel hypoplasia (Dobney and Goodman, 1991; May et al., 1993). General socio-economic status may also affect the occurrence of hypoplasia, although many factors may be considered when assessing status, even for modern populations (see Dobney and Goodman, 1991: the Bradford study). Diet may only be one factor contributing to the development of enamel defects but it is not known whether it is the overriding factor. Furthermore, when compared with other stress indicators (see Chapter 8), enamel defect frequency may be very similar or can be different, suggesting that many factors may be influencing the development of these defects. For example, Kolaridou (1991) found no correlation between Harris line formation and other stress indicators (including enamel defects) in a group of French Medieval individuals (but see Chapter 8 for a discussion of the problems of recording and interpreting Harris lines). However, Mittler et al. (1992) found a strong association between enamel hypoplasia and cribra orbitalia (see Chapter 8) in an ancient Nubian population. Some studies, however, have noted a reduced age at death for individuals with enamel hypoplasia (Duray, 1996), thus indicating 'stress' in its broadest sense influencing poor health. Duray suggests damage to the immune system during pre- or post-natal development may be operating to induce the defects.

A number of studies have also looked at the most common time for enamel defects to develop during a child's growth (weaning stress?). As the chronology of tooth formation is well known, measuring where the defect occurs on the tooth has been used to assess when it occurred in the person's life (Goodman and Rose, 1990). All these studies have to assume that standards for tooth crown formation (usually those of Massler et al., 1941; and Sarnat and Schour, 1941) were the same in the past as they are today and that there is no variation between and within populations of different time periods and geographic areas. This cannot, however, be assumed (Hillson, 1997). Corruccini et al. (1985) examined children's teeth from a population of Barbados slaves dated to the seventeenth to nineteenth centuries AD and found that the majority of the defects occurred at the age of 3–4 years rather than between 2 and 3 years as found in non-industrialized populations. The suggestion was that children of slaves were weaned later than normal. Moggi-Cecchi et al. (1994) were able to correlate documentary records for nineteenth-century Florence with data on enamel hypoplasia from eighty-three skulls of unclaimed indigents dating from 1870 to 1874. At this time weaning occurred between 12 and 18 months of age, and most defects occurred between 1.5 and 3.5 years, suggesting that these individuals were suffering stress following weaning. However, as Larsen (1997: 49) states, 'weaning may be a cause of stress leading to poor enamel (but) . . . the link . . . is coincidental'.

Recording of defects is usually undertaken macroscopically or using a binocular microscope with good lighting, but some researchers have developed more sophisticated methods (Hillson and Jones, 1989) or use casts to record the defects (Hillson, 1992). Furthermore, Hillson (1997) advocates histological analysis to gain some degree of accuracy. An important study by Propst et al. (1994) showed that recording defects on casts rather than on the teeth themselves was easier, more productive and more accurate. The Federation Dentale Internationale (FDI) has developed a classification system for defects in enamel which Hillson (1997: 132) advocates as a standard. Number and type of teeth affected, number of defects, appearance and severity are all standard data which should be recorded.

DENTAL PROBLEMS AND ASSOCIATED DISEASES

Several other dental problems may be associated with specific disease processes. Of course, any person who has a health problem may develop dental enamel defects on his or her teeth if the disease affects the person while the teeth are developing, but there are specific patterns of dental involvement in certain diseases. For example, the more severe form of leprosy (lepromatous leprosy – see Chapter 7) can induce malformation of tooth roots, especially in the central incisors (Danielsen, 1970; Roberts, 1986b). Most of this work has been carried out on the Medieval leprous skeletons from Naestved, Denmark, although no evidence has been reported from other leprous cemetery sites (e.g. at Chichester, Sussex, England, where a number of Medieval skeletons were suffering from lepromatous leprosy). Likewise, the treponematoses (and more specifically congenital syphilis) can affect the normal development of the teeth, producing 'mulberry molars', Moon's molars and 'Hutchinson's incisors' (Hillson et al., 1998; also see treponemal disease in Chapter 7). Moon's molars are normal in appearance, but the tips of the cusps are very close together (Hillson *et al.*, 1998). Hutchinson's incisors occur because one of the three cusplets on the incisor edge is poorly developed and therefore a notch occurs. Mulberry molars are characterised by the cusps of the first molar being small nodules, which results from a defect in the surrounding tooth structure. A number of sites have reported the occurrence of these dental anomalies (e.g. see Dutour *et al.*, 1994) but care should be exercised in diagnosis, especially in the case of molar malformations, when severe enamel hypoplasia could be considered as a differential diagnosis.

DENTAL ATTRITION

The predisposition of teeth to dental caries from dental attrition has already been discussed. Although not a dental disease *per se*, dental wear is the 'natural result of masticatory stress upon the dentition in the course of both alimentary and technological activities' (Powell, 1985: 308), and it can occur on the biting or occlusal surfaces of the teeth during grinding of the crowns of the teeth against each other (Fig. 4.6). Another form of wear is erosion, where, for example, an acidic polluting environment or high acid–content foods may erode the tooth enamel. Abrasion is defined as wear from contact with objects other than the teeth (Hillson, 2000: 257) and usually occurs away from the occlusal surface and may be the result of cultural activities, e.g. brushing the teeth with an abrasive substance or smoking a pipe. A recent report of a male skeleton from Kent in England (Turner and Anderson, 2003) describes marked dental abrasion, possibly related to holding nails in the teeth during carpentry. Attrition can predispose to other dental pathological conditions, e.g. caries and abscesses. As the teeth wear, secondary dentine is produced under the worn enamel to protect the pulp cavity.

Modern westernized diets tend to be much softer and easier to chew and digest than those in the past and therefore wear on the teeth is not significant. One major factor affecting wear on the teeth in past populations was the processing of foods (Hillson, 1986: 183–4). For example, grinding grain on a stone mortar (Fig. 4.7) incorporates tiny particles of the stone into the grain and food produced from it; this will accelerate wear on the teeth. However, attrition may be somewhat beneficial to teeth in that it removes the fissures and pits on the biting surfaces of the molars which may trap food particles.

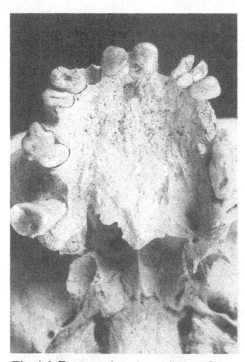

Fig. 4.6. Extreme dental attrition on the teeth of an individual from Indian Knoll (290069), Kentucky, United States.

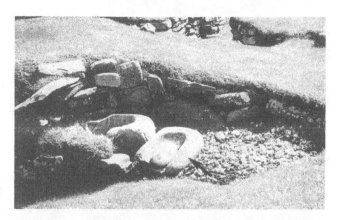

Fig. 4.7. Stone mortars and pestles (Jarlshof, Shetland Islands, Scotland).

Experimental work, nevertheless, supports the suggestion that a diet incorporating stone-ground cereals can lead to an increased rate of tooth wear. Teaford and Lytle (1996) found that, by adding a large component of stone-ground maize to Lytle's diet and taking dental impressions at relevant points in the experiment, molar wear rates increased by approximately thirty times on the sandstone-ground maize diet. This, of course, has implications for the use of dental wear for adult age estimation, with one of their conclusions being that it would take as little as 10–15 years to wear the enamel on a molar facet. While this was an experimental study on one person, various other factors could also increase or decrease the rate of wear.

Many methods of recording attrition have been developed for archaeological human groups as an age indicator, i.e. observation of the patterning and rate of dentine exposure (Murphy, 1959; Miles, 1963; Molnar, 1971; Scott, 1979; Brothwell, 1981; Smith, 1984; Santini et al., 1990; Kambe et al., 1991; Walker et al., 1991), although attrition, as we have seen, also reflects cultural factors within those groups. Clearly, attrition will vary between groups, time periods and geographic areas, and therefore one method of recording developed on a particular group may not be applicable to another population. What is also clear is that the teeth compensate for wear and maintain their height by 'continually erupting' (Levers and Darling, 1983; Whittaker et al., 1985). Levers and Darling measured the height of worn teeth from the inferior alveolar canal and found that worn occlusal surfaces maintained a more or less constant distance from the canal at all ages in the archaeological populations they studied.

The cause of severe attrition may be reflected in two other areas of the oral cavity. Degeneration of the temporomandibular joint may occur and has been observed in association with attrition in some archaeological populations. Richards (1990) considered two groups of Australian Aboriginal skulls and found significant differences in patterns of tooth wear and frequency of temporo-mandibular joint changes between the two groups and sexes. Hodges (1991) also found an association of temporomandibular joint disease and attrition in 369 individuals from British populations and suggested that attrition predisposed to joint disease at this site. Furthermore, Merbs' (1983) study of the Eskimo Inuit

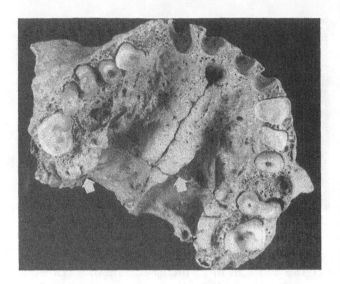

Fig. 4.8. Maxillary and palatine tori, and severe dental attrition on maxillary teeth (early Medieval, eighth–tenth centuries AD, Raunds, England).

population found a correlation between the two conditions, especially in females; this, he suggested, reflected the use of the jaws and teeth for cultural activities such as stretching and softening animal skins to make into clothing. Another condition seen in the oral cavity which may be present with heavy wear and temporomandibular joint disease are the mandibular, maxillary and palatine tori which, it is believed, reflect high levels of masticatory stress, producing a bony reaction (Fig. 4.8). New bone forms along the lingual aspects of the mandible and maxilla, usually around the molar region, and along the midline of the palatal bones. Interestingly, they occur in high frequencies in Iceland and Greenland today (Halffman et al., 1992).

CULTURALLY INDUCED DENTAL ALTERATION

As previously discussed, dental diseases have been strongly associated with cultural behaviour. To complement this account, the final area of study in this chapter focuses on evidence of direct cultural behaviour on the dentition, i.e. artificially produced abnormalities (e.g. Ikehara-Quebral and Toomay Douglas, 1997). A large literature exists both for modern and archaeological populations on how people use (and might use) their teeth for performing activities necessary, for example, in their subsistence economy. In addition, deliberate intervention (dentistry) for the treatment of dental disease is also occasionally seen.

Behaviourally induced dental modification may be evident macroscopically (Milner and Larsen, 1991) or may be seen as microscopic striations (Teaford, 1991; Larsen, 1997). Microscopic analysis of tooth wear can provide us with data on diet, use of the teeth as tools and the mechanisms of chewing (Teaford, 1991). Scanning electron microscopy allows the analysis of the intricacies of tooth wear in the form of pits and scratches. Summaries of research on microwear in various populations of human and non-human groups are provided by Larsen (1997:

262–7). Differences in food textures and abrasiveness, methods used for processing of foods, and types of diet have all been explored. For example, the adoption of pottery and its use in cooking allowed softer diets to develop with subsequent declines in scratches and pits on the tooth surface. Trauma to the teeth may also be identified in the form of fractures and chipping of the enamel, reflecting use of the teeth as tools for processing foods, and the quality of the foods consumed (Larsen, 1997: 268). Macroscopic alteration of teeth may be intentional, due to trauma or oral surgery (Milner and Larsen, 1991: 357). Direct alteration of tooth shape, extraction of teeth and inlaying teeth with precious stones may also be part of the behaviour of specific populations. For example, in the New World the Mayan culture developed the art of inlaying the (mainly) incisor and canine teeth using stones such as jade significantly between AD 460 and 600 (Aufderheide and Rodríguez-Martín, 1998: 411), and lip plugs (labret) in the lower lip are known archaeologically and ethnographically as a body modification. A recent study of the impact of labret use in a burial from pre-Columbian Chile (AD 400–900) found abrasion on the mandibular incisor teeth indicating double labret use, periostitis of the mandible and poor general dental health. Modern studies have shown that labret use can be particularly detrimental to dental health (Torres-Rouff, 2003). Dental modifications may represent a specific time or event in a person's life or may be used purely for decorative purposes (e.g. see Robb, 1997 on intentional tooth removal in the Italian Neolithic).

Unintentional alteration relates to the use of the jaws and dentition as tools. Probably the most common alteration to teeth is that caused by activity. Patterns of tooth wear and alteration from normal shape may be induced by activities such as habitually pulling flexible materials through and over the teeth, e.g. plant fibres for basketry work (Larsen, 1985; Lukacs and Pastor, 1988) or holding materials static in the teeth to allow manipulation (e.g. see Merbs, 1983). Differences in tooth wear between groups with different subsistence economies may be striking, allowing differentiation of hunter-gathering from agricultural groups. Hinton (1981) showed this in his study of aboriginal human groups where hunter-gatherers had labially rounded wear and individuals practising agriculture had little or no rounding but high frequencies of heavy cupped wear, the latter indicating heavy mastication. Some studies (both archaeological and ethnographic) have suggested that a considerable amount of pressure may be exerted on the teeth and associated structures when using them as tools which may lead to alterations in these structures and eventual loss (Molnar, 1972). In addition, dental changes will be induced not only by activities essential for survival but also by activities related to leisure, particularly in modern populations, such as habitual pipe smoking or Scottish bagpipe playing (Pindborg, 1970). All surfaces of the tooth may be affected, but it is only by comparing patterns of tooth alteration from modern populations with past populations that suggestions for their modification through cultural behaviour may be made, and often there may be no available comparative data.

Evidence for dental surgery in archaeological populations is rare but has been reported. Zias and Numeroff (1987) describe an individual from Israel, dated to 200 BC, with a 2.5mm-long bronze wire implanted in a tooth. Bennike and Fredebo (1986) also noted a skeleton dated to between 3200 and 1800 BC from a

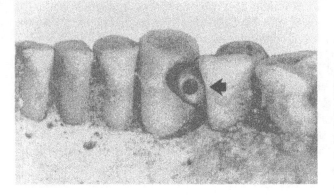

Fig. 4.9. Rosary bead placed in carious tooth in a late Medieval, twelfth–sixteenth centuries AD, Danish individual. *(With permission of the Museum of Medical History, Copenhagen, and Pia Bennike)*

passage grave in Denmark (Middle Neolithic period). The individual had a drilled cavity between the roots of the upper second permanent molar and another between the first and second molars; these teeth had evident carious cavities. Other examples of tooth drilling come from AD 1300–1700 in Alaska (Schwartz *et al.*, 1995), where observation of the alveolar bone around a central incisor revealed a hole that appeared to have been drilled deliberately to treat an abscessed tooth, and from AD 1025 in Colorado, where an occlusally drilled canine tooth was associated with a dental abscess (White *et al.*, 1997). A more direct possible treatment for a carious tooth was described from Denmark by Møller-Christensen (1969a). Here a mature adult dated to the fifteenth century AD had dental caries in a mandibular tooth which was filled with a bone rosary bead (Fig. 4.9). With respect to identifying deliberate extraction of teeth, although there is abundant evidence in written records and artistic representation in the past, determining whether a tooth has been extracted or lost ante-mortem is very difficult.

Direct primary evidence for dental care is rarely observed, even though documentary and art evidence suggest that some populations in antiquity did practise dentistry. Primary evidence for dental hygiene is also rare, but evidence of grooves on adjacent teeth (Bahn, 1989) suggests that tooth-picks may have been used as early as the French Middle Palaeolithic, 1.84 million years ago, although this is controversial. There is further evidence of dental care, particularly from Etruscan populations living in Italy over 2,500 years ago (Becker, 1994), where gold bridges, dentures and individual false teeth are noted. Whittaker (1993: 53–9) also found evidence, in the Christ Church, Spitalfields, post-Medieval crypt population in London, for gold-foil fillings and dentures in nine individuals; the dentures were composed of porcelain, ivory or bone and fitted using metal base plates and other stabilizing features such as gold pins.

METHODS OF RECORDING DENTAL DISEASE

Dental disease and modification of the dentition, through whatever means, provide the palaeopathologist with a wealth of information on diet, oral hygiene, dental care and occupation. However, use and comparison of these data are only possible when researchers utilize the same methods of analysis. Therefore, as standardized methods of recording develop and are accepted, these comparisons can be made. Dental data are often presented in a variety of forms, as already discussed, but they are summarized here:

1. Teeth/tooth sockets affected as a percentage of the total teeth/sockets available for examination.
2. Individuals affected as a percentage of the total individuals examined; this assumes all teeth and sockets are preserved.
3. Number of pathological lesions per individual (again, assuming all teeth and sockets are preserved).

It is also essential to present these data with reference to the age and sex of the populations being studied. If a person lives longer, dental disease will naturally be more likely to occur, and therefore a population composed mainly of older people would be expected to have higher rates of dental disease than a younger group. However, it has to be emphasized that, especially in the older age classes, the age at which the person developed the dental disease cannot be surmised. Differentiating the prevalence of dental disease on the basis of sex is also essential if sex differences are to be established. These differences, when put into context, e.g. access to diet or status of the person in the population, allow inferences to be made more easily. Lukacs (1989) also advocated the use of the Dental Pathology Profile to indicate general differences in dental pathology between different subsistence groups, but, for comparisons to be made, the demographic profile of each population must be similar. As Buikstra and Mielke (1985) have indicated, differences between subsistence groups and urban and rural environments will affect the demographic structure of the population and hence its propensity to develop not only dental disease but also other pathological conditions to be discussed in the following chapters.

While dental disease is probably the one health indicater that, on the face of it, allows the easiest comparisons between populations, there is still much to be done in developing and accepting recording methods. Buikstra and Ubelaker (1994), Lukacs (1989) and Hillson (2000) have perhaps made the most impact on attempting to introduce some standardization to recording. However, for other classifications of disease in palaeopathology there is much more work to be done.

CHAPTER 5

Trauma

Life without injury can hardly be imagined. (Wells, 1964a: 45)

INTRODUCTION

Trauma can be defined as any bodily injury or wound. It can be further subdivided into four categories (Ortner and Putschar, 1981: 55): partial or complete break in a bone (fractures); abnormal displacement or dislocation of a bone; disruption in nerve and/or blood supply; and artificially induced abnormal shape or contour (e.g. deliberate skull deformation; Fig. 5.1). The first category also includes amputation and trepanation (surgical removal of a piece of the skull). Fractures and dislocations will be the main conditions considered in this chapter. The evidence for trauma in a population may reflect many factors about the lifestyle of individuals, for example their material culture, economy (e.g. hunting and gathering versus agriculture), living environment (e.g. urban versus rural), occupation and interpersonal violence, and the state of healing of the injuries may indicate dietary status, availability of treatment and the occurrence of complications. Trauma (especially fractures) is one of the most common pathological conditions seen in human skeletal remains, along with the dental and

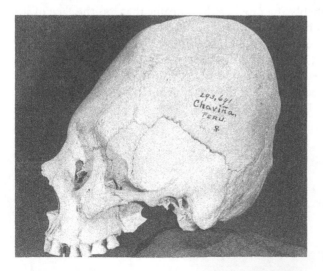

Fig. 5.1. Skull deformation: National Museum of Natural History, Washington DC, United States, 293691, adult female, probably prehistoric, Chavina, Peru, South America. *(With permission of Don Ortner)*

joint diseases, and it appears regularly in the palaeopathological literature (e.g. Steinbock, 1976; Ortner and Putschar, 1981; Merbs, 1989a; Larsen, 1997; Lovell, 1997; Aufderheide and Rodríguez-Martín, 1998; Roberts, 2000b). Susceptibility to injury is a characteristic of all life forms. The increase in the complexity of life, both in biological and in social terms, results in an increase in susceptibility to, and complexity of, injuries sustained. For example, road-traffic accidents are a major cause of fractures today.

The bones of the skeleton are important as they provide a supporting framework, store minerals, make blood cells, allow movement and protect the delicate areas of the body. Damage to the skeleton will therefore affect these functions. What is of interest to the palaeopathologist is not merely the presence of isolated traumatic features but the change that has occurred in the pattern of human trauma with the passage of time. The precise morphological characteristics of these traumatic features indicate the cause and clinical severity of the injury. Indeed, they throw light upon the everyday activities of the afflicted individual. The palaeolithic hunter, the Medieval farmer and the modern factory machine operator will all exhibit traumatic evidence of their trade. Young and old alike are subject to injuries characteristic of their age group, and the influence of biological sex on fracture patterns is clear (see below). Trauma may not, of course, be accidental, whether domestic or industrial. Notwithstanding the suggestions of some that people are not innately aggressive, warfare on an ever-increasing scale and complexity seems to have been a recurring theme throughout history. Even in very recent times, conflict in Afghanistan, Africa and Iraq reminds us that human populations have not learnt to live in harmony. The Neolithic arrowhead, the Medieval battleaxe and the later musket-ball may leave their evidence in the palaeopathological record (e.g. see Novak in Fiorato et al., 2001 for cranial wounds suffered by soldiers at the Battle of Towton). Surgical practice also does, of course, result in intentional inflicted wounds, albeit without aggression, and the orthopaedic and neurosurgeons of antiquity also left their mark in the record (Mays, 1996a; Arnott et al., 2003).

Before considering the bone injuries themselves, it must be appreciated that the palaeopathological evidence of trauma is but a small part of the total spectrum of injury affecting populations. By and large it is the gross injury which is in evidence; the multitude of commonplace cuts, abrasions and bruises so familiar to us all are lost in the archaeological record. Evidence of soft-tissue injury is sparse and merely inferential in skeletal remains, although more obvious in fleshed remains. For example, trauma in the form of strangulation is often seen in association with the 'bog bodies' of north-western Europe, where a ligature may be found around the neck (Brothwell, 1986). In order to recognize soft-tissue injury in skeletal remains, it is necessary for new bone formation to have occurred within the haematoma produced as a result of damaged soft tissue (myositis ossificans). Such an example is seen on the pelvis of a seventeenth-century Royalist soldier from England in whom a severe muscle tear must have occurred (Fig. 5.2) (Manchester, 1978b). Clearly, any injury that penetrates bone must also involve the surrounding soft tissues, even though the damage to these cannot be seen in skeletal remains. One may also infer damage to soft tissues by examining the

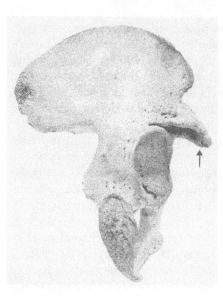

Fig. 5.2. Soft tissue injury. Ossification following injury to muscle. Male 18–20 years (Sandal Castle, Yorkshire, England).

location of the injury closely. Some fractures at specific sites in the body may lead to damage to blood vessels or nerves. For example, a fracture to the mid-shaft of the humerus (upper arm) often damages the radial nerve (Shaw and Sakellarides, 1967); obviously this would have implications for the individual's normal function.

Likewise, fractured ribs could cause damage to the lungs, a fractured spine could also cause nerve damage, while pelvic fractures and cranial trauma could injure the abdominal organs and brain respectively (see Crawford-Adams, 1983; Paton, 1984; Resnick and Goergen, 1995 on complications of fractures).

Destructive (or lytic) lesions may also occur as a result of stress or strain in an associated soft tissue structure. For example, in the postero-medial aspect of the distal femur, Resnick and Greenway (1982) identified cortical defects, irregularities and excavations (Fig. 5.3). The most common of these lesions in clinical contexts, cortical irregularity, was found to be more common in children and adolescents and associated with stress of the adductor muscle. Less common in modern populations but seen archaeologically is the cortical excavation, again associated with stress of the medial head of the gastrocnemius muscle.

Before discussing fractures in more detail, three examples of deliberate artificial deformation of the skeleton will be considered. Deformation of the skull was first described in written texts in the fifth century BC by the Graeco-Roman writer Hippocrates (Gerszten and Gerszten, 1995), and the earliest recorded case in a skeleton comes from Shanidar Cave, Iraq and is dated to 45,000 BC. Social status and

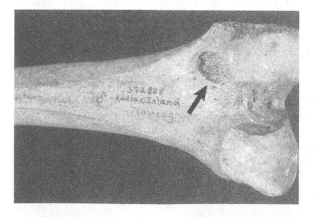

Fig. 5.3. Male individual from Alaska, United States, with cortical defect on the posterior aspect of the femur (curated in the National Museum of Natural History, Washington DC, United States).

a desire to make warriors more ferocious (Gerszten and Gerszten, 1995), plus ritual and religious purposes (Aufderheide and Rodríguez-Martín, 1998), have been indicated as reasons for deformation. It has been noted in skeletal remains in Europe (e.g. Beñus *et al.*, 1999; Özbek, 2001), the Near East (e.g. Meiklejohn *et al.*, 1992), Asia, the Americas, Africa, Australasia and the Pacific Islands, and probably developed as a practice independently at various times. It is a practice that can be effective only if undertaken in infancy when the bones of the skull are 'plastic' and easily deformed, and methods include the application of boards, pads and stones to the head of the newborn. The application of boards is believed to be the most effective and usually involved applying them to the frontal and occipital bones, while the use of stones placed around the child's head while in its cradle was less effective. Deforming devices were usually kept in place for three years and then removed, with growth of the skull then continuing in the direction established by the deforming apparatus (Aufderheide and Rodríguez-Martín, 1998: 35–6). Many resulting different shapes have been documented. Some associated 'pathological' conditions have been recorded, for example, alteration of the normal closure pattern of the skull's sutures, and overlapping of the temporal bones leading to a prominent border and necrosis of bone (Gerszten and Gerszten, 1995), but nothing of a serious nature, and certainly with no indications of reduced mental function. One study investigating the relationship of suture closure and cranial deformation found that there was a frequent association of deformation, premature sagittal suture fusion, and wormian bones in the lambdoid suture, in adults from the Lamanai site, Belize, Central America (White, 1996). Other work, examining casts of the endocranial surfaces of deformed and undeformed skulls, also indicates that the sinus and meningeal vessel pattern can change with deformation. Dean's (1995, 1996) study indicated vessels flattened in areas of deformation, and some individuals had enlarged occipital/marginal sinuses. She hypothesized that this indicated increased intracranial pressure. In a more recent study, Dean (2004) examined the relationship between the presence of wormian bones and deformation. She found that there was an increased frequency of wormian bones in the lambdoid suture in all forms of cranial deformation, but was unable to say whether deformation affected initial presence or absence of wormian bones. Another study by Kohn *et al.* (1995) of deformed skulls from a North American Hopi site dated to AD 1300–1680 (Kuchaptavela) found that there was a significant effect of deformation on the growth of the cranial vault, but not the face or base of the skull.

While cranial deformation has frequently been reported in past populations, other forms of deformation have rarely been noted. Of relevance here can be included the changes of female footbinding, which apparently began in China in the tenth century AD (Levy, 1967 in Mann *et al.*, 1990) as an indication of high social status, beauty and femininity (walking on bound feet would lead to enlargement of the abdomen, a vertical groove in the back and accentuated buttocks). Although no archaeological examples of footbinding have been reported to date, it is worth noting that changes to the tarsals, metatarsals and phalanges are inevitable and may potentially be seen archaeologically. For example, in a known (non-archaeological) case of footbinding described by Mann *et al.* (1990) the heads and shafts of the metatarsals were atrophied and deformed,

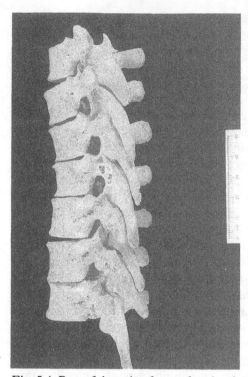

Fig. 5.4. Part of the spine from a female of late Medieval date (twelfth–sixteenth centuries AD); Ripon Cathedral, Yorkshire, England. Note the spinous processes are flattened, which may be the result of compression treatment for a sternal deformity. *(Photograph by Trevor Woods, Department of Archaeology, University of Durham)*

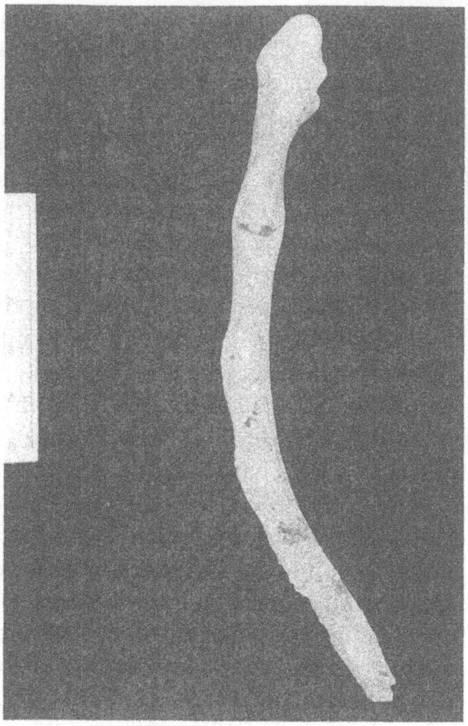

Fig. 5.5. Bowing of sternum (*Pectus carinatum*) in the same individual as Fig. 5.4. *(Photograph by Trevor Woods, Department of Archaeology, University of Durham)*

and the phalanges had constricted shafts, while the metatarso-phalangeal joints were partially dislocated. The practice was usually performed by mothers on their daughters every two weeks using silk bandages up to ten feet long until the full growth of the foot had been achieved (Mann *et al.*, 1990). A final example of deformation can be seen in the case of a late Medieval female skeleton from Ripon Cathedral, England (Groves *et al.*, 2003). Here it was hypothesized that a congenital sternal deformity (*Pectus carinatum*) was treated by compression of the upper chest, which led to flattening of the spinous processes of some of the thoracic vertebrae (Figs 5.4 and 5.5).

TYPES AND CAUSES OF FRACTURES

It is with the damage to bone that the palaeopathologist is mainly concerned. Except for small accumulations of blood that become ossified beneath the

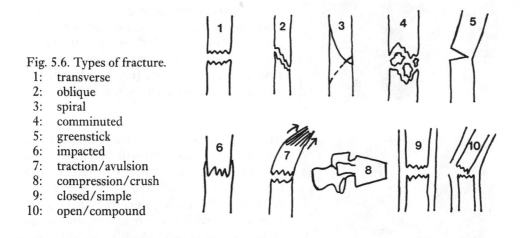

Fig. 5.6. Types of fracture.
1: transverse
2: oblique
3: spiral
4: comminuted
5: greenstick
6: impacted
7: traction/avulsion
8: compression/crush
9: closed/simple
10: open/compound

periosteum, recognized as fairly circumscribed swellings on the bone surface, the results of trauma to the skeleton are bone fractures. A fracture can be defined as the result of any traumatic event that leads to a complete or partial break of a bone. In theory, then, injuries to the skull caused by a bladed weapon, piercing injuries and surgical procedures, such as trepanation, to bone are all classed as fractures under this definition. The fractures that occur a short time before death or maybe coincident with it, and which show no evidence of healing, are often very difficult to distinguish from post-mortem breaks of bone (see Figs 5.20, 5.21 and 5.22 showing ante-mortem (healed), post-mortem and peri-mortem (unhealed) fractures). It is with the healed fracture or the ununited but healing fracture that the palaeopathologist is usually concerned, because the majority of fractures observed from archaeological contexts are healed.

All fractures belong to one of two categories, closed or open (Fig. 5.6: 9 and 10). Closed fractures are those in which there is no connection between the outer skin surface and the fractured bone itself. Open (or compound) fractures are those in which there is an open connection between the fracture site and the skin surface. This connection is a ready opportunity for bacteria to enter the bone from outside the body, and therefore all these fractures can potentially be infected, a problem even in modern medical practice. In the past, without the benefit of antibiotics, such an infection in a severely injured person was probably fatal in many cases. However, well-healed infected fractures have been noted. Those individuals fortunate enough to survive may have been left with a chronic discharging osteomyelitic bone.

The absence of soft tissues in skeletal remains clearly means that the placing of a fracture in one or other category is largely inferential unless clear evidence of infection associated with the fracture is present. Skeletal evidence for an open fracture is the superficial infection, osteitic pitting and irregularity of bone surface around the fracture site, or osteomyelitis; however, care should be exercised in inferring an open fracture when infection may have been present before the fracture occurred.

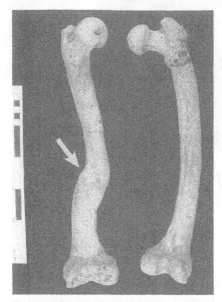

Fig. 5.7. Healed fracture to the left femur in a male with underlying Paget's Disease, and non-fractured opposite femur (early Medieval, eighth–tenth centuries AD, Jarrow, Tyne and Wear, England).
(Photograph by Trevor Woods, Department of Archaeology, University of Durham)

There are three major causes of fractures: acute injury (e.g. a skiing accident in a modern context); underlying disease, which weakens the bone and makes it more susceptible to fracture (e.g. tumour of the bone); and repeated stress, e.g. in an athlete today (see Resnick *et al.*, 1995: table 67–3 for stress fractures and associated activity). In stress fractures there is often no history of direct injury and pain will increase if the activity continues. Many stress fractures are hairline in nature and are difficult to diagnose, even by radiography; once they heal there may be no evidence left to see, and in an archaeological context identifying these types of fracture may be difficult, if not impossible. Pathological fractures may be induced by general or localized disease in the body. For example, osteoporosis (decrease in bone quantity) may affect the body generally and a tumour may affect an individual bone in the skeleton, but both lead to a weaker structure which makes the bone more susceptible to fracture. An archaeological example from Jarrow (Wells and Woodhouse, 1975), an early Medieval cemetery in the north of England, revealed Paget's disease and a fracture to the femur (Fig. 5.7). This is of course an assumption but one has to consider the possibility that the disease occurred after the fracture happened.

A further subdivision of fractures, and one that throws light on the mechanism of the injury, is the type (and by inference direction) of the break in the bone (Fig. 5.6). Direct and indirect injuries cause fractures. The simplest fracture in mechanical terms is transverse, which is a horizontal break across the bone. A force applied at right angles to the bone, either by accident or by direct blow, is necessary to create this fracture. Oblique or spiral fractures are due to indirect and/or rotational force. A further feature of fractures may be the multiple splintering of the broken bones. These comminuted fractures (i.e. more than two fracture fragments) are common in road-traffic accidents today and are less likely to heal in a functionally satisfactory manner. In the young, immature bone, transverse fractures may be incomplete and are termed greenstick, bowing or torus (Resnick *et al.*, 1995: 2570). Impaction fractures result in the two fractured ends being forced together, producing a rather stable fracture which may heal readily, even though some length may be lost on the affected limb. A traction/avulsion fracture is the result of a sudden strain of a muscle associated with a bone or a ligament or joint capsule. In this case it pulls a small piece of the bone away. A rather special type of fracture is the crush fracture of a vertebra (Fig. 5.8); crush or compression fractures are also commonly found on the joint surfaces. Often associated with osteoporosis causing weakness of the bone structure, the individual vertebra collapses in a wedge-shaped manner. A further type of direct trauma is that of penetration where the cortex is completely or partially penetrated and fractured, possibly into many pieces; this is then also called a comminuted fracture (Lovell, 1997: 141). These injuries are the result of the impact of a 'large force to a small area' (Lovell, 1997: 141) and may represent the blade of a weapon or a projectile point.

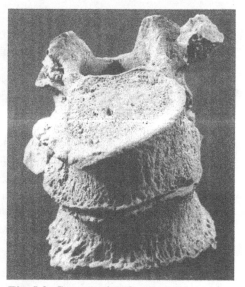

Fig. 5.8. Compression fractures to vertebrae (late Medieval, twelfth–sixteenth centuries AD, France).

HEALING OF FRACTURES

After a fracture, the healing process normally consists of three phases of differing duration. In general terms, the time taken for a fracture to heal depends on the bone element fractured and the type and position of the fracture, severity, apposition of the fractured fragments, stability of the fragments during healing, age and nutritional status of the individual, presence or absence of infection or other pathological process, a good blood supply and access to treatment. Fractures in young individuals tend to heal faster and more efficiently than in older adults, and upper limb fractures heal faster than those of the lower limb.

The three phases of healing are: circulatory or **cellular**, **metabolic** and **mechanical**. The **cellular** phase begins with closure of the fracture and formation of primary callus or woven, immature new bone (Latin: *callum*, hard). Initially blood seeps out from the fractured ends of the bone and forms a haematoma or collection of blood around and between the fracture (Sevitt, 1981). Severed blood vessels contract and become sealed with blood clots; this occurs within 12 hours of the fracture. Bone adjacent to the fracture dies (necroses), and fibrous granulation connective tissue forms through the action of fibroblasts (Ortner and Putschar, 1981: 62); the haematoma is eventually absorbed. Fibrous union of the fracture occurs by about 15 days. The blood supply to the fractured area develops, the granulation tissue matures and the fibroblasts are transformed into osteoclasts and osteoblasts which create an unmineralized intercellular matrix of collagen and carbohydrate (osteoid) by about 21 days. Calcium salts impregnate the osteoid and this leads to the formation of callus by between 3 and 9 weeks. The callus occurs between the fracture at the cortex, endosteum and periosteum, and its quantity is determined by the type and level of the fracture, associated soft-tissue damage and deformity present, for example.

The **metabolic** phase involves replacement of the immature bone of callus with more mature lamellar bone. The final **mechanical** phase contributes over two-thirds of the total healing time and involves realignment and remodelling of bone along the lines of stress. Remodelling occurs over many years, with eventual restoration of the normal architecture of the bone to its original appearance, even on a radiograph. The healing process is completed at different times for different bones of the body. Lovell (1997: 145) points out that cancellous bone heals faster than cortical bone because there is a larger area of contact between the fractured bits of bone, and the spongy nature of this type of bone allows 'easy penetration of bone forming tissue'. Radiography aids considerably in the interpretation of fractures (Roberts, 1989), particularly in assessing the mechanism behind the injury (type of fracture), and the state of healing of the fractured bone (Fig. 5.9). In archaeological contexts, taking accurate measurements of angulation, apposition (how much of the fractured fragments are apposed to each other) and overlap of the fragments is possible using radiographs (see Grauer and Roberts, 1996 for an example of a population study).

FRACTURE COMPLICATIONS

There are several fracture complications which can occur at the time of the injury or years later, some of which can be determined by analysis of skeletal remains. Compound fractures can lead potentially to **infection** of the fracture site and cause delay in healing, typically periostitis or osteomyelitis (see Chapter 7). If a fracture is not adequately reduced, i.e. the bone ends are not pulled apart and 'set' in the correct anatomical position, **shortening** of the affected limb and **malalignment** are possible, which could lead potentially to adjacent joint degeneration and **osteoarthritis**. However, care must be taken to try to determine whether infection or joint degeneration was not already present before the fracture. A further point to make is that it is possible, when examining skeletal material, to confuse an osteomyelitic sinus associated with a fracture with a hole that has been left as a result of decay of soft tissue that was originally incorporated into the fracture at the time of the injury (i.e. while the body was buried). Associated damage to the soft tissues, including **blood vessels and nerves**, can occur in relation to fractures in certain parts of the body (Crawford-Adams, 1983: figs 67 and 68). For example, a fracture to the neck of the femur can affect the blood supply to its head and cause problems with the normal healing process, and a fracture to the humerus can damage the radial nerve and lead to paralysis of the forearm.

In archaeological contexts many of these fracture complications cannot be observed directly and are only surmised from the position of the fracture. For example, in some fractures fat globules can be released from the medullary cavity into the bloodstream and may lead to obstruction of vessels in the brain or lungs. **Non-union** of fractures in antiquity has been observed but care must be taken in differentiating between true non-union and **delayed union** (i.e. not healed in the time expected) at the time of death, the latter suggesting that there had been insufficient time for the fracture to heal. Non-union is commonly seen in fractures to the femoral neck and in the shafts of the forearm bones, and the most common causes include: inadequate nutrition, infection, poor blood supply, inadequate immobilization or apposition. The most frequent bone to suffer from non-union is the ulna shaft, probably because of imperfect immobilization

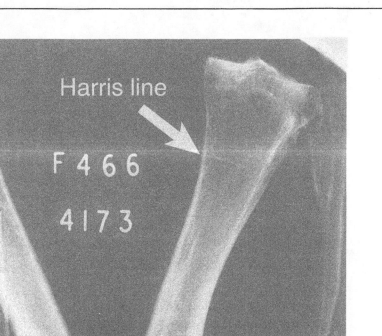

Fig. 5.9. Radiograph of bilateral fractures to tibiae and fibulae from a male adult showing healing, but associated angulation deformities and a sinus from osteomyelitis (see Chapter 7) (Romano-British, fourth century AD, Baldock, Hertfordshire, England); note also the Harris lines of arrested growth in tibiae (see Chapter 8).

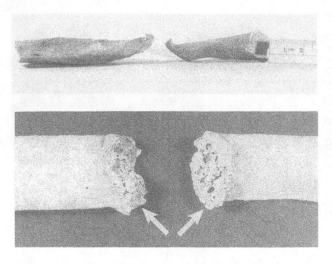

Fig. 5.10. Non-union of fractured radius from Ala 329, San Francisco Bay, California (500 BC–AD 1700). *(With permission of Robert Jurmain)*

Fig. 5.11. Non-union of rib fracture; note the formation of new bone at the rib ends, which suggests that the person died before the rib had chance to heal (late Medieval, twelfth–sixteenth centuries AD, Kirk Hill 14, Scotland).

(Crawford-Adams, 1983: 159), but other bones can be involved (Figs 5.10 and 5.11). In antiquity recognition of non-union is possible, with fracture fragments displaying some opacity of the fractured ends on a radiograph, indicating attempts at healing. There may also be a false joint or pseudoarthrosis. Stewart (1976) and Jurmain (1991) have described non-union of fractures in New World populations; it is, however, possible that many cases of non-union of fractures are not identified and are mistaken for post-mortem breaks.

LIMITATIONS OF TRAUMA STUDY

There are a number of limitations in the interpretation of fracture data. Modern population studies can look at the real age distribution of fractures, but in archaeological groups this is not possible. Even though an individual died at a certain age and had a healed fracture, this does not mean that it was sustained at that age; the fracture could have occurred many years before the death of the individual. Therefore, it is not possible to look at age and susceptibility to fracture unless the fracture occurred around death and illustrates the very early stages of fracture healing. However, the older a person is the more likely they would be to suffer trauma and therefore older people would be expected to have more fractures. In addition, very few fractures are seen in juveniles from archaeological contexts. This cannot be accepted as the true prevalence of fractures in this age group, and it is likely that many of these fractures are invisible to the palaeopathologist probably because they were greenstick fractures which healed so efficiently and quickly that they are not even visible on a radiograph. However, Glencross and Stuart-Macadam (2000) have indicated ways of identifying childhood fractures in adult skeletons. There are also problems in identifying peri-mortem (around death) fractures if there had been no time for healing to start to take place when the individual died; these fractures may appear to be post-mortem breaks and may not be identified as ante-mortem injury. Examining the patterning of fractures and comparing the pattern observed in modern cases may help to identify these peri-mortem fractures. For example, the pattern of injury in child abuse is characteristic, with fractured ribs and localized new bone formation on some bones of the skeleton. Indeed, some biological anthropologists have started to identify this patterning in archaeological contexts (Walker et al., 1997).

FRACTURES: LIVING POPULATION STUDIES

Both human and non-human primates can of course sustain fractures to the bones of their skeletons, and, while the activities they perform may be different, the underlying forces causing particular fracture types will be the same. Fracture patterns in non-human mammals from archaeological sites have received relatively little attention from archaeozoologists, but some work has been carried out on relatively modern primates (e.g. Lovell, 1990; Jurmain, 1997). For example, Jurmain (1997) studied fractures in chimpanzees, lowland gorillas and bonobos. Cranial fractures were much more common in the gorillas and least common in bonobos. Post-cranial trauma was found in 21.7 per cent and 30.8 per cent of two chimpanzee groups, 17.7 per cent of the gorillas and 13.3 per cent of the bonobos, and most were found in the upper appendages. The conclusions of the study indicated serious risks of falling in the chimpanzees and bonobos, and inter-individual aggression in chimpanzees and gorillas. Studies of trauma in earlier humans have also been limited, possibly because of the relative lack of skeletal remains recovered for these time periods. However, there have been some focused studies of Neanderthal populations. For example, Berger and Trinkaus (1995) looked at trauma pattern data from all available Neanderthal skeletal remains and compared the patterns seen with recent modern samples and a highly selected group of athletes, that of North American rodeo performers. The high rate of head and neck trauma seen in both the Neanderthals and the rodeo performers provided the greatest similarity, and close encounters with large animals were suggested as a cause for the trauma seen in the former.

Fracture prevalence rates in both ancient and modern populations reflect both intentional violence and accidental injury (see Judd, 2004 on a comparison of past and present injury). Technology has changed through time and today many more severe fractures are related to high-impact road-traffic accidents. Furthermore, many fractures may be directly the result of repetitive occupationally induced stress or pure accidents, such as falling. A recent study of admissions for fractures in England in people aged 45 years or above considered the time period 1989–90 to 1997–8 (Balasegaram et al., 2000). It found admission rates increased with age, especially for women. It was estimated that these rates would increase by 41 per cent for men and 21 per cent for women by the years 2021–2 because of the increasing numbers of elderly people in the population.

Age and sex determine many of the fracture patterns seen in modern populations; for example, older individuals, especially females, suffer fractures with underlying osteoporosis. Many population studies of trauma reveal age and sex distribution of fracture prevalence in defined populations (Fife et al., 1984; Sahlin, 1990; Prince et al., 1993), and the data is compared between populations from different environments. For example, Jónsson *et al.* (1993) studied lifestyle and fracture prevalence in Swedish populations from urban and rural environments and found a lower fracture rate in the urban environment; this was explained by the increased risk rural populations would have been exposed to during their everyday activities. However, another study (Jónsson *et al.*, 1992) showed the opposite result; the lower rate in the rural population was explained by the maintenance of physical activity in that population and its preventative effects against osteoporosis development and fracture. In a further study, of a Minnesotan population in the United States between 1980 and 1989, Madhok *et al.* (1993) found that hip fractures were 36 per cent more common in the urban group. This, they explained, was probably because of a multitude of factors. It may be that urban populations are less healthy generally and have more medical problems, which might lead to osteoporosis and the risk of falls. Alternatively, less physical activity in urban situations may have led to reduced bone mass. Osteoporosis-related fractures are a major concern confronting contemporary populations, although in antiquity it is unknown how common osteoporosis was, and whether it predisposed to a high frequency of fractures. What can be observed is that the classic sites in modern populations for osteoporosis-related fractures – the hip, wrist and spine – are affected. Furthermore, Mensforth and Latimer (1989) recorded the prevalence of fractures of the distal radius, hip, spine and sacrum in 938 individuals in the Hamann–Todd Collection (a modern documented skeletal collection). White females were most frequently affected by fracture at all sites compared to white males and both black males and females; osteoporosis was probably the main underlying cause.

In all the modern studies published, each fracture usually represents one individual and rates of fractures per 1,000, 10,000 or 100,000 individuals can be produced. In an archaeological context, fracture rates are usually calculated as a percentage of the total bones examined; presenting data as a percentage of individuals affected is problematic because it assumes complete survival of all the bones of the skeleton. For example, it is difficult to know whether, if an individual has a fractured radius, there was an associated fracture to the ulna if this bone has not survived burial to be examined. There is then a problem with comparing fracture prevalence between ancient and modern populations in that for modern groups all the bones of the skeleton are present to observe, whereas in an archaeological population they are not.

POST-CRANIAL FRACTURES: PAST POPULATION STUDIES

In order for fracture frequencies to be compared between skeletal populations on a global scale, methods of recording need to be the same for all researchers (as with any other pathological lesion). First, a detailed description of the fracture should be made, including the bone affected, side if appropriate, position of fracture, type of fracture, evidence of healing, problems with healing (linear angulation, spiral deformity, poor apposition and overlap of fragments) and evidence of complications. Linear angulation is measured on a radiograph using a protractor and ruler (along the longitudinal axis of the bone), and the degree of angulation of the distal fragment is measured in relation to the proximal fragment. The direction of angulation of the distal fragment (laterally, medially, anteriorly or posteriorly) should also be assessed. Spiral or rotational deformity can only be assessed by comparing the affected bone with its opposite side, or a normal anatomical specimen, and recording whether the distal fragment is rotated internally/medially or externally/laterally. Apposition, again, is measured on a radiograph, and the measurement is of the amount of bone apposed between each fragment as a percentage of the 100 per cent of total possible apposed bone; in effect this horizontal displacement of the bone fragments can occur in a medio-lateral or antero-posterior direction. Overlap of fracture fragments (which means that there would be no apposition at all) is also measured on a radiograph. However, by measuring the maximum length of the bone (and its opposite if available) it is also possible to see how much length has been lost on healing of the fracture (see Grauer and Roberts, 1996 for illustrations and discussion). Blunt or sharp force trauma in the skull are the two basic classificatory types of head trauma (see below for more detailed discussion), but a detailed description will reveal more specifically the type of force directed at the skull and whether the trauma is healed. Descriptions of the bones of the skull involved and the characteristics of the fracture lines, including any deformation, should be provided.

The above are basic variables that would be recommended for recording. However, more detailed methods of analysis of long bone fractures have been described and tested by Judd (2000, 2002a), studies that have particular relevance for recording fractures in fragmentary bones. When testing five different methods of recording long bone fractures, she found that some methods allowed for differential preservation and raised the fracture frequency compared to methods that did not. All methods focused on the 'bone count' – i.e. counting the numbers of bones and identifying those with fractures. However, Judd also noted that fracture frequency would decline, as more fragmentary long bones without trauma were included in the sample. Judd (2002a: 1263) found that if only complete undamaged bones were included in the assessment then 21 per cent (6 of 28) of the fractures would be excluded. This study, and the selection of a specific method of analysis for long bone fractures, has implications for final analysis and interpretation of population samples (and their comparison with others). It also indicates that using a method that takes into account differential preservation, for example, in cremated remains, will produce more information about trauma patterns in a wider variety of population samples.

In addition to knowing how many bones are fractured out of how many were observed for each bone element, most researchers also present the data on fractures according to the number of individuals affected. This, however, assumes that all bones of the skeleton were present to be observed, as we have seen before; what we cannot say is how many of the bones not preserved or excavated were fractured. Nevertheless, related to the individual experience of trauma, the distribution pattern of injuries may tell us something of the nature of their causes. Additionally, people who are older tend to have more injuries and therefore older ages at death should correlate with more fractures. However, this may not necessarily be the case for all populations. Judd (2002b) examined a Sudanese Nubian population dated to *c.* 2500–1500 BC and found people with violence-related injuries had more fractures than those with fractures associated with accidental injury, and that young males had most of the former.

Notable studies of trauma in past populations are seen in work in both the Old and New Worlds. In the Old World Angel (1974) considered rates of fractures through long periods of time in Greece and Turkey (seventh millennium BC to second century AD). The prevalence of fractures for males and females (i.e. the number of individuals affected) was given; males were affected more than females in all periods and the prevalence rate ranged from 1.0 to 3.6 per cent. Further east, Judd (2000) found at Kerma, Nubia (1750–1500 BC) 47 fractured bones from a total of 1,771 bones observed (2.7 per cent), compared to a study (Alvrus 1996, 1999) from Semna South (300 BC–AD 300), where 48 bones were fractured from a total of 3,013 bones (1.6 per cent), and a study by Kilgore et al. (1997) from Kulubnarti (550–1450 AD), where 4.3 per cent (66) of 1,526 bones were fractured (Table 5.1). Judd (2000) also compared fracture patterning between the rural skeletal population from Dongola and the urban population from Kerma, 70km away (Table 5.2). Again, radius and ulna fractures were some of the most frequent of all the long bones affected in the rural population, although the tibia was also affected at 11.1 per cent. In the urban population, however, even though radius and ulna were the most frequently fractured bones, the rates were lower than for the rural population, and also lower for lower limb fractures. It is suggested that the fractures in the rural population were the result of cultivation and herding activities. This was also found in the study by Judd and Roberts (1999) at Raunds, in Northamptonshire, England, a Medieval farming village, where 2.9 per cent of the long bones (clavicle omitted) were fractured (27 of 944). This was much higher than urban fracture frequency rates for England (Table 5.3), apart from the figure for St Nicholas Shambles and Chichester, a late Medieval leprosy hospital.

Table 5.1 Frequency of fractures in different populations, Old and New World data (clavicles excluded)

Site	Fracture No.	Total Bones	%	Sources
Old World				
Kerma, Nubia	47	1,771	2.7	1
Semna South	48	3,013	1.6	2
Kulubnarti	66	1,526	4.3	3
Denmark	36	4,518	0.8	4
New World				
San Pedro de Atacama, Chile	46	2,471	1.9	5
Libben, Ottawa County, Ohio, USA	57	2,123	2.7	6
Central California Ala 329	36	2,047	1.8	7
Central California SCI-038	23	1,018	2.3	8

Sources: 1. Judd (2000); 2. Alvrus (1996, 1999); 3. Kilgore *et al.* (1997); 4. Bennike (1985): note, these data cover prehistoric and historic samples; 5. Neves *et al.* (1999); 6. Lovejoy and Heiple (1981); 7. Jurmain (1991); 8. Jurmain (2001).

Table 5.2 Frequency of fractures in different long bones, Old and New World data (% of total bones observed)

Bone	1	2	3	4	5	6	7
Humerus	0.0	1.0	0.1	0.2	0.7	0.3	2.1
Radius	7.8	2.4	1.5	4.2	5.4	4.3	3.7
Ulna	13.8	8.3	2.1	4.1	3.1	5.2	6.9
Femur	0.0	1.5	0.1	0.7	2.6	0.0	1.7
Tibia	11.1	0.9	0.7	0.7	1.4	1.6	0.6
Fibula	5.8	0.9	0.5	0.7	3.5	0.0	0.8

Sources: 1. Dongola, Nubia – rural (Judd, 2000); 2. Kerma, Nubia – urban (Judd, 2000); 3. Denmark (Bennike, 1985): note, these data cover prehistoric and historic samples; 4. San Pedro de Atacama (Neves *et al.*, 1999); 5. Libben, Ohio (Lovejoy and Heiple, 1981); 6. Ala-329, California (Jurmain, 1991); 7. SCI-038, California (Jurmain, 2001).

A recent study (Grauer and Roberts, 1996) examined fracture prevalence rates from Medieval British sites and found very similar rates between them (Table 5.3), ranging from 0.3 to 6.1 per cent of bones observed. All the cemetery sites served urban communities; those with the highest prevalence rates were from St Nicholas Shambles, London, and the late Medieval hospital cemetery from Chichester. It is likely that the higher rates in London may be explained by the small number of bones available to examine, or perhaps this prevalence represents the hazards of urban living in a big city. The rate for the Chichester group may reflect its use as a hospital and therefore the likelihood of people being admitted for care following fracture.

Table 5.3 Fracture prevalence in six late Medieval British urban populations

Site	Fracture No.	Total Bones	%	Sources
Whithorn, Scotland	27	9,563	0.3	1
Blackfriars, Gloucester	11	1,861	0.6	2
St Helen-on-the-Walls, York	41	4,938	0.8	3
St Andrew, Fishergate, York	26	3,235	0.8	4
Chichester, Sussex	41	1,554	2.6	5
St Nicholas Shambles, London	18	296	6.1	6

Sources: 1. Cardy (1997); 2. Wiggins *et al.* (1993); 3. Grauer and Roberts (1996); 4. Stroud and Kemp (1993); 5. Judd and Roberts (1998); 6. White (1988).

Examination of the pattern of fractures in the skeleton for these sites reveals that the arm (especially the **radius** and **ulna**, Table 5.4) was the most frequently affected limb, except at Whithorn, Chichester and Fishergate where the fibula rate was higher. Rates for the **femur** are particularly low in all groups; today, fractured femurs at the neck or trochanteric region are common in elderly females, i.e. 60 years plus, who usually have underlying osteoporosis (Crawford-Adams, 1983), and fractures in the shaft of the femur follow severe violence (for example in a road-traffic accident). This probably explains their relative absence in the fracture prevalence record for antiquity, when motorized vehicles were not the norm and people living into old age are believed to be rare (but see Chapter 2). Fractures to the **patella** are caused by direct or indirect trauma but are not commonly seen in skeletal populations. Fractures to the **tibia** were also rare in all groups. In Britain today motor-cycle accidents are 'by far the commonest single cause of major fractures to the shafts of the **tibia and fibula**' (Crawford-Adams, 1983: 251), causing an angulatory/rotational force. The low frequency of such fractures in ancient populations could be explained again by this lack of technological advance. Fractures to the tibia and fibula today tend to be focused on the ankle so the very distal parts of these bones are those most fractured, often associated with soft tissue injury (Lovell, 1997: 163). Fractures of both bones may be at the same level if there is a direct blow to the bone, but if it is a spiral indirect injury then the opposite ends of the bones are affected (Lovell, 1997: 163).

Table 5.4 Fracture prevalence by bone element for six late Medieval British urban populations (%)

Bone	1	2	3	4	5	6
Humerus	0.0	0.3	0.8	0.4	4.2	5.3
Radius	0.5	1.4	1.3	0.8	3.2	8.8
Ulna	0.1	0.5	1.5	0.8	2.8	8.2
Femur	0.2	0.5	0.1	0.2	0.4	3.8
Tibia	0.4	0.5	0.7	0.5	2.3	6.0
Fibula	0.8	0.3	0.8	1.7	7.2	1.1

Sources: 1. Cardy (1997); 2. Wiggins *et al.* (1993); 3. Grauer and Roberts (1996); 4. Stroud and Kemp (1993); 5. Judd and Roberts (1998); 6. White (1988).

If we turn now to the ancient New World data (Tables 5.1 and 5.2), Lovejoy and Heiple's study of the Libben site in Ohio, United States (1981) revealed a 3 per cent fracture prevalence rate (72 of 2,383 bones; includes clavicle) and they indicated that most of the fractures were accidental rather than due to interpersonal violence; again, most of the fractures occurred in the arm. Further west in North America, Jurmain (1991, 2001) has focused on two prehistoric central Californian skeletal populations: Ala–329 on the east side of the San Francisco Bay (AD 500–AD 1700), and SCI-038 (240 BC–AD 1770) in the Santa Clara Valley, 14 miles south of Ala-329. At Santa Clara 23 of 1,018 long bones were fractured (2.3 per cent) and at Ala-329 36 of 2,047 bones had fractures (1.8 per cent). At both sites, as seen in many other studies, the forearm bones were most frequently fractured. Craniofacial trauma was also observed in 7 of 159 individuals (4.4 per cent). Other studies of trauma patterning in the New World, this time in South America, have focused on

144 individuals from a Northern Chilean population of 4,000 years BP Chinchorro culture (Standen and Arriaza, 2000). Here, hunting and gathering concentrated on coastal resources, complemented by wild plants and camelids. Only one of the 55 non-adults showed any evidence of trauma (a quartz lithic point tip in a vertebra), but 27 of the 89 adults (30 per cent) had some evidence of trauma, mainly to the skull (17 people), with three times more seen in the males. This was interpreted as being the result of interpersonal aggression more than accidental or work-related trauma. Unfortunately, the 'bone-count' data for this study were not provided, and therefore frequencies could not be compared with other studies presented here. However, another study of a prehistoric population from the region of San Pedro de Atacama in the same country and dated to AD 250–1240 did provide some useful data. Here, 244 individuals (161 adults) who relied on camelids and small garden cultivation in oases were examined (Neves et al., 1999); 1.9 per cent of the 2,471 bones observed (humerus, radius, ulna, femur, tibia and fibula) were fractured (Table 5.1). The most frequently fractured bones were the radius and ulna as for the British populations (Table 5.2).

Overall the extant data for Old and New Worlds for long bone fracture frequency indicate that late Medieval London, England, has the highest rate (6.1 per cent), with Kulubnarti in the Sudan at 4.3 per cent. It is possible that the high urban rate for London reflects the complex nature of living in a large Medieval city, and Kilgore et al. (1997) suggest that the rugged terrain where the people from Kulubnarti resided put them at risk from falls. The 2.9 per cent rate for the rural site of Raunds, England, may indicate accidents associated with farming (Judd and Roberts, 1999), and that of 2.7 per cent for Kerma is interpreted as the result mainly of non-lethal violence (Judd, 2000). This rate was also seen for the Libben (US) sample, and Lovejoy and Heiple (1981) also indicate accidents as the major cause of fractures here. At the Medieval leprosy hospital at Chichester a 2.6 per cent fracture frequency rate was recorded; Judd and Roberts (1998) suggest that a number of factors may have been influencing the occurrence of fractures here, including the hazards of the urban environment and the presence of lepromatous leprosy in some individuals creating sensory deficiencies and accidental falls (see Chapter 7), and the effect of poor health generally on the senses, making people more susceptible to having accidents. The Santa Clara, California, population had the next highest fracture frequency rate at 2.3 per cent, and this rate was termed 'moderate' when compared to other sites in North America and elsewhere (Jurmain, 2001: 21). The rest of the sites considered here had frequencies ranging from 1.9 per cent down to 0.3 per cent, with two sites in England (St Helen-on-the-Walls, York, and Blackfriars, Gloucester) and one in Scotland (Whithorn) having the lowest rates; all these sites were associated with complex urban environments, which is surprising considering the higher rate in a similar environment seen in London (St Nicholas Shambles). Perhaps there were different factors at work in London that contributed to this higher rate. While the reader is directed to the specific papers documenting age and sex differences, it should be noted that, generally speaking, all these studies noted a higher male fracture rate. One main factor to bear in mind is that some of these figures do not take into account the preservation status of the skeletal samples (some skeletons may not have all bones preserved to be observed).

In modern studies fracture prevalence rates for different parts of the body vary, but there are larger numbers of fractures to the bones of the leg, while the radius and ulna together contribute significantly to the fracture prevalence rate. A number of population studies in the following summary illustrate the complex nature of the variables underlying the patterns of trauma seen today in different populations. Donaldson *et al.* (1990) studied 850,000 people from urban and rural Leicestershire, England, over three years and found over 12,000 males and 10,000 females had been seen at one accident and emergency department. Males had a fracture frequency of 100/10,000 and females had a rate of 81/10,000. Females over the age of 55 years had more fractures than males, due to osteoporosis and falls. Most fractures overall were of the distal radius and ulna (especially in females), but males had more fractures of the metacarpals and skull. Buhr and Cooke (1959: 512) looked at fracture patterning in over 8,500 admissions to a hospital in Oxford, England, between 1953 and 1957 using a different approach. They found four different groups and named them according to the shape of letters the patterns displayed on the curves plotted on a graph. The A group showed the 'wage-earners' fracture pattern, which consisted of a preponderance of males with fractures to the hands and feet. The J group characterized older people of both sexes (the 'post-wage-earners'), with a high frequency of proximal humerus and femur fractures. The L group comprised mainly young people (the 'pre-wage-earners'), especially males, with a preponderance of tibial shaft fractures. Finally the 'Composite group' had two groups mainly affected, people in their youth, and older males and females. This study confirms that people of both sexes will be differentially affected through their lifespan by fractures, for various reasons.

Shaheen *et al.* (1990) considered dislocations and fractures in people in Saudi Arabia (52 per cent were Saudi) during 1986. Only 4 per cent of the total injuries were dislocations (over 50 per cent were of the shoulder), but 80 per cent of the injuries were to males. In all, 86 per cent of the injuries were not induced by road-traffic accidents and the most frequent fractures were to the radius and ulna (27 per cent of the total). Females rarely had fractures as a result of road-traffic accidents, probably because most were housewives and rarely ventured outside their homes. In females children had the most fractures (53.7 per cent), while young adult males had the highest frequency for that age group (55 per cent). Despite fractures to the spine being relatively rare (3 per cent of the total injuries), 24 per cent had spinal cord complications, a possibility to bear in mind when considering fractured spines in archaeologically derived populations.

In a study during 1977 by Fife and Barancik (1985) of 8,177 people from north-east Ohio, United States, there were 877 people with fractures (517 males), and rates of 26 per 1,000 males and 16 per 1,000 females were identified. Two peaks of age-related trauma were found, in 10–14 year olds and people over 60 years, although male fractures exceeded female fractures until the age of 50 years. Some 46 per cent of the injuries were caused by falls, but in the over 65 year olds this rose to 87 per cent of the fractures. Other causes were road-traffic accidents (9 per cent and mostly in the younger age groups), occupationally related accidents (8 per cent), assaults (5 per cent) and cycle accidents (3 per cent). However, 18 per cent were sustained in the context of sports (by falls or being struck by objects). While age and sex, and 'occupation' in its broadest sense, clearly have an effect on fracture patterns, the climate and the weather may also cause problems. While one could argue that people in countries with particularly hazardous climates have probably adapted to these situations by introducing measures to prevent accidents, people who do not usually experience those hazards may be 'caught out' by freak climatic conditions. For example, in Cardiff, Wales, in 1978 and 1979 there were occasions when the streets were covered with ice and hard-packed snow, which predisposed people to falls (Ráliš, 1981). During that time forearm and wrist fractures were 16.5 times more common, and fractures overall were three times more common when compared to a control group.

While we can use some of these clinical data as a comparison for our archaeological populations to try to understand why they sustained fractures, specific data that relate to the causes of fractures in the past are harder to access because modern technological advances causing fractures are not relevant. However, fractures that are due to extremes in weather are certainly worth considering, as are occupations that may have been practised in the past. For example, the interaction of animals with humans must also have been hazardous at times, from the hunting of animals to the domestication of them. Studies of injuries in populations as a result of animals also appear in the clinical literature. For example, Björnstig et al. (1991) studied animal-related injuries of 628 people over a two-year period in Umeå, Sweden, and found 58 per cent of them were in females. Dogs (42 per cent), cats (9 per cent), horses (31 per cent), cattle (8 per cent) and moose (6 per cent) accounted for the majority of encounters. Although most of the injuries were to the soft tissues, for example, bites, bruises and scratches, 34 fractures were caused by falls as a result of walking a dog, 3 fractures were a result of cat encounters, 43 fractures occurred in upper and lower extremities from falls from horses (and less commonly from being kicked or trampled), 11 had fractures from handling cattle (the most severe injuries of all), and 5 had metacarpal or forearm fractures from car accidents involving collisions with moose. Jones (1990) also found in a study of three years of admissions in the Amish community of mid-eastern Ohio, United States, that 26.7 per cent of the trauma observed was cattle or horse related. The Amish are a group of people whose religious beliefs disallow the use of many modern conveniences, including cars and electricity, and thus they may be very similar to our archaeological communities in terms of their health. Yet another study in the United States of agricultural injuries in Wisconsin over twelve years found that a majority of trauma was caused by animals (30 per cent) as a result of falls from horses and assaults from uncontrollable horses and cattle. Some 22 per cent of the 739 individuals were left with significant permanent neurological, pulmonary or orthopaedic disability (Cogbill et al., 1991).

Fractures to parts of the skeleton other than the major long bones are also observed in modern and ancient groups. However, fractures to the **hands and feet** were particularly infrequent in the past; this may be explained by the relatively poor survival of these bones in archaeological contexts. The scaphoid bone can be fractured (usually in young adults) by falling on an outstretched hand, but the rest of the carpals are rarely fractured (Crawford-Adams, 1983: 182). However, a fracture of the hamate bone of the wrist in a late Medieval male from

Abingdon, Berkshire, was suggested to be a united fracture (Wakely and Young, 1995); these fractures are usually caused by a fall onto the hand, as a result of a crushing injury, or from 'gripping and swinging a club', for example, when playing golf (Wakely and Young, 1995: 53). The base of the first metacarpal can be fractured as a result of boxing, as can the other metacarpals, but fractures through their bases and shafts can also occur (with similar fractures of the phalanges). Fractures to the tarsal bones may include compression injuries to the talus and calcaneus caused by a fall from a height and landing on the feet (Crawford–Adams, 1983: 277). Wells (1976a) describes some examples from the palaeopathological record. The metatarsals can be fractured through their shafts, usually as a result of something falling on the foot, a twisting injury, or by repeated stress (the stress or March fracture). Fractures to the shafts of the phalanges of the foot are usually caused by heavy objects landing on the toes. None of these hand and foot injuries is, however, seen much archaeologically, but the metacarpo-phalangeal fractures may indicate defence wounds as a result of interpersonal violence.

Fractures involving the **pelvis** are also rare, probably because today they occur most frequently following high–impact road–traffic accidents. Damage to the abdominal structures is a potentially serious complication. **Sternal** (especially associated with anterior rib fractures) and **scapula** fractures are rare, but when seen in an archaeological population they may indicate the results of a blow to the back or chest of the individual and interpersonal violence (Fig. 5.12). Unfortunately, the scapula is often damaged, especially in the blade area (where the majority of fractures occur), during burial or excavation, and therefore the frequency of this fracture is probably underestimated for past populations. Fracture to the acromion of the scapula has been recorded in archaeological contexts (Miles, 1994) but there may be confusion between a true fracture (and non-union) or non-fusion of the acromial epiphysis – *os acromiale* (see Chapter 6), perhaps because of a specific activity (Stirland, 2000). In the Medieval population from Ensay, Scotland (Miles, 1989), 11 examples of separation (non-fusion?)of the acromial tip were recorded in 220 scapulae (10.0 per cent), and Stirland (2000) recorded a 13.6 per cent prevalence in the group of individuals from the Tudor warship the *Mary Rose*. In the latter case it was suggested that non-union

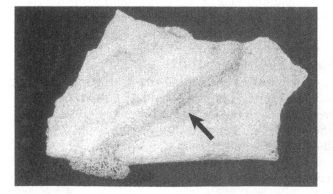

Fig. 5.12. Fragment of scapula blade with healing fracture (Romano–British, fourth century AD, Cirencester 338, Gloucestershire, England).

was the result of the movements necessary for archery, and practising this from an early age may prevent fusion of the epiphysis.

Fractures to the humerus are not very frequently seen archaeologically, as we have observed, but in modern populations the shaft (usually mid-third and caused by indirect twisting/direct injury) and neck (seen in elderly women with osteoporosis and caused by a fall on the limb) are most commonly affected (Crawford-Adams, 1983). Fractures to the shaft of the **ulna** may represent interpersonal violence, i.e. defending a blow to the head but could equally be caused by a fall on the arm (see Jurmain, 1999). Colles fractures to the **radius**, often with underlying osteoporosis, may have been the result of falling on the outstretched hand; they have posterior displacement and are quite commonly seen. Fractures of both these bones are commonly identified in archaeological contexts (see above). The **clavicle** is usually broken in accidents involving falling and is also seen regularly in palaeopathology. Along with **rib** fractures (again, commonly observed), even in modern contexts, clavicle fractures are often left to heal without therapeutic intervention. The ribs are fractured as a result of a fall or a direct blow to the rib cage, although constant coughing or sneezing can also break the ribs (Lovell, 1997: 159). Damage to underlying soft tissues such as the lung may be a problem.

Trauma in the vertebral bodies of the **spine** can result from a vertical force induced hyperflexion injury, such as jumping from a height onto the feet, leading to compression fractures, scoliosis and kyphosis (Crawford-Adams, 1983: 98); often underlying osteoporosis may lead to weakness and fracture. Merbs (1983) reported that thirty-six of eighty adult Sadlermiut Eskimo vertebral columns suffered from vertebral compression fractures from the third thoracic vertebra down to the fifth lumbar vertebra. The frequency was higher in females; the suggested reason was that females rode on sleds and toboggans over rough terrain, allowing compressive forces to be transmitted through the spine. Females also carried their offspring on their backs, and older females may have had underlying osteoporosis. Compression fractures can also occur in the cervical spine and, although less frequent, are more serious (Crawford-Adams, 1983: 86); they are often associated with subluxation or partial dislocation and there is an increased risk of damage to the spinal cord at this level. Fracture-dislocation to the second and/or third cervical vertebrae has been consistently referred to, since 1965 when it was named as such (Pathria, 1995), as the 'Hangman's Fracture' (James and Nasmyth-Jones, 1992: 82), but, as Pathria (1995: 2853) notes, 'Despite its popular name, the injury [today] typically results from a motor vehicle accident or a fall.' While no cases have been reported archaeologically, it is indicated, as a result of the examination of three series of criminals executed by hanging between 1882 and 1945 (thirty-four bodies), that a fracture-dislocation of C2/C3 (or traumatic spondylolisthesis of the axis) is the 'exception rather than the rule' (James and Nasmyth-Jones, 1992: 91). Fractures at the levels of the seventh cervical and first thoracic vertebrae are termed 'clay-shoveller's fractures' (Knüsel et al., 1996). Fig. 5.13 shows an unhealed example from the Romano-British site at Baldock, Hertfordshire, England. The combination of the actions of the trapezius and rhomboid muscles during shovelling initiate this fracture and may help identify occupation, although there have been few reports to date in palaeopathology.

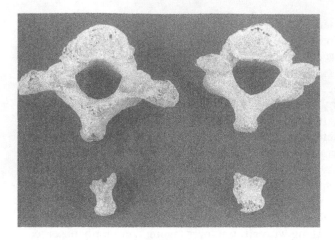

Fig. 5.13. Unhealed 'clay-shoveller's' fractures to the spinous processes of the seventh cervical and first thoracic vertebrae (Romano-British, fourth century AD, Baldock, Hertfordshire, England).

A rather special type of vertebral fracture, which is particularly common in all periods of antiquity, may have its roots in a congenital weakness of a small area of bone. This condition, known as **spondylolysis**, is recognized in skeletal remains as the separation of a single vertebra into two parts. The weakness of the bone is present at the position between the upper and lower joint surfaces on the neural arch, or that part of the vertebra lying behind the solid central body and surrounding the spinal cord. It is only seen in hominids and is related to bipedalism and an erect posture (Merbs, 1996). It develops after a child starts to walk, and is more common in males. It is suggested that the recurrent stresses and strains of bending and lifting in the upright posture create a gradual series of small stress fractures at the site of weakness (Fig. 5.14); it is probably caused by stress or fatigue at the site but also by acute injury. Modern studies (cited in Merbs, 1996) indicate that spondylolysis results from repetitive, vigorous movements of the lower back, for example in weight lifting, dancing, kayaking and wrestling. It also appears to be a condition associated with gymnastics. For example, Jackson et al. (1976) found an 11.0 per cent incidence in 100 female gymnasts, and many had associated spina bifida occulta. Ultimately the bone at that site fractures partially or entirely and the neural arch may separate from the vertebral body. The only attachment remaining is by ligament and fibrous tissue. Generally speaking, healing of these fractures does not take place, probably, as Merbs (1989a: 170) suggests, because of continual stress at the site, although evidence of healing has occasionally been found (Eisenstein, 1978; Merbs, 1995). Most cases of the condition occur at the fifth lumbar vertebra, less commonly at the fourth, and occasionally elsewhere. Merbs (2002a: 156) also notes that asymmetrical spondylolyis can occur and is 'part of the earliest picture of spondylolysis'. If this occurs, the right side is most affected and this, he suggests, may be related to handedness. The end result of an asymmetrical spondylolytic lesion may be development into a bilateral lesion, healing of the asymmetrical lesion, or development into spondylolisthesis (see below). The modern incidence of the condition is around 3.0 per cent of Caucasian populations (Merbs, 1989b), but there is considerable ethnic variation. The incidence in Eskimos may be up to 50 per cent, a feature that is attributed to their physically arduous existence. In a recent study by Merbs (2002b) 22 per cent of 417 skeletons from Arctic Canada had spondylolysis, with a ratio of males to females affected of 2.4:1. Interestingly, the condition increased with age, and then declined in the middle and older age categories.

Arriaza (1997) has also noted a high frequency of this condition in skeletons dated to *c.* 1200–1521 AD from Guam. A rate of 21 per cent of individuals was observed (8 of 38 skeletons with complete spines). In this case, there was evidence at the site of house building using very large stone pillars, and the author suggested that transporting these pillars might have led to spondylolysis. Both males and females were affected (29 per cent of males and 14 per cent of females), which may illustrate that both were involved with this occupation.

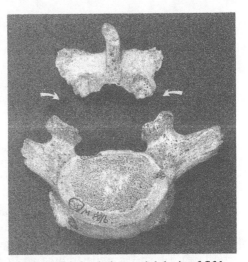

Fig. 5.14. Unhealed spondylolysis of fifth lumbar vertebra (Romano-British, fourth century AD, Gambier-Parry Lodge 552, Gloucester, England).

Apart from slight, constant, lower back discomfort, the condition causes no symptoms unless it is associated with a dislocation of the now unstable vertebral body. This condition, termed spondylolisthesis, is a serious abnormality which may therefore justly be regarded as a complication of trauma. Although uncommon, it was no doubt present in the past. The recognition of the abnormality in skeletons from archaeological sites is difficult and rests upon the observation of bone formation along the rims of the displaced vertebral bodies (Congdon, 1931). Fusion by bone of the displaced vertebra upon its neighbour may also occur. A rare case of spondylolisthesis (Fig. 5.15) shows the condition in an Anglo-Saxon individual from Kent, England, in which bony fusion between the displaced vertebra and its neighbour has occurred (Manchester, 1982). This natural process of antiquity has achieved, albeit in a poor position, what modern orthopaedic surgical practice endeavours to do.

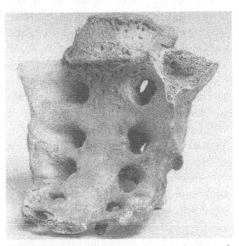

Fig. 5.15. Spondylolisthesis with fusion of the fifth lumbar vertebra to the sacrum (early Medieval, sixth–eighth centuries AD, Eccles, Kent).

INTERPERSONAL AGGRESSION AND TRAUMATIC LESIONS

In the twenty-first century we are all familiar with aggressive society. Even within a single population group, one section of a society may live in peace with only sporadic and infrequent episodes of aggression, while in a neighbouring area an undercurrent of continuous violence may be the norm. Often the most dramatic injuries are to the skull as, certainly in interpersonal/intergroup violence, the head is often the main target for blows; if head protection is not worn then the skull may suffer injury. In crime scene investigations where the cause and manner of a victim's death are being evaluated, it is usually the head and neck which reveal most of the trauma identified. As Knight (1991: 156) states, it is the head which is usually the target for violence as the brain and skull are the most vulnerable areas of the body when damaged, and injury to the brain is often a consequence of skull fracture due to increased intercranial pressure from bleeding. However, if a person falls to the ground, the head can also be damaged. In addition to skull injuries (including the face), rib and scapula trauma and defence injuries to the forearms and hands may be an indicator of interpersonal violence, and patterning of injury should always be considered (see Jurmain, 1999; Judd, 2002b). Injuries to the neck through strangulation and severe trauma or suffocation may also lead to fractures of the hyoid bone and/or calcified thyroid cartilage (Ubelaker, 1992). As these elements of the skeleton are rarely excavated this type of injury has not been documented. The subject of 'Parry' fractures has recently received some attention in the literature. Indeed, these fractures of the mid or distal third of the ulna can be caused by different events such as a fall on the forearm, or indeed from parrying a blow to protect oneself from injury. Jurmain (1999: 217) describes interpreting Parry fractures as the result of interpersonal violence as 'obviously straightforward and neat; they *might* even be correct'. He further suggests that such patterning of fractures could be 'made to fit the hypothesis', but indicates that in most contemporary contexts ulnar shaft fractures are caused by falls. To determine whether the fracture was due to a fall, it would be, he suggests, wise to inspect the radial head to see whether there is evidence of dislocation, which usually accompanies an ulnar shaft fracture that is due to a fall (Monteggia fracture).

Since, as noted, skull injury probably represents intentional blows, the enumeration of such injuries may indicate the peace or otherwise of communities. Although injury in general is often more common in the male both past and present (e.g. Bennike, 1985 in multiperiod Danish skeletons; Wells, 1982 in a Romano-British cemetery; Jurmain and Bellifemine, 1997 in a central Californian skeletal sample; Stodder, 1994 in New Mexico pueblo populations), the sex difference in skull injury is perhaps the most striking (e.g. see Walker, 1989 and summary in Jurmain, 1999). Assessing sex differences in the study of injury may provide insights into social organization, occupational roles and of course interpersonal and intergroup violence. Generally speaking, males, both today and in the past, often performed heavy manual work and composed a society's fighting forces. Therefore their risk of injury may have been greater, although this assumption can never be certain.

Injuries to the skull are often seen in past populations. Usually they are the result of hand-to-hand fighting with the opponents facing each other, resulting in injuries to the frontal and parietal bones. Many cranial injuries are found on the left side of the skull, and a blow from a right-handed aggressor engaged in face-to-face and hand-to-hand combat would indeed result in a left-sided head injury. Only occasionally are blows delivered from behind, and, accepting that 90 per cent of the world's population is right-handed (Coren and Porac, 1977 in Ruff, 2000), an occipital bone injury, at the back of the head on the right side, would be expected in this scenario. The skeletal material from the Battle of Wisby showed frequent occipital wounds, suggesting that blows were delivered to a fleeing enemy (Courville, 1965) or that people were struck while lying face down on the ground. Wounds of the facial skeleton are infrequent, suggesting that blows to the skull, which are observed in past groups, were purposefully delivered to the cranium to produce maximum damage; it may be, however, that the facial bones, being commonly damaged during burial, do not survive well or often enough to identify injury to this part of the body. Nasal injuries are sometimes seen and these, no doubt, are due to fist-fighting, an age-old and continuing method of solving minor disputes. For example Walker (1997) found a 7 per cent rate (106 of 1,506 individuals) of nasal fractures in populations from the United States, Europe and Asia. He also found nasal fractures to be more common than other cranial injuries. It has also been demonstrated from the Battle of Wisby skeletons (Courville, 1965) that the majority of cutting wounds were the result of obliquely directed downward blows. Less frequent is the vertically directed blow and, even more rare is the horizontal blow. This merely reflects the ease with which a heavy sword or axe is wielded. As would be expected with fatal wounds sustained in combat, many cranial injuries consist of a single cut. In those skulls possessing several cuts, the direction of the blows is often variable, but work using scanning electron microscopy on skull wounds has been able to suggest the order and direction of injury in individuals from an early Medieval cemetery from Kent, England (Wenham, 1987).

The type of skull fracture produced will be dependent on the direction, force and time taken to produce it, the area of skull involved, and the size, shape and velocity of the weapon used to produce it (if a weapon is involved) (Gurdjian *et al.*, 1950; Polson *et al.*, 1985; Leestma and Kirkpatrick, 1988; Merbs, 1989a). In addition, the individual characteristics of the skull, hair and scalp can ultimately affect the resulting fracture pattern (Gordon *et al.*, 1988). Whether the person was moving or stationary, on horseback or on foot, or wearing protective armour (Boylston, 2000) are other factors to consider in the interpretation of head injuries, but these are often forgotten in archaeological contexts (Polson *et al.*, 1985; Leestma and Kirkpatrick, 1988; Merbs, 1989a). Each fracture may be caused by direct (e.g. a blow to the back of the head) or indirect (e.g. jumping from a height, leading to skull fracture) trauma; Lovell (1997: 149) notes that the most common fractures to the skull are from direct low-velocity injuries which are usually linear or depressed (blunt trauma) or penetrating (such as from a projectile). In blunt trauma the skull vault curve flattens and the force is distributed over a large area; the area around the impact bends outwards and the centre is depressed inwards. In some cases associated fracture lines develop, usually in the weakest areas of the skull. The position of the fracture lines may indicate the impact point; star-shaped fracture lines occur at the point of impact, while radiating lines run away from it (Lovell, 1997: 154). The penetrating

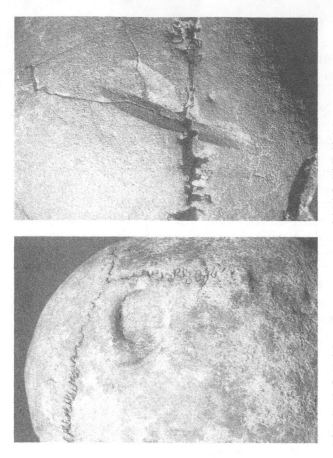

Fig. 5.16. Unhealed peri-mortem blade wound to the skull (late Iron Age/early Roman, first century BC–first century AD, Beckford, Hereford and Worcester, England).

Fig. 5.17. Healed depressed fracture to the parietal bone (late Medieval, twelfth–sixteenth centuries AD, St Oswald's Priory, Gloucester, Gloucestershire, England).

injury has a much higher velocity and the entry wound is small, circular and discrete, with inner table bevelling (the skull has an inner layer (table) and an outer layer and in between is the diploic space). The exit wound, however, is larger and irregular, and may have comminution and loss of some bone fragments, with outer table bevelling (Aufderheide and Rodríguez-Martín, 1998: 28). Forensic experiments conducted on cadaveric material have produced useful data on the type of cranial fracture pattern produced when forces are applied from different directions (Gurdjian *et al.*, 1950); this work is important for archaeological applications.

Three types of head injury may be seen archaeologically: the **sharp**, **blunt** and **projectile**. Sharp injuries are usually the result of an edged weapon (Fig. 5.16), while the blunt injury, caused by a blunt instrument or a fall, usually results in a depressed fracture (Fig. 5.17). The projectile injury is characterized by the velocity with which the weapon contacts the body (Novak, 2001: 91); in this type there are very obvious entry and exit wounds and extensive fracturing. All these injuries can produce radiating fractures away from the site of impact; this occurs when the impact distorts the bone beyond its maximum elastic properties (Novak, 2001: 91). In addition, a study of the intersection of the fracture lines allows a reconstruction of the sequence of injuries. In head injuries the outer table of the skull is compressed and the inner table is under tension (Berryman and Haun, 1996), although this is reversed for projectile injuries. Bone is nearly twice as strong in compression as it is in tension (Curry, 1970 in Berryman and Haun, 1996), and if force is applied slowly then the bone can withstand a greater load (Evans, 1973 in Berryman and Haun, 1996). The configuration of the cortical and cancellous bone and structural buttressing result in lines of lesser and greater resistance, and fractures will develop along the former.

A blunt force injury can be recognized by concentric radiating fractures on the external surface first (Fig. 5.18), a light blow producing a linear fracture and a higher force resulting in a comminuted injury with radiating fractures in the immediate area of the injury, or on the opposite side of the skull (Boylston, 2000). A very useful classification of blunt force trauma has been highlighted by King (1992), who collated data from a number of authors to show the different types of cranial fracture patterns according to force, velocity and type of weapon used; she subsequently used the data to interpret cranial trauma from a French Roman context.

Projectile injuries are rare in the archaeological record, although examples of such injuries have been noted from as early as prehistoric contexts, and Jurmain (1999: 211–14) summarizes a number of reports. Gunshot wounds, for example, consist of high impact force, with rapid loading applied to a relatively small area (Berryman and Haun, 1996). The entry wound will be bevelled on the internal surface and circular with radiating fractures away from the wound, but the exit wound will often be irregular and bevelled externally. The weapon used to produce the projectile injury may also be interpreted from the injury observed, as we have seen, but only rarely is the weapon found *in situ* in the wound. With the weapon in place, it may be possible to surmise the direction of flight, and even associated soft tissue damage and complications (see Polet *et al.*, 1996; Schutkowski *et al.*, 1996).

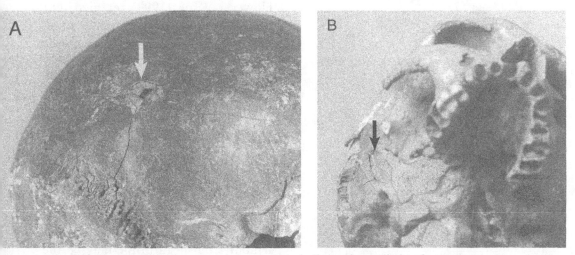

Fig. 5.18. A: unhealed blunt force injury to the skull showing radiating fractures; B: endocranial (internal) aspect of A showing 'flap' of bone. *(Photographs by Jeff Veitch, Department of Archaeology, University of Durham)*

Armed with this knowledge, and with an understanding of anatomy, the soft tissue and skeletal damage can be assessed and the clinical effects of the injury reconstructed. Consider, for example, the Neolithic arrowhead in the anterior aspect of a lumbar vertebra (Wells, 1964a). This weapon, entering the body of the victim from the front, would, on reaching the abdomen, perforate the gut and transfix the aorta, the largest artery of the body, lying immediately in front of the vertebra at this level. The resultant haemorrhage would have been catastrophic, and death would have ensued within minutes.

In contrast is the early Medieval example of an arrowhead which came to rest on the posterior aspect of the third lumbar vertebra (Manchester and Elmhirst, 1980). Clearly, its horizontal position suggests that the arrow was shot at the upright victim, probably from fairly close range to his right (Fig. 5.19). The injury did no more damage than create great pain, some bleeding and, in this instance at least, a minor opening in the spinal canal. This was insignificant, because the victim became subject to a tremendous blow to the right side of the back of the head. Of course, the availability of different materials to produce projectile weapons changed through time from the production of flint arrowheads to the development of metals; this would have affected the type of resulting injury. Therefore, as we move later in time we will see more injuries resulting from metal weapons, and even gunshot wounds. Bennike (1985) reports *in situ* weapons in the pelvis, palate, cervical vertebrae and sternum of skeletons of various dates from the Neolithic (4200–1800 BC) to the Viking Period (AD 800–1050). All the injuries were unhealed and the presence of these weapons suggests they contributed to the death of the individuals concerned. With reference to gunshot wounds, although common in forensic contexts, archaeological examples are rare. However, King (1994) revealed four lead-shot balls with a skull with evidence of fracture from a post-Medieval cemetery at Glasgow Cathedral, Scotland, and Willey and Scott (1996) report six of ten skeletons from the Battle of the Little Bighorn with gunshot wounds to either the cranium or the postcranium. Here, radiographic analysis provided evidence of metal fragments at the site of some of the wounds, and the direction of the shot was also ascertained by the characteristics of the wounds. The Medieval knight encased in metal armour from head to toe may be the classic, or rather popular, soldier of antiquity (e.g. see Gurdjian, 1973 for a

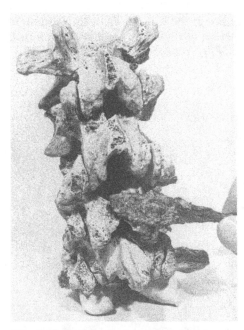

Fig. 5.19. Lumbar spine found with iron arrowhead adjacent to the third lumbar vertebra (early Medieval, sixth–eighth centuries AD, Eccles, Kent, England).

discussion of head protection through time). The rank and file, the ancestors of our armies today, were rather less fortunate. Body and skull protection for these people may have been no more than leather garments, although there are more sophisticated examples. However, even these would have afforded some protection against an aggressive blow. The protection or otherwise of the victim must be borne in mind when examining skeletal remains of victims of suspected interpersonal violence.

The potential resulting brain damage in a head injury, will vary according to the fracture type. Depressed fractures often lead to brain damage, both directly underneath the fracture and at a distance from the site, while a linear, blade injury has potential for causing brain damage directly below the fracture. Of course, brain tissue, in the majority of archaeological contexts, is not preserved, and therefore the extent of brain damage can only be inferred on the basis of the type, pattern and position of the fracture on the skull. Brain damage may include necrosis of some of the tissue; this is due to increased pressure from a collection of blood inside the skull leading to lack of oxygen supplied to the tissue (subdural or extradural haematoma). Infection of the brain is also a potential hazard in cranial trauma, and would have been a problem in antiquity; it is probable that individuals in the past who suffered infection of the brain tissue would have died before bony change had time to develop at the fracture site.

Not only do cranial wounds throw light on the actions of the fighter; they may also give an indication of the type of weapon used. A sharp blade will produce a clean cut, usually with smooth, straight, polished edges, and a blunter type of instrument may cause splintering of the edges of the wound. The battle-hammer or mace tends to produce depressed fractures (Moodie, 1927; Wells, 1964a), and one of the most malicious hand weapons of all times was the Medieval 'morning star' or 'holy water sprinkler'. This flailing weapon consisted of a wooden ball with protruding metal spikes. It is often the case that palaeopathologists try to assess the type of weapon used to make the injury on the skull, and forensic research can help in assessing this aspect of the injury. For example, Andahl (1978) considered the effect of different saws on different materials, including bone. More recent work (Humphrey and Hutchinson, 2001; Tucker et al., 2001) examined the characteristic macroscopic and microscopic effects of machetes, axes and cleavers on fresh pig bone, with different appearances being confirmed. In archaeological contexts there have also been attempts to determine the weapon type that produced the wound. For example, Novak (2001), by comparing injuries observed at the Medieval battlefield site of Towton, Yorkshire, England, with likely weapons for that period, indicates that war hammers, poleaxes, crossbow bolts, blades, arrowheads and swords caused the puncture wounds observed.

Of course, a cranial wound may be healed (Fig. 5.20) or unhealed, the latter suggesting that the wound may have contributed to the cause of death. Skull fractures usually heal with fibrous union, but bony union is also found. Bone formation during the healing process is present but is less important than in fractures of the postcranium (Sevitt, 1981: 231). A detailed study of 135 crania from Civil War victims, curated at the National Museum of Health and Medicine, Armed Forces Institute of Pathology, Washington DC, considered the evidence of

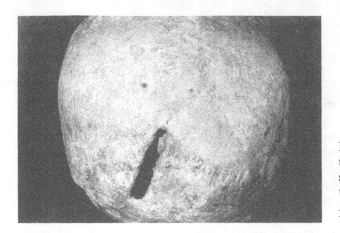

Fig. 5.20. Healed injury to the occipital bone of the skull (late Medieval, twelfth–sixteenth centuries AD, St Helen-on-the-Walls, York, England).

healing of cranial traumatic lesions (Sledzik and Barbian, 1997). These specimens have an associated documented history, so that it is known when the injury occurred and how long it was before the person died. They found that the earliest bone response to cranial fracture was five days, but in most cases no osseous response was evident during the first week following the trauma. By the fourth week all injuries had some osteoblastic response and by the sixth week all had osteoclastic response. The expression of these responses was similar on both the endocranial and the ectocranial surfaces, but, generally speaking, the more severe expression was on the latter. Other features noted were lines of demarcation establishing a boundary between dead and living bone (probably where the periosteum had been torn away from the bone during the injury), and sequestration, or the formation of dead bone. Often one of the most common questions asked of chronic bone lesions in palaeopathology is 'how long did the person have the disease or trauma before they died, and how long had the lesions been forming?' Unfortunately, it is usually impossible to say, although studies such as these may help in archaeological contexts to add a time dimension to suffering, bearing in mind that many factors can affect healing rates. Healing, identified as rounding of the wound edges, indicates survival of the person following the injury, but little can be said of what complications were present. Distinguishing recent ante-mortem or peri-mortem unhealed injury from post-mortem breaks may also be difficult, requiring detailed observation (see Figs 5.21 and 5.22 as a comparison). Lovell (1997: 145) provides a useful summary of how to distinguish between ante-mortem and peri-mortem injuries or breaks, illustrated in Table 5.5 (peri-mortem is defined as around the time of death or the recent ante-mortem period – or up to three weeks after the injury or before death).

It is worth noting features described by other researchers with reference to the distinction between peri-mortem and post-mortem fractures. Hutchinson (1996) notes that fractures occurring in fresh bone are usually uniform in their cortical and non-cortical coloration and the edges of the wounds have acute or obtuse angles, while dry bone fractures are usually perpendicular to the long axis of the bone and have irregular surfaces, because the collagen has disappeared from the bone, leading to it being more brittle and shattering on impact (Kaufman *et al.*, 1997). Ubelaker and

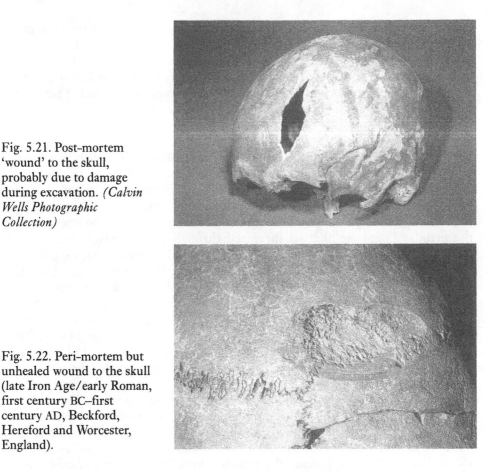

Fig. 5.21. Post-mortem 'wound' to the skull, probably due to damage during excavation. *(Calvin Wells Photographic Collection)*

Fig. 5.22. Peri-mortem but unhealed wound to the skull (late Iron Age/early Roman, first century BC–first century AD, Beckford, Hereford and Worcester, England).

Table 5.5 Differences between ante-mortem, peri-mortem and post-mortem trauma

Ante-mortem/peri-mortem	*Post-mortem*
Any evidence of healing/inflammation	Smaller fragments
Uniform presence of water/soil stains or vegetation on broken/adjacent surfaces	Non-uniform coloration of fractured ends and adjacent bone surface
Presence of greenstick/spiral/depressed/compressed fractures	Squared fracture edges
Oblique angles on fractured ends	Absence of fracture patterning (dry brittle bone shatters on impact)
A pattern of concentric circular, radiating or stellate lines	

Source: Lovell (1997: 145).

Adams (1995) and Quatrehomme and Iscan (1997) emphasize that the ends of the bones fractured have a lighter colour if there is a post-mortem break, and Kaufmann *et al.* indicate that, if there is evidence of healing of a fracture to the skull, then the evidence would be seen by just over one week following the fracture (although within forty-eight hours there will be proliferation of the osteogenic layer of the periosteum microscopically (Ham and Harris, 1956 in Kaufmann *et al.*, 1997)).

Specific studies of cranial trauma reveal interesting information both temporally and geographically. Walker (1989), studying 774 crania from the North Channel Islands in southern California, identified 144 individuals (19.3 per cent) with one or more fractures to the cranium; they were commonly seen on the left side of the head and on the frontal and parietal bones. Males were more affected than females (12:5), with the differences being highly significant. More injuries were seen on the island groups (perhaps because of competition for scarce resources) than on the mainland, and frequencies increased through time (possibly the result of increased population density). Both accidental and interpersonal injuries were identified. Injury was rarely seen on the occipital bone, suggesting that interpersonal injuries were sustained by 'frontal' combat, not during flight.

Three sites in Britain with particularly high prevalence rates of unhealed cranial blade injuries come from Eccles, Kent (Manchester and Elmhirst, 1980), Fishergate, York (Stroud and Kemp, 1993), and Towton, Yorkshire (Novak, 2001). Eccles, dated to the sixth to eighth centuries AD, revealed seven individuals with unhealed blade wounds suggesting interpersonal violence; some of the victims also sustained postcranial injuries. At Fishergate a total of sixteen males had similar injuries, many multiple, with some also having traumatic lesions to the spine and limbs. Most of the injuries occurred on the left side of the body and most were to young individuals. At the Battle of Towton in AD 1461 there were many victims, but only around forty individuals have been found and excavated (Fiorato *et al.*, 2001). Novak (2001) considered the evidence for cranial and postcranial trauma. Thirteen of thirty-nine discrete burials had postcranial trauma, with an average of 2.2 wounds per individual. Most of the trauma occurred in the forearms (both blunt and sharp force trauma), and defence injuries are suggested as the mechanism behind these injuries. There were twenty-eight crania available for examination of trauma and nine (32 per cent) had healed trauma, with twenty-seven having evidence of peri-mortem trauma (4.2 wounds on average per cranium). Some 65 per cent were sharp injuries, 25 per cent blunt and 10 per cent puncture wounds. Most of the sharp and blunt injuries were interpreted as being the result of blows from the front in face-to-face combat. The twelve puncture wounds in eight people were mostly square-shaped (three sharp, two projectile and seven blunt), and arrowheads, poleaxe top-spikes, war-hammers and crossbow bolts were suggested as weapons that could have produced the injuries.

DECAPITATION AND SCALPING

Another type of sharp force injury may be the result of decapitation; evidence may be identified either from cut marks on the cervical vertebrae or from the context of deposition of the body, although the former is safer. The latter may involve a buried body whose skull is placed elsewhere in the grave. We assume that in the past most evidence for decapitation was deliberate and the result of corporal punishment by another person, although self-decapitation has been noted in a modern context (Prichard, 1993). A number of other reasons for decapitation have been suggested; these include interpersonal aggression with trauma to the neck region leading to decapitation, mismanaged hanging, as a means to trophy collection, a form of bloodletting and as a means for reliquary collection (Boylston *et al.*, 2000). Two examples of decapitation serve to illustrate the evidence. At Cirencester, a Romano-British cemetery in Gloucestershire, England (Wells, 1982), six individuals had been decapitated through their cervical vertebrae; the crania were excavated in the correct anatomical position and, as suggested, this may represent partial maintenance of the soft tissues around the neck, following severance of the head. At Kempston, Bedfordshire, also in England, Boylston *et al.* (2000) found that twelve of the ninety-two third- and fourth-centuries AD Romano-British burials had been decapitated. Four were definitely female and five were definitely male, with one being a child (rare). In all cases the skull had been placed near the tibiae or feet in the grave, and eight had been buried in the main cemetery (with four being placed in a ditched enclosure and classed as 'special'). Five of the twelve were buried in coffins and five had evidence of cut marks on their cervical vertebrae. It was hypothesized that the decapitations were performed on incapacitated individuals or on already dead individuals and that some may have been casualties of armed conflict (Boylston *et al.*, 2000: 250)

The culturally induced practice of scalping, resulting in cut marks to the head, is defined as 'the forcible removal of all or part of the scalp' (Owsley, 1994: 335). A sharp implement was used on living (but mostly dead or dying) people, leaving short, straight or slightly curved cut marks on the frontal and parietal bones of the skull. In some cases fragments of the implement used for scalping have been found in the resulting wound (Olsen and Shipman, 1994). During scalping, the periosteum and covering skin were removed from the skull, usually across the forehead, thus depriving the skull of its periosteal blood supply. This resulted in death of the bone of the skull's outer table. If the person survived the process, which has been noted, inflammatory granulation tissue develops in the diploic space and the dead bone becomes separated from the living tissue by it (Smith, 2003: 308). These changes were seen in three individuals from Late Mississippian sites in the south-eastern United States (Smith, 2003). New bone formation eventually occurs if the person survives and the healed surface appears depressed, smooth and variable in thickness (Ortner, 2003). Another feature that has been identified is a groove around the circumference of the cranium which indicates the area of skin and scalp incision (Hamperl, 1967: 632). As Bueschgen and Case (1996) point out, the changes seen on the skull will vary according to whether the whole or part of the scalp is removed, and whether it is removed in bits or in one piece.

Events that may have led to scalping include violent interpersonal aggression, the collection of human trophies, intragroup sacrifice, medical treatment of a head wound, primitive autopsy, the removal of the scalp as a keepsake before burial (Bueschgen and Case, 1996) and even an accidental encounter with a wild animal, identified because of the irregular margins of the area involved (Ortner and Ribas, 1997). The practice was first described by the Greek writer Herodotus in the fifth century BC, but it has been seen worldwide in both prehistoric and historic periods. Bueschgen and Case (1996) indicate that the earliest evidence for scalping in North America dates from 5000–1500 years BP, and the majority of the evidence comes from the North Plains of the mid-west, where tribal warfare is evident; men, women and children were all affected. The Old World has also produced evidence for scalping, summarized in Murphy *et al.* (2002), with the earliest cases coming from Neolithic Denmark (4500 BC).

'DOMESTIC' VIOLENCE: INFANTICIDE, CHILD ABUSE, DEFLESHING AND CANNIBALISM

The presence of cut marks elsewhere on the skeleton may represent other cultural practices, such as infanticide, child abuse, cannibalism and defleshing. Distinguishing ante-mortem and peri-mortem from post-mortem cut marks in all these possible scenarios is important. **Infanticide** can be defined as the practice of killing unwanted infants (Elmahi, 2000), and today is undertaken usually before the infant has the status of a real person (Scrimshaw, 1984). Infanticide in the past could have occurred because the child could not be provided for; it was also done to contribute to birth spacing. It was undertaken preferentially on females because males were preferred (males being more valuable and strong), or it may have been practised on deformed or diseased children. As Elmahi (2000) notes, contemporary hunter-gatherer and pastoral groups still practise infanticide, although accurate data on the number of victims are virtually non-existent. Scrimshaw (1984) has identified two main methods of disposing of infants, deliberate infanticide and passive infanticide. The latter may involve placing an infant in a dangerous situation, severely burning or battering a child so that it eventually dies, and decreasing emotional and biological support in the form of food and drink. Archaeologically speaking, infanticide has not been identified very often on the basis of the interpretation of skeletal remains. However, it has been suggested following the analysis of the age at death distribution for perinatal individuals and their burial context (Smith and Kahila, 1992; Mays, 1993). The remains of the 1–2-day-old infants from Ashkelon, Israel, found beneath the fourth century AD Roman bathhouse in a sewer (Smith and Kahila, 1992) have also been subject to ancient DNA analysis to identify the sex distribution of the victims. Faerman *et al.* (1997) obtained nineteen successful results from the forty-three individuals analysed and fourteen of them were male at this site, while Mays and Faerman (2001) analysed thirty-one individuals from Romano-British burial sites in England and found that, of the thirteen successful analyses, nine were males and four were females. It is likely that it will be a long time before it will be possible systematically to explore whether males or females were preferentially selected for infanticide in various societies in the past using ancient DNA analysis. This is mainly because of the problems of survival of ancient DNA in many environmental conditions, and the cost of analysis.

The identification of **child abuse** in the archaeological record on the basis of injury to the skeleton is another area of investigation that is seeing some interest. Clinical data tell us that today an abused child is usually less than 3 years old, with an average age of 18 months (Walker *et al.*, 1997). The pattern of injuries could include fractures to the long bones (metaphyseal, and spiral due to twisting forces), rib fractures (bilateral and close to the spine, and caused by grasping the child's chest), skull fractures and widened sutures as a result of subdural haematomas causing pressure inside the skull, and subperiosteal haematomas (and new bone formation) as a result of ripping of the periosteum from the bone if a child is grabbed forcibly and/or swung around (this may also be a result of hitting the child). Burns, scars, lacerations and a failure to thrive and grow normally are also features that may be observed in the living child, but the key feature to the recognition of child abuse is the occurrence of injuries in several locations in different stages of healing, which indicates repeated episodes of abuse (Walker, *et al.*, 1997). They also suggest that Harris lines of arrested growth, dental defects and shorter than normal long bones for the age of the child may also be indicators of child abuse in both the present and the past. Related to child abuse is the evidence of the abuse of women in the past. While little research has been undertaken in this area, the reader is referred to Martin (1997) and Wilkinson (1997), where violence against women in prehistory in North America is considered, while Walker (1997) takes a wider view.

Defleshing of soft tissue from the skeleton may also leave marks on the bone, and distinguishing between scalping and defleshing may be undertaken by examining the distribution of cut marks. Cut marks located on the skull can usually be attributed solely to scalping (e.g. see Williamson *et al.*, 2003), while cut marks located more widely over the body could be due to defleshing, the latter indicated by cut marks around the joint surfaces, indicating disarticulation. A complicating factor may be post-mortem erosion of areas of the skeleton with cut marks before and after defleshing which may indicate that the body had been exposed prior to mutilation (Olsen and Shipman, 1994).

Cannibalism as a cultural practice also has to be differentiated from defleshing as part of secondary burial. Most evidence comes from the American south-west and especially the late prehistoric Anasazi (see the special issue of *Int. J. Osteoarchaeology* 10(1) for 2000). The sites concerned date from AD 900–1650, and a small proportion of the burials are multiple interments with many disarticulated and broken skeletal elements (Larsen, 1997), but representing males, females and juveniles. Turner (1993) provides useful criteria for identifying cannibalism in the archaeological record, based on an assemblage of eight Anasazi individuals from Chaco Canyon, New Mexico. Peri-mortem cranial and postcranial bone breaks, cut marks, anvil-hammerstone abrasions, burning, bone fragment end polishing and missing vertebrae were suggested as evidence of cannibalism. White (1992) also provides detailed data on the Mancos Canyon skeletal remains where human-induced toolmarks (indicating defleshing, percussion, chopping and disarticulation) and thermal modification were identified on bone. Long bones were also extensively longitudinally fractured with patterns of fractures similar to those seen in animal bones where defleshing, disarticulation and marrow extraction had been undertaken. Other data from elsewhere in the world include those reported from Fiji (50 BC–AD 1900) (DeGusta 1999, 2000), and Europe (e.g. Cook, 1986; Villa *et al.*, 1986; Boulestin and Gomez de Soto, 1995, Fernando-Jalvo *et al.*, 1999).

TRAUMA AND CAUSE OF DEATH

Usually it is not easy to establish cause of death when faced with the examination of a skeleton from an archaeological site. However, the presence of a weapon *in situ* in a bone (e.g. see Buckley, 2000 on a possible fatal wound by a bone point in a child from the south-east Solomon Islands in the Pacific), an unhealed injury and decapitation will, at least, suggest how the death came about, if not its absolute cause in all cases. Of course, the preservation of a body will allow a more specific attribution of cause of death to be made, purely because of the presence of soft tissues. For example, the evidence from many of the north-western European bodies buried and preserved in anaerobic acidic peat bogs suggested that asphyxia had been the cause of death (Brothwell, 1986). For example, Lindow Man, the Iron Age body discovered in a Cheshire peat bog in England in the 1980s, had a sinew thong around his neck with the knot in the sinew biting deeply into the soft tissues; two of the cervical vertebrae were fractured and the throat had been slit. In skeletonized individuals, strangulation, hanging or severe trauma to the neck, as we have seen, may be revealed in fractures to the hyoid bone, second cervical vertebra or calcified cartilages, all located in the neck region. Although hanging and strangulation are only two causes of death, the preservation and retrieval of the hyoid bone and neck cartilages may aid in reconstructing cause of death for archaeological populations. The context of burial may also help.

Indications of live burial, deduced from the examination of bodies during excavation, have been seen in the Danish 'bog burials' (Glob, 1973). Evidence of cause of death based on skeletal posture has also been revealed in England (Rahtz, 1960; Hawkes and Wells, 1975; Manchester, 1978a; Powlesland, 1980). In the case of live burials, the posture of the skeleton within the grave fossilizes the moment of death, with the individual struggling to free himself or herself from certain asphyxiation. An unusual possible cause of death may be attributed to a skeletonized individual from Israel, where the right calcaneum (heel bone) had an 11.5cm iron nail through its body, which also incorporated traces of wood (Zias and Sekeles, 1985). It was hypothesized that this was evidence for crucifixion; a likely scenario of the use of ropes to suspend the upper body from the horizontal part of the cross, and nailing the feet to the vertical part of the cross was proposed, with asphyxia suggested as the cause of death. Selection of the method of dispatch must surely have been dictated by the cultural attitude of society to pain and death. In the absence of documentation the reasons for judicial executions in antiquity are forever unknown.

DISLOCATION

Another traumatic lesion is that of dislocation, where there is loss of contact between two osseous surfaces which are normally a joint. This can also be associated with a fractured bone – for example, the Monteggia fracture – dislocation where the ulna fractures and the radial head dislocates (Resnick and Goergen, 1995). A dislocation may be total or partial (subluxation) and, in archaeological contexts, is recognizable only if the bones remain unreduced, i.e. out of alignment. This may be why so few dislocations are identified in palaeopathology. Should a joint remain dislocated for long enough, then a new joint surface may develop away from the original joint or adjacent to it. Joint degeneration later in life, and also damage to bones, ligaments, tendons and joint capsules at the time of the dislocation, may also be recognized. The cause of dislocations may be trauma (acquired and most common), but people can also be born with, for example, a dislocated hip (see Chapter 3 and Fig. 3.8). A dislocation may also be a complication of another condition, for example, rheumatoid arthritis of the metacarpophalangeal joints (knuckles) where loss of bone at the joints allows the joints to dislocate partially (Resnick and Niwayama, 1995a). Dislocations generally tend to affect the hip and shoulder joints, but of course potentially any other joint could be affected. Sometimes a joint can 'reduce itself', especially if it is an unstable joint such as the shoulder, where the anatomical structure makes it particularly susceptible to dislocation anyway.

OSTEOCHONDRITIS DISSECANS

Apart from the obvious case of trauma-induced fractures, there is another relatively frequently occurring condition in skeletal material, that of osteochondritis dissecans. It is classified with other, so-called, osteochondroses, such as Scheuermann's disease of the spine, Osgood-Schlatter's disease of the knee and Perthes disease of the hip (Resnick, 1995a). All these conditions involve fragmentation and collapse of part of the joint of the skeleton. They all affect young individuals, especially males in their first decade of life, and are the result of death of bone tissue from significant obliteration of the affected area's blood supply. The knee is affected in 80 per cent of cases, usually with an underlying traumatic aetiology. The necrotic fragment of bone separates and may remain loose in the joint, may become absorbed or may heal back into the defect (Fig. 5.23). There are few specific reports on osteochondritis dissecans in the palaeopathological literature (Wells, 1974a; Loveland *et al.*, 1984). It is important to appreciate that there are also defects in the joints which may be mistakenly attributed to osteochondritis dissecans (Fig. 5.24) and there is a danger of overinflating prevalence rates if these are counted as such. A true osteochondritic lesion consists of a well-defined, porous, often circular, defect, usually lower than the normal joint surface.

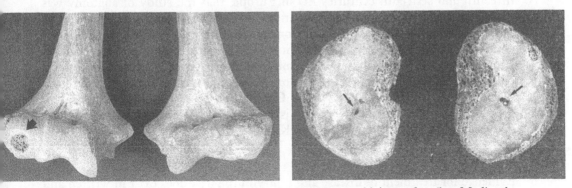

Left: Fig. 5.23. Osteochondritis dissecans in the distal humeral joint surface (late Medieval, twelfth–sixteenth centuries AD, France). *Right:* Fig. 5.24. Joint lesions that may be confused with osteochondritis dissecans (proximal articular surfaces of the first metatarsals).

TREATMENT OF TRAUMA

Trauma is painful, visible and debilitating; today people afflicted with trauma try to seek help and have their injuries treated. Fractures, like childbirth, have faced all societies in the past and may have presented problems. However, the treatment of a broken leg with a simple fracture by reducing and splinting just needs a little common sense. The evidence for the treatment of trauma is plentiful in historical data but direct evidence on the skeleton is more rare. The availability of such treatment, however, for all people of whatever status, age or sex is generally unknown, although in Britain today island populations may have poorer access to health care (Gould and Moon, 2000). While the more obvious treatments of trauma such as splinting of fractures, trepanation for head injuries, or amputation of traumatized limbs may be seen in skeletal remains, the complementary medical treatments so commonly resorted to today (e.g. maggot therapy for wound infection (Bonn, 2000)) and drug therapy may only be seen in historical written and illustrated data (e.g. see Rawcliffe, 1997 on late Medieval English medicine). Nevertheless, some archaeological sites have produced indicative evidence of, for example, various medicines (e.g. Ilani *et al.*, 1999; Ciaraldi, 2000).

To be able to treat trauma and disease today needs some knowledge of the anatomy and physiology of the human body; this knowledge was not always evident in past communities and was often based on dissection of animals. Likewise, today, many developing societies often rely on applying knowledge of animal anatomy to human problems (Lucier *et al.*, 1971). In fact, over much of the past, dissection of the human body was not allowed (for example, the Church in Europe banned dissection for a long period of time). The discovery of the shape, structure and physiology of the brain took some time to master and was rather neglected until Vesalius, working in the sixteenth century AD, described its surface anatomy. Aristotle also believed that the brain cooled the heart, the latter being the seat of intelligence (Backay, 1985). However, in some cases very detailed anatomical knowledge allowed the development of what would be recognized today as very successful methods of treatment. However, it was not until the work of artists such as Leonardo Da Vinci, Vesalius and Michelangelo, during the fifteenth and sixteenth centuries AD in Europe, that the study of anatomy was placed on a firm foundation of observations. As dissections and autopsies became more commonplace (with evidence from the skeletal record – e.g. in fifteenth-century France – Valentin and d'Errico, 1995), and illustrated anatomy texts became more freely available and disseminated, there were advances in anatomical research (Schultz, 1985: 23). Furthermore, recognition that anatomy needed to be learned was emphasized by Guy de Chauliac, a fourteenth-century French surgeon, who said, 'the surgeon who is ignorant of anatomy carves the human body as a blind man carves wood' (MacKinney, 1957: 402).

Amputation

Evidence for treatment of disease and injury in the past does exist in written and artistic form (e.g. Porter, 1997), and there are useful comparative data from ethnographic and non-human primate studies of treatment (e.g. Huffman, 1997 on self medication in primates), but the direct evidence consists of amputation, splinting of fractures and trepanation of the skull. Amputation of limbs has been carried out since very early times and for various reasons. Apart from the traumatic amputation of a limb during battle or domestic accident, the deliberate removal of part or the whole of a limb has been carried out as a surgical procedure for the treatment of disease, such as infection, or injury, or for punishment. For example, three probable cases of foot amputation have been documented from Peru, dated to AD 100–750, correlating well with Moche ceramic depictions of people without feet (Verano *et al.*, 2000). A particularly macabre reason for amputation in early Egypt was for ensuring statistical accuracy. Introduced in the XIX Dynasty and certainly pictorially portrayed in the Temple of Rameses III, is the practice of hand amputation of prisoners of war. Apparently this was carried out to assist in the counting of numbers of prisoners (Brothwell and Møller-Christensen, 1963). One of the earliest examples of amputation, dated to the IX Dynasty, but one which has nevertheless been disputed, is the loss of the distal half of the right radius and ulna (Brothwell and Møller-Christensen, 1963). In this case a bridge of bone between the stump ends and obvious healing and remodelling of the ends indicate that the individual survived the surgical operation of amputation.

Evidence for amputation, however, is rare in the archaeological record (Fig. 5.25), probably because unhealed amputated limbs could be mistaken for post-mortem breaks of bones. In both cases, whether amputated or damaged post-mortem, there would be no evidence of healing, i.e. in the former the person died at the time of or very soon after the amputation, probably due to massive uncontrolled haemorrhage. Another differential diagnosis for bones which may appear to have been amputated is a fracture where there has been no attempt (or very little) at healing, i.e. an ununited fracture; if the distal fragment is missing an incorrect diagnosis may be made. However, microscopic examination of the cut surface of the unhealed bone may reveal marks indicative of the instrument used, thus differentiating between post-mortem breakage, an unhealed fracture and an unhealed amputation. Differentiating between peri-mortem and post-mortem cuts has been discussed above and is highly relevant here. Nevertheless, it may be possible to extend the diagnosis of amputations by assessing

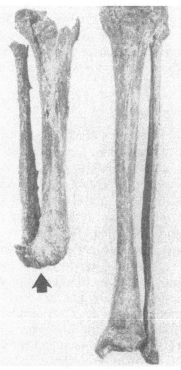

Fig. 5.25. Healed amputation of the tibia and fibula.

the rest of the skeleton and observing abnormal bone change. If a limb has been amputated, a particular scenario could be envisaged. A person will not be able to use the affected limb, with resultant disuse atrophy, i.e. reduction in the size of the limb compared to the opposite, unaffected side, associated with reduction in the prominence of muscle attachments. Lazenby and Pfeiffer (1993) describe overall size, cross-sectional geometry and mid-shaft histological features in an historically identified nineteenth-century below-knee amputee, which supported the scenario described above. Individuals may also have had a false limb and crutches, and although these artefacts are generally lost to the palaeopathologist, they are described and illustrated (e.g. Epstein, 1937). Mays's (1996a) paper very adequately reviews the evidence for amputations in the Old World, detailing a case from the late Medieval English site at Blackfriars Friary, Ipswich. Bloom *et al.* (1995) also describe the first case of an amputation from a site in Israel. The skeleton was that of an adult male, dated to 3,600 years old, and the amputation showed clear evidence of healing. More recently, a rather unique case of amputation of the big toe in an older adult female mummy from the necropolis of Thebes-West, Egypt (tomb dated to *c.* 1550–1300 BC) also revealed replacement of the toe with a wooden prosthesis (Nerlich *et al.*, 2000). Evidence from the New World is not as great, although Ortner (2003) and Aufderheide and Rodríguez-Martín (1998) describe some cases from South America.

The skeletal evidence of amputation is rather scant, but relatively speaking records of trepanation are abundant, albeit geographically biased. When the surgical risks of the two procedures are compared, it is perhaps surprising that, on the evidence available, trepanation appears to have been a more common surgical manoeuvre than amputation. The figures may, however, be clouded by the ease of recognition of trepanation and the likely difficulty of recognition of amputation.

Trepanation

Trepanation is a practice known since very early times, being first recorded by the Greek medical writer Hippocrates in the fifth century BC (Mariani-Costantini *et al.*, 2000); it is also seen in developing countries (Ackerknecht, 1967). The operation involves, for whatever reason, incision of the scalp and the cutting through and removal of an area of skull (Fig. 5.26). The result is the exposure of the membranes (dura) covering the brain. Survival of the patient, for he or she must be regarded as a patient in this surgical operation, probably depended upon the skilful avoidance of perforation of these membranes and the avoidance, either by luck or good judgement, of the major blood vessels within the skull. It should be noted that the proportion of survivors of this operation in antiquity was high (Piggott, 1940). The evidence for survival is, of course, the healing and remodelling of the bone around the operation site. Several examples exist of individuals having undergone more than one trepanning operation, having survived a preceding one. A notable specimen, the Cuzco skull from Peru, shows no fewer than seven trepanned holes, all showing signs of healing (Oakley *et al.*, 1959). Perhaps equally surprising is the size of trepanned areas, particularly where survival has occurred. For example, a Neolithic skull from Latvia

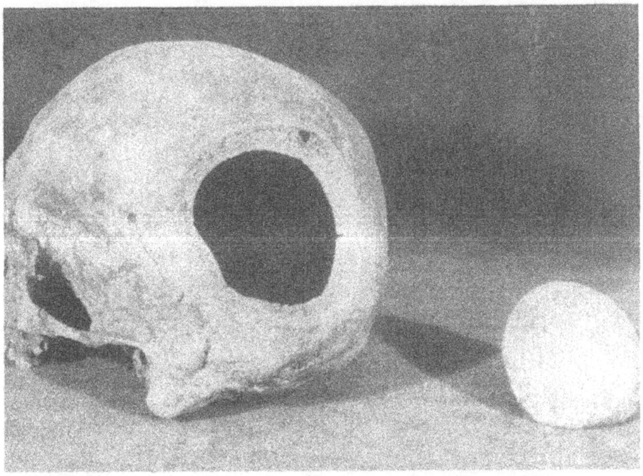

Fig. 5.26. Unhealed trepanation of the left parietal bone (early Bronze Age, 2600–800 BC, Crichel Down, Dorset, England).

possessed three trepanning defects in the skull. The largest single hole measured 68 × 55mm, and all three merged to produce an opening 120 × 60mm in size. This individual survived his horrific surgical trauma and died over a year later, possibly from some other disease unrelated to the trepanation (Derums, 1979).

Ancient examples of trepanation number well into the thousands and their distribution is worldwide (Arnott et al., 2003). Perhaps because of the excellence and extent of archaeological excavation and post-excavation skeletal analysis, Europe affords many of these examples (e.g. Bennike, 1985; Roberts and McKinley, 2003), and Piggott (1940) suggests that central and northern Europe may be the original home of trepanation. The Americas (Stone and Miles, 1990; Richards, 1995), Australia (Webb, 1988), Asia, Africa and Melanesia have also produced examples, and Aufderheide and Rodríguez-Martín (1998) detail the evidence worldwide. A late Palaeolithic origin has been claimed and certainly in the Neolithic period it was an active practice. Although flourishing in the Neolithic period in Europe, perhaps more than at any other time, the operation has been performed during all periods since.

The technical object of the operation was clear, but the actual surgical procedure adopted was variable. Dependent upon the era and the technologies available, the operation may have been carried out with a flint scraper or blade, or a metal implement which may or may not have been adapted specifically for the purpose. Recent work has provided evidence for the type of instrument used in one case. Stevens and Wakeley (1993) used scanning electron microscopy to examine a trepanation and, by experimental analogy, suggested that the tool used had been a shell. Initial incision of the scalp is a very bloody procedure, but the haemorrhage can be minimized by turning back the scalp flaps created; no doubt this was realized and carried out by early surgeons.

After cutting the soft tissues, the outer skull surface was exposed. At this point the type of trepanation varied. Five types of trepanation have been identified from skeletal material worldwide. The scraped type involved the bone surface being removed and bevelled edges to the wound were created towards the central hole in the skull. The gouge method removed a larger piece of skull by delineating a circular area on the skull and gouging the area with an implement. The bore and saw method usually involved the use of a drill-type implement in which a series of holes were made in a circle between which saw marks were subsequently made. The saw method consisted of the creation of four saw marks in a square to enable a piece of bone to be removed from the skull. The final method involved the creation of a small hole with a drill (which should strictly be called a trephination or a hole made by a trephine).

These types of trepanation appear in differing frequencies in different parts of the world and in different eras. For example, the scraping method appears more frequently in Europe and Britain especially (Roberts and McKinley, 2003), and the sawing method in South America. Studies of the site of trepanation indicate that many were performed on the left side of the frontal and parietal bones; rarely were these operations performed over the skull sutures. Hippocrates (and many other authors) recommended not to trepan over the sutures for fear of lacerating a major vein (Lisowski, 1967). One can imagine the agony suffered by the patient in antiquity. Such agony may not have been physical, since after cutting the soft tissues the operation is relatively painless, particularly if pain relief is assisted by alcohol or by herbal preparations; drugs such as opium, henbane and mandrake have all been quoted as substances used for inducing anaesthesia and analgesia in particular population groups.

During all of these processes the bone dust created may have been collected. In more recent periods human skull dust has been used among developing societies as a magical remedy (Janssens, 1970); it is known that trepanation was also undertaken to produce amulets. Whatever method was employed by whichever society, the end result was the removal of a piece of skull and the exposure of the membranes covering the brain. The post-operative care of this bloody and potentially infected area of operation is equally impressive, particularly in view of the survival of many victims. A study by Stewart (1958) found that over 50 per cent of 214 skulls with trepanation from Peru had healed. In Britain it is apparent that the scraping method was accompanied by better survival than the other methods (Roberts and McKinley, 2003). Perhaps the gradual scraping of the skull allowed more precise and controlled penetration of the inner table of bone and hence less likelihood of brain injury. Osteitis and bone scarring surrounding the hole in the skull has been attributed to chemical irritants applied post-operatively. These features are, however, more likely to be due to sepsis of the wound (Stewart, 1958). Doubtless some closure of the skin wound must have been made, either by drawing together the skin flaps or by the application of a pad, possibly of vegetation. It was noted, for instance, in historic times in Melanesia that the operation site was covered with materials such as wood bark, banana leaf and coconut shell.

The technique of operation is plain to see. The motive for the operation is not known for certain in most cases (see Roberts and McKinley, 2003; but see Fig. 5.27), and most likely lies in the culture of the societies who practised it. The popular and somewhat romantic notion that trepanation was carried out solely for magico-ritual reasons is hardly credible. Such a reason there may have been for carrying out the operation on a corpse, and this undoubtedly did occur. In these cases no healing would be expected and post-mortem damage could be implicated for the lesion, although the discussion about differentiating peri-mortem from post-mortem wounds (above) is relevant here. The absence of documentation from the long periods of prehistory permits only speculation. It is difficult to imagine living people submitting themselves willingly to such an horrific operation with a high mortality merely for ritual reasons, although they may have had no choice. And yet, as Oakley *et al.* remarked (1959), so many trepanned skulls have been found in the chambered tombs of the Seine–Oise–Marne area of France that it is probable that the operation had some ritual significance; roundels of human skull bone have also been found in early prehistoric graves, suggesting that such objects were treated as fetishes by prehistoric people.

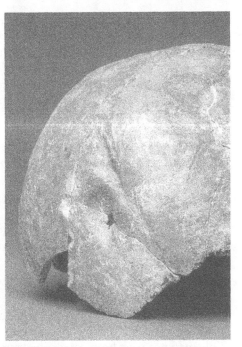

Fig. 5.27. Healed (scraped) trepanation and skull injury (early Medieval, fifth–seventh centuries AD, Broughton Lodge, Willoughby-on-the-Wolds, Nottinghamshire, England).

To the contemporary mind, however, the bizarre behaviour of the schizophrenic, the strange uncontrollable fits of the epileptic, and the incapacitating head pain of migraine may have seemed sufficient justification to 'let the evil spirit out of the brain'. These illnesses are without skeletal manifestation and must, therefore, remain speculative. Nevertheless, recent research has documented the funerary context of trepanned individuals from British burials to explore whether these people were buried in different ways from the normal rite for the period and geographic location (Roberts and McKinley, 2003). The hypothesis was that people who had been trepanned might have been regarded as being different in some way (for example, they may have had some mental impairment). However, there was no evidence that this was the case from this study. There is clear documentary evidence, at least from Hippocratic times, that the operation was also carried out for justifiable clinical reasons, even by modern standards. Hippocrates recommended trepanation for wounds of the head and the release of haematomas. Celsus also proposed the operation for cranial injuries (Lisowski, 1967). It has been noted in some examples that trepanation may be related to the site of cranial fracture (Haneveld and Perizonius, 1980; Wells, 1982; Parker *et al.*, 1986), and some evidence suggests infection of the sinuses may have initiated trepanation (Zias and Pomeranz, 1992); here a skull with two healed and one unhealed trepanations also had frontal sinusitis and intracranial infection. More recent cases from the literature suggest other reasons for trepanation. Mogle and Zias (1995) report a possible case of scurvy in an 8–9-year-old Middle Bronze Age (*c.* 2200 BC) child from Israel with an unhealed trepanation, while Smrčka *et al.* (2003) describe a late Medieval (AD 1298–1550) male skull from the Czech Republic with a trepanation probably undertaken to treat a meningioma (tumour) which probably led to increased intracranial pressure.

Whatever the ailment being treated in the past, it is certainly clear that the association of increased intracranial pressure and head wounds was recognized. There are several other lesions of the skull that may be considered in a differential diagnosis for trepanation; thinning of the parietal bones resulting in a hole (usually in old age), tumours producing holes in the tables of the skull, enlarged parietal foramina and post-mortem damage (Steinbock, 1976; Kaufman *et al.*, 1997). However, with the advent of the use of sophisticated methods of analysis such as the scanning electron microscope, these differential diagnoses should be easily eliminated.

Treatment of fractures

Satisfactory healing of fractures in adults is a long process taking perhaps many weeks or months, during which time total rest of the injured part is essential. This may not have been too difficult to do in the case of an upper limb fracture in the past, when the afflicted individual would have been able to perform some tasks with the opposite limb. It would have been much more difficult in the case of a person from a small community who fractured a lower limb bone. There must have been little room for 'passengers' in the work-centred groups of the past, particularly in hunter-gatherer populations. In such cases the injured, if he or she survived, would have been dependent for welfare upon kinspeople. And what reorganization of lifestyle of the group would be required if the injured person was a member of a nomadic group, for surely he or she would be totally incapacitated for perhaps three months with a badly fractured femur? Bone fractures healing in a position of poor alignment are a common finding in skeletal remains from the past. The large bones such as the femur, which is surrounded by powerful muscles which will contract strongly around the site of fracture, and the tibia and fibula are the most common sites for this malalignment. Satisfactory bone healing in a position of good alignment is even less likely in the case of the comminuted fracture. Add to the intense pain of the leg fracture the long period of total immobility and dependence upon others and the subsequent crippling because of a grossly shortened leg, and it may be possible to gain an insight into the sufferings of the injured victim of antiquity. This is not to say that all fractures of the past had such appalling results.

The successful treatment of fractures is suggested in both art and written records contemporary with many historically documented populations worldwide. This is in contradiction to the statement by Wells (1974b: 220) that 'with very few exceptions they [Anglo-Saxons] made virtually no difference to what the natural healing powers of the body would have achieved unaided'. The study of developing societies also supports the fact, already discussed, that treatment of fractures by reduction and splinting is a very simple and logical process to learn. Reduction by manipulation, or sometimes traction, and splinting of broken bones with natural products such as bark, reeds (Huber and Anderson, 1995) (Fig. 5.28), bamboo (Carroll, 1972), animal skins (Fortuine, 1984) and clay are observed in some societies, suggesting that at least some thought is being channelled into caring for the injured. Herbal concoctions and bandages, and the use of animal hair and plant fibres, comprise methods of treatment of associated wounds. The Yoruba of Nigeria (Oyebola, 1980) were conversant at that time with the clinical features of fractures (pain, swelling, deformity and loss of function) but, having no radiography facility, they missed the diagnosis of hairline greenstick fractures, identifying only the major breaks. Herbal dressings and splints were applied and reapplied daily following hot fomentations. The results varied but observations suggest that patients were mobilized too early, reduction was not maintained consistently and that this delayed healing.

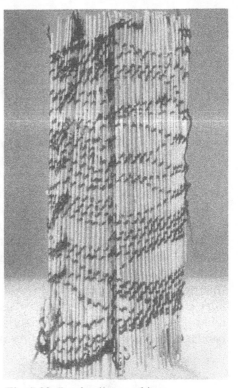

Fig. 5.28. Reed splint used in some developing countries to stabilise fractures once reduced. *(With permission of the Science Museum, Science and Society Picture Library)*

However, despite these shortcomings, it is clear that relatively effective treatment was practised in this and other developing societies and there is no reason to suggest that this was not the case in past communities.

Hippocrates (fifth century BC) had an intimate knowledge of the bones and joints, and described several methods of treatment of dislocations and fractures, some of which are still used today. Reduction and splinting of fractures, and maintaining the fracture in reduction, with pads and bandages reinforced by clays and starches, including the adjacent joints, and using the other elements of the limb anatomically to splint the broken bone, e.g. radius/ulna and tibia/fibula, were all recommended as methods of treatment for fractures by Hippocrates. He also suggested consuming a healthy diet. During later eras in Europe similar fracture treatment methods were advocated by surgeons such as Guy De Chauliac (1300–70, France), who was the first to reduce fractures by traction (Clark, 1937: 53), Ambroise Paré (1510–90, France) and Hieronymus Brunschwig (1450–1533, Germany).

In addition to surgeons, who would inevitably have become involved with the treatment of fractures, bonesetters were a group of people who developed specifically for this purpose; they appear to have been present in many countries around the world, particularly in the sixteenth and seventeenth centuries AD, and still are today (e.g. see Huber and Anderson, 1995). The 'natural' bonesetter was the forerunner of the orthopaedic surgeon. He or she met the needs of the majority of the population when they had an illness involving bone, joint or muscle. The bonesetting skill was believed to descend in families. Herbal remedies such as comfrey ('knitbone') and 'bonewort' (violet/pansy) mixed with egg white were also recommended for fractured bones (Bonser, 1963) in early Medieval England, but the treatment of wounds associated with fractures varied from the relatively sensible (wine, honey) to the need to make the wound septic (the 'laudable pus' of Galen; Knight, 1981). Stitching wounds was also practised, the earliest evidence dating to 1100 BC in an Egyptian mummy (Black, 1982: 620), and linen, catgut, silk, wool and metal clips were used, in addition to the less conventional wound treatment in the form of cautery (application of hot irons).

Splints made from natural products, such as those identified in developing societies, were probably used for fracture treatment but rarely are they preserved in the archaeological record attached to fractured bones. Interestingly, most fractures found archaeologically are healed, which would preclude the need to bury a body with splints. However, some direct examples of splinting have been identified. Elliot-Smith (1908) described splints of bark held in place with linen bandages on broken, unhealed limbs of mummies from Egypt dated to 5000 BC

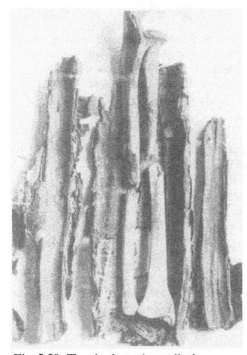

(Fig. 5.29). Although there is evidence in Egypt for limbs being broken post-mortem during the embalming process and splints being attached, it is known from documentary evidence that splinting as a form of treatment for fractures was practised at that time. Nevertheless, assessing the state of healing of fractures, including their alignment and presence of complications, does go some way to suggesting whether people's fractures were treated in the past without the presence of a splint (e.g. see Grauer and Roberts, 1996; Neri and Lancellotti, 2004).

Other direct evidence for treatment comes from the humeri and a knee joint of four skeletons from different sites and periods in Europe. Copper plates were found around the humerus of a skeleton of late sixteenth- or early seventeenth-century date in Belgium, but with no evidence of disease underneath the plates (Janssens, 1987).

Fig. 5.29. Tree bark used as splinting material on a mummified arm in Egypt 5,000 years ago.

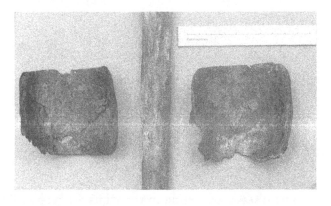

Fig. 5.30. Copper plates
(lined with ivy leaves) applied
to a humerus with non-
specific infective changes
(early Medieval,
fifth–seventh centuries AD,
Jack-of-both-Sides, Reading,
Berkshire, England).
*(Photograph and permission
from Reading Museum)*

Copper plates lined with ivy leaves were also found around the humerus of an early Medieval skeleton from Reading in Berkshire, England (Wells, 1964b) (Fig. 5.30). The final case, also of copper plates on a humerus, is that of a late Medieval Swedish skeleton (Hällback, 1976). The latter two cases had evidence of ante-mortem disease/trauma. The infected knee of an individual from the late Medieval cemetery of Fishergate, York, England (Knüsel *et al.*, 1995), also appeared to have had copper plates applied to it. All these cases indicate that copper was probably known to have a therapeutic effect.

Any assessment of whether a society treated fractures or not in the past should be undertaken using multidisciplinary forms of evidence (Roberts, 1988a, 1989, 1991), and data should be compared with modern clinical data on success of healing of fractures treated by simple external reduction and splinting. The study of skeletal remains from archaeological sites provides a large data set for considering trauma and its implications for lifestyle in the past, as shown in this chapter. Like trauma, the joint diseases were also common in the past and will be covered in the next chapter.

CHAPTER 6

Joint Disease

> The diseases occurring in the joints are responsible for a great deal of pain and disability and are an increasing burden for modern ageing populations. The potential hardships caused by joint diseases make them a very important part of palaeopathological studies. (Rogers, 2000: 163)

INTRODUCTION

Degenerative diseases are a group of separate and yet in some ways related abnormalities. Gradual deterioration with advancing age is a phenomenon of both animal and plant worlds. In long-lived organisms, there is more time for degenerative disease to appear, advance and become clinically manifest with approaching senility. Degenerative processes affect all the major body systems. The confusion and memory loss of senile dementia due to cerebral degeneration; the dizziness, 'stroke' and coronary thrombosis of arterial degeneration; and the pain, limp and stiffness of degenerative arthritis are examples of age-related degenerative diseases. Joint problems are estimated to represent 20–30 per cent of a doctor's workload (Shipley et al., 2002: 511). It is a phenomenon most obvious in humans possibly because, in contrast to many non-humans, people live longer, especially today. Developments in health care, preventive medicine and health education, in the western world particularly, now allow people to live well into their 70s and 80s, but along with the benefits go risks such as the development of diseases of old age. For example, a study in 1999 of life expectancy in 191 countries found that average life expectancy in the United Kingdom was 71.7 years (Mather et al., 2000); by the year 2021 life expectancy at birth in males is predicted to be 78.8 years and for females 82.9 years (Anon., 2001). That is not to say that non-humans do not suffer from degenerative diseases; many examples of joint disease in other mammals occur in the literature (e.g. Lovell, 1990). Joint disease is a very old problem; it has even been diagnosed in the fossilized spine of a Comanchean dinosaur of 100,000,000 years ago (Karsh and McCarthy, 1960). Degeneration of joints is also observed in earlier humans who may not have lived as long as later groups (Trinkhaus, 1983). However, age is not the only factor in the development of joint disease (see below).

Of the multitude of symptoms and signs due to the degenerative process known in clinical practice today, only the degeneration of bones and joints are obviously recognizable in the skeletal remains of the past. The soft-tissue degenerations may, of course, be found in mummified soft tissues, but evisceration during the mummification technique may also destroy this evidence. Arterial degeneration, however, has been found in Egyptian mummies through microscopical examination of their soft tissues (Ruffer, 1911), and in the Utqiagvik mummies of Barrow, Alaska (Zimmerman and Aufderheide, 1984 in Aufderheide, 2003). This disease, for long assumed to be a problem of our modern lifestyle, has thus been shown to have a history of several thousand years. Whether the inhabitants of that time suffered the same frequency of 'strokes' or coronary thrombosis – the complications of arterial degeneration – is regrettably not known. These problems of such increasing social and economic importance may not be new phenomena at all.

The common diseases of degeneration affecting the skeleton are then the joint diseases. Over the years the literature which contains the terminology used for these diseases has often appeared confusing to both amateur and professional; the simultaneous use of osteoarthrosis, osteoarthritis, degenerative joint disease, arthropathies and rheumatism is seen. Changes occurring in joints of different anatomical and functional type have often all been considered as one, and thus early descriptions of joint disease in skeletal remains were probably imprecise. These different joint diseases, to a large extent, have now been clarified, and, using a clinical base, their characteristics, causes and clinical symptoms have been established; there is, however, still much research to be done.

Along with dental disease and trauma, the joint diseases comprise most of the evidence for disease in past human groups; 1–5 per cent of US citizens under the age of 45 years and 15–85 per cent of those older than 45 years were afflicted in studies in the 1980s, especially with osteoarthritis and rheumatoid arthritis (Cotran *et al.*, 1989: 1346). The joint diseases affect one or more joints of the body, usually in a clearly defined distribution pattern (Fig. 6.1); they may destroy or form bone or promote both. The problem with diagnosing specific joint diseases in palaeopathology is that many of these numerous diseases leave identical marks on the skeleton and some are known to develop subsequent to others – for example, osteoarthritis complicates rheumatoid arthritis; this means that a complete skeleton is a prerequisite to even attempting a

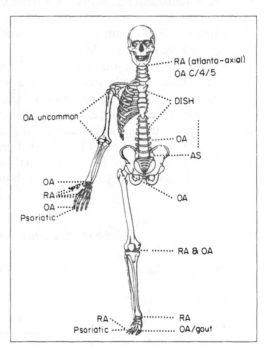

Fig. 6.1. Distribution pattern of some of the joint diseases. *(From Rogers* et al., *1987 and with permission from Juliet Rogers)*
Key
RA   Rheumatoid arthritis
OA   Osteoarthritis
AS   Ankylosing spondylitis
DISH Diffuse idiopathic skeletal hyperostosis

diagnosis of the different joint diseases. Resnick (1995b) provides a useful view on the diagnosis of joint diseases from a clinical standpoint. His 'Target Area Approach' is a good reference point for assessing distribution patterns of joint lesions. However, even with modern technological advances in medicine, diagnosis may not be easy, even in living populations.

JOINT ANATOMY AND PHYSIOLOGY

The joints of the body can be classified by joint movement and by histological features. A synarthrosis is a fixed or rigid joint (e.g. sutures of the skull), an amphiarthrosis is a slightly movable joint (e.g. the pubic symphysis) and the diarthroses are freely movable joints (e.g. the hip). A fibrous joint may be a tooth in its socket, while cartilaginous joints include the intervertebral articulations, and a synovial joint (one whose cavity is lined by synovial membrane, and contains synovial fluid) may be the hip, knee or elbow; this latter type tends to be affected more frequently by the joint diseases. A joint's function depends on the geometry of the bone surfaces which meet each other, its functional integrity in terms of surrounding muscles, tendons and ligaments, the strength, resilience and elasticity of the articular cartilage covering the joint surfaces, and the underlying bone; any changes to these structures may lead to subsequent degeneration. For example, damage to ligaments holding the knee stable may lead to malpositioning of the joint and degeneration.

Cartilage covers the joint surfaces and has a number of functions: transmission and distribution of loads, maintenance of contact between the bones of the joint with little friction, and absorption of shock. The first stages of joint disease usually involve the cartilage; repeated stress leads to breaking up of the cartilage structure by fissuring, flaking and pitting, and loss of cartilage leads to exposure of the bone underneath it. The joint diseases are classified in many different ways, but basically the bone abnormalities observed are proliferative (bone formation), erosive (destruction of bone) or both. Table 6.1 shows one

Table 6.1 Classification of joint diseases

Type of joint disease	Examples to be discussed

Neuromechanical	Osteoarthritis
	    primary (with increasing age)
	    secondary (any age in a previously damaged joint)

Inflammatory*	Septic arthritis
Immune	Rheumatoid arthritis Psoriatic arthritis Ankylosing spondylitis Forestier's disease (DISH)
Metabolic	Gouty arthritis

* May also include gout, rheumatoid arthritis, ankylosing spondylitis and psoriatic arthritis.

classification and includes those joint diseases to be covered in this chapter. The term 'sero negative spondyloarthropathies' can be used to define psoriatic arthritis, ankylosing spondylitis and Reiter's syndrome (not covered here), where there is a tendency for spinal involvement of tendon and ligament insertions and the absence of rheumatoid factor, which is found in the blood of people with rheumatoid arthritis (Rogers *et al.*, 1987).

JOINT DISEASE: PATHOLOGICAL PROCESS

Skeletal involvement in the joint diseases potentially consists of two processes, as we have noted above: formation and destruction of bone. Formation of bone is in the form of bony outgrowths from joint surfaces and their margins, called osteophytes (Fig. 6.2); these represent the body's attempt to spread the load at the joint and compensate for the stress to which the joint is being subject. Osteophytes may occur on the joint surface, marginal to it or away from it, e.g. at insertions of ligaments and tendons (entheses); in addition, new bone may form in the periosteum as a reaction to changes in the joints themselves (Rogers *et al.*, 1987: 180). The extent and character of this new bone formation varies on and around the joint, and this may be characteristic of a particular joint disease.

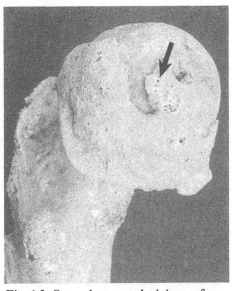

Fig. 6.2. Osteophytes on the joint surface and around the margins of a femoral head (late Medieval, twelfth–sixteenth centuries AD, France).

Once cartilage is destroyed, if the individual continues to use the joint, the underlying bone can become very hard (sclerosis) and polished (eburnation – Fig. 6.3). If osteophyte formation is extensive a joint may become fused. Ossification may occur in cartilage away from the joint itself in some joint diseases; for example, the disease abbreviated to DISH (see below) usually involves ossification of costal (rib) and neck cartilages. Bone may also be destroyed in the joint diseases, on the joint surfaces themselves, on their margins or distal to the joint; the

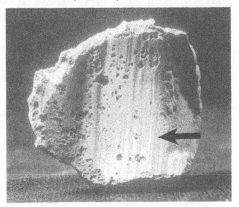

Fig. 6.3. Eburnation of the patella (Kulubnarti, Nubia). *(With permission from Lynn Kilgore)*

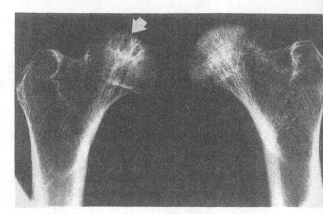

Left: Fig. 6.4. Porosity of joint surfaces of the shoulder joint (Romano-British, fourth century AD, Gambier-Parry Lodge, Gloucester, England); note also the osteophytes and eburnation. *Right:* Fig. 6.5. Subchondral cysts (arrow) illustrated on a radiograph of a femur.

patterning and character of these lesions may aid in diagnosis. The destruction of the cartilage on the joint surface allows the bone to degenerate and become porous (Fig. 6.4). In a synovial joint, synovial fluid can then infiltrate into the bone directly under the cartilage; the lesions formed are called subchondral cysts and are readily visible on radiographs (Fig. 6.5).

Resnick and Niwayama (1988: 1914) suggest that 'an accurate radiological diagnosis of joint disease is based on evaluation of two fundamental parameters; the morphology of the articular lesions and their distribution in the body'. The same can be said for macroscopic examination of the dry-bone lesions in the skeleton. However, comparison between archaeological and modern population groups in terms of the prevalence of osteoarthritis is difficult, largely because many of the diagnostic methods are different. For example, the occurrence of relevant symptoms, and changes in radiography, such as joint space narrowing, seen in a living patient, would not be possible to assess for an archaeological joint. It has also been shown, for example, that radiography may not identify all the degenerative joint changes visible macroscopically (Riddle *et al.*, 1988; Rogers *et al.*, 1990), and that quite subtle joint changes may be missed if radiography is used for diagnosis (of course, this is not an option for modern diagnosis); this may explain, as Rogers *et al.* (1990) suggest, why the signs and symptoms of living patients do not always correlate with the severity of the radiographic findings.

NEUROMECHANICAL JOINT DISEASE: OSTEOARTHRITIS

The most commonly occurring joint disease seen in archaeologically derived human skeletal remains and in clinical contexts is osteoarthritis (Jurmain and Kilgore, 1995); this disease is non-inflammatory and affects the synovial joints (see Rogers and Waldron, 1995: 2, for the structure of a synovial joint). Diagnosis of osteoarthritis rests on the identification of the abnormalities already described, but it cannot be diagnosed purely on the basis of one of these features. For example,

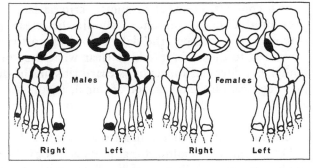

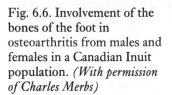

Fig. 6.6. Involvement of the bones of the foot in osteoarthritis from males and females in a Canadian Inuit population. *(With permission of Charles Merbs)*

the formation of osteophytes can occur merely as a result of the ageing process. Waldron and Rogers (1991) recommend that, if eburnation is not present on the joint surface (a sure sign of osteoarthritis), then two other features of osteoarthritis must be present, e.g. osteophytes and a porous joint surface. The recording of joint disease on skeletal material has resulted in many different methods being proposed by different authors. The basic point to make is that, as with any palaeopathological lesion, recording the basic data in a standardized format is essential so that comparisons can be made. Additionally, photographs and definitions of severity must be included in reports so that another researcher can be sure that, for example, their 'severe' grade of osteoarthritis is the same as that of another study (for some examples of recording formats see Walker and Hollimon, 1989; Jurmain, 1990; Lovell, 1994). Furthermore, generation of the distribution pattern of joint changes in the different bones of a joint in males and females (Fig. 6.6) may help in assessing the different loading patterns across a joint surface, how these may differ between the sexes and what the aetiological factors might have been (Merbs, 1983). Clearly every joint, and all parts of it, should be assessed to ensure a realistic picture of joint disease in groups of skeletons.

Bearing these factors in mind, it is useful to consider the study by Waldron and Rogers (1991) where people with varying degrees of expertise were given the opportunity of recording presence and absence of osteoarthritis in a series of joints. Presence and absence of eburnation, osteophytes, new bone on the joint surface, pitting of the joint and deformation of the joint contour were recorded, along with the severity of lesions. There was little overall difference in agreement between beginners and experts, but there was disagreement as to whether or not the bony changes were present and their degree of severity. The presence of eburnation and new bone formation on the joint were the most agreed-on bone changes. Interestingly, all ten specimens had osteoarthritis according to the authors' criteria, but there were only three specimens unanimously agreed upon by the experts and only one by the beginners. This reflects the problems in recording osteoarthritis; if the basic data are not recorded accurately then any interpretations will be invalid. This makes comparison of population osteoarthritis in different geographical contexts and time periods impossible. For example, Roberts and Cox (2003) came across a considerable problem with interpreting, first, what was meant by osteoarthritis in many skeletal reports from

British contexts, i.e. what diagnostic criteria had been used, and, secondly, the presented data. Researchers should be clear how they have diagnosed osteoarthritis, present the data according to the numbers of joints affected compared to those observed, be clear what they mean by a joint (one bone or both?), consider the impact of osteoarthritis on the different compartments of the joint, be clear on the discussion of spinal, as opposed to extraspinal, osteoarthritis, and also when talking overall about affected individuals in the population to describe them clearly in terms of whether they have spinal or extraspinal osteoarthritis, or whether both areas are affected.

Osteoarthritis is multifactorial in its aetiology. Increasing age, a strong genetic predisposition (an influence of 35–65 per cent – Shipley *et al.*, 2002: 534), obesity (leading to stress on the joints), underlying trauma and congenital hip dislocation, a range of diseases causing joint damage, activity/lifestyle, even posture and furniture use (Arce, 2003), and environmental factors such as climate may all contribute to its development. Urbanized, as opposed to rural, environments may produce different prevalence rates and skeletal distribution patterns in populations, both today and in the past. Pain, limitation of movement, swelling of the joint, wasting of muscles and deformity of joints may be clinical features associated with osteoarthritis, but some studies have shown no association between severity of joint involvement and symptoms (see above). Of course, any joint of the body can be affected, and some have characteristic epidemiologies. For example, shoulder osteoarthritis usually follows severe trauma or is related to a specific activity; it is also associated with damage to the rotator cuff soft tissues of this joint.

OSTEOARTHRITIS: SKELETAL INVOLVEMENT

In both archaeological and living population studies, the hip and knee are often the most commonly affected joints of the body in osteoarthritis; these are the major weight-bearing joints. Waldron (1997a) found in his study of 1,198 skeletons from British sites dated from AD 1200 to 1850 that about 3 per cent of individuals had hip osteoarthritis, a figure similar to modern studies; it was seen more in males, and affected one hip (usually the right). Waldron (1995) also found osteoarthritis of the knee became more common in England in the post-Medieval and later periods. In the upper body, osteoarthritis of the elbow is rare today, except in people with particularly stressful occupations such as mining or pneumatic drilling (Resnick and Niwayama, 1988: 1406); osteoarthritis of the shoulder is also rare without a history of trauma. However, the acromioclavicular and sternoclavicular joints are affected in many elderly individuals today. The hands and feet are affected by osteoarthritis with varying rates in living populations, with the joints of the hand (interphalangeal, metacarpophalangeal and some of the wrist bones) being commonly involved, especially in middle-aged post-menopausal women (Resnick and Niwayama, 1988: 1398). Osteoarthritis of the ankle is rare, but significant change in the first metatarsophalangeal joint (big toe) is seen frequently. Joint disease of the temporomandibular joint (TMJ) has already been mentioned in Chapter 4. Its frequency in living populations can be high and is discussed in Hodges (1991). This study examined the occurrence of osteoarthritis at the TMJ and its association with attrition, tooth loss, age and sex in five British skeletal populations. Only attrition and joint disease were significantly associated. Although attrition was probably a major predisposing factor to the development of joint disease in the jaw, structural abnormalities in the anatomy and physiology of the joint may also be a factor in its development.

In archaeological studies, osteoarthritis of the upper extremities can be more common than for living populations (Merbs, 1983: 99), which is surprising because increasing age is a strong correlate of shoulder and hip osteoarthritis rather than elbow and knee osteoarthritis (Jurmain, 1980: 144). If people live longer today then a higher frequency of joint disease in the shoulder would be expected. However, it is likely that osteoarthritis in the upper limb suggests a lifestyle predisposing these joints to degeneration, a lifestyle which was quite different from that of today. Skeletal studies have also shown a stronger side difference in size of upper compared to lower limbs, probably reflecting activity (Constandse-Westermann and Newell, 1989).

Relatively little work has been carried out on osteoarthritis of the hand and foot in archaeological groups, perhaps because these smaller bones often do not survive burial and excavation. Hand osteoarthritis is a common finding in modern population studies, especially in females (Resnick and Niwayama, 1995) and may be related to occupation; in fact, one of the few studies of osteoarthritis of the hands suggests a similar frequency in past populations (Waldron, 1993a). Waldron and Cox (1989) also examined the hand bones of 367 skeletons from the crypt excavations at Christ Church, Spitalfields, London, dated to between AD 1729 and 1869. The occupations of these individuals were obtained from historical sources; twenty-nine of the males were weavers, and the hypothesis proposed was that this occupation could induce hand osteoarthritis. However, of the thirteen males with osteoarthritis in their hands, only three were weavers, and there appeared to be a strong correlation with increased age in those affected.

SPINAL JOINT DISEASE

One of the penalties paid by humans for their adoption of the erect bipedal posture is an increased susceptibility to vertebral osteoarthritis, a direct consequence of spinal stress (Bridges, 1994). It might be thought that the mechanical stress and strain upon each segment of the spine is constant in the upright posture. However, the spine is not just a straight line and exhibits a backward curve in the chest or thoracic region and a forward curve in the lumbar and cervical regions, leading to the fifth cervical, eighth thoracic and fourth lumbar vertebrae being most affected in joint disease. It is suggested (Nathan, 1962) that because of these curves there are points of maximum and minimum stress, and that this is responsible for the variation in frequency of osteoarthritis in the spine.

The intervertebral discs consist of a fibrous 'capsule' containing a gelatinous internal substance. With advancing age a chemical and degenerative change occurs in these tissues. The constant stress to which these discs are subject, for example in the bending and lifting of everyday activity, causes the internal nucleus pulposus to invade the annulus fibrosus. The rupture of this fibrous

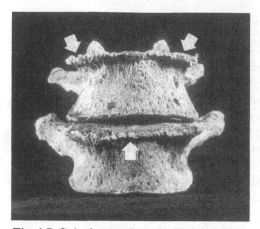

Fig. 6.7. Spinal osteophytosis (Kulubnarti, Nubia). *(With permission of Lynn Kilgore)*

capsule stimulates the growth of bone from the margins of the vertebral body itself (osteophytes or osteophytosis – see Fig. 6.7). This is a compensatory reaction to injury just like many other body reactions to trauma. For reasons of pure mechanics, the anterior area of the annulus and vertebral body are more liable to the process of osteophytosis development than the posterior area. With increasing stress and annulus rupture, the size of osteophytes increases. At the extreme, the osteophytes from contiguous vertebrae grow together and unite, so fixing the spinal segment and preventing movement. This localized and restricted fixation, or ankylosis, is not to be confused with the more generalized diseases of spinal fixation which will be considered later. The inexorable advance of time results in all people developing the clinical symptoms and signs of vertebral osteophytosis. Intermittent backache, stiffness and an inability to touch the toes are the all too familiar features of this ageing process. Just as today, so it was in antiquity.

In reviewing relatively modern vertebral columns, Nathan (1962) found that by the third decade of life a large proportion of individuals studied had vertebral osteophytosis, and by the fifth decade all of them had the condition. Since this is a mechanically induced condition there is, naturally, variation among individuals. The man or woman engaged in heavy manual work is more liable to develop osteophytosis than the sedentary worker. Quite probably, therefore, the more active lifestyle of people in antiquity will have led to vertebral osteophytosis at an earlier age than in their modern office-working descendant. Certainly the condition is almost universal in adult skeletal remains of the past, although its frequency varies between groups.

Along with osteophytes developing around the vertebral body margins, the body surface, a cartilaginous joint, also degenerates, and both these changes are referred to as spondylosis (degenerative disc disease) (Rogers, 2000). The body surfaces become porous and pitted and there may be new bone formed (intervertebral osteochondrosis); this occurs most frequently on the mid-lower cervical spine, upper thoracic and lower lumbar areas (Rogers, 2000: 169). As well as the vertebral body surfaces, the posterior apophyseal joints and transverse process joints of the vertebrae (synovial joints) are also affected in joint disease (Fig. 6.8). Associated with degeneration of the intervertebral discs are Schmorl's nodes (Fig. 6.9), where the disc contents exert pressure on the vertebral body surfaces. These nodes are seen in the lower thoracic and lumbar spine, and in many cases their specific aetiology may be unknown (Saluja *et al.*, 1986). Trauma has been implicated as one of the major causes of this condition, with underlying

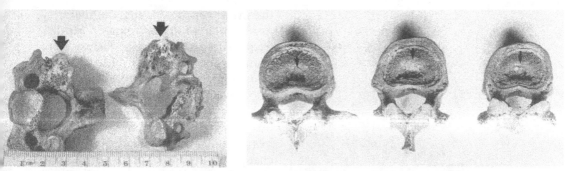

Left: Fig. 6.8. Osteoarthritis of the apophyseal joints of cervical vertebrae (500 BC–AD 1700, Ala 329, San Francisco Bay, California, United States). *(With permission of Robert Jurmain) Right:* Fig. 6.9. Schmorl's nodes of the superior surfaces of vertebral bodies. *(Calvin Wells Photographic Collection)*

infection, osteoporosis and neoplastic disease weakening the bone structure, enabling Schmorl's nodes to develop (Resnick and Niwayama, 1988: 1528).

A pioneering study by Sager (1969) set some precedents for recording spinal osteoarthritis for archaeological populations. Sager examined 100 cervical spines (52 males and 48 females) of a Danish modern urban population and skeletons from Medieval monastic and hospital cemeteries from Denmark; the characteristic osteoarthritic changes already discussed were recorded. This study concluded that the modern material had a higher prevalence rate in all age groups than the archaeological material. Sager's descriptions and photographic records of the stages in the disease were exemplary.

Spinal joint disease seems to be ubiquitous in past human groups of all periods (Trinkhaus, 1985) but in varying degrees of severity and distribution through the spine, perhaps reflecting the influence of activity on its development (Figs 6.10 and 6.11 show modern examples of carrying loads). For example, Bridges (1994) reports a high frequency of neck osteoarthritis in 125 skeletons from north-west Alabama, United States; carrying loads through the use of a tumpline around the forehead was considered as a cause. A study by Lovell (1994) examined joint changes in the spines of individuals from a Bronze Age site in Pakistan (4,000–5,000 years ago). The results showed that, although the pattern of osteoarthritis in the neck vertebrae was unusual, this patterning may have been reflecting activity such as carrying heavy loads on the head. As there was no increase in prevalence with age in this study, an occupation-related aetiology was suggested.

Activity of a specific kind was also suggested by Stirland (2000) and Stirland and Waldron (1997) when they studied the spines of individuals from the Tudor warship the *Mary Rose*, excavated off the south coast of England. Dated to AD 1545, when the ship sank, the minimum number of individuals was 179 based on skull and mandible counts; this was 43 per cent of the historically documented crew. The contextual data for this site were very specific and it was known that 200 mariners, 185 soldiers and 30 gunners were on board, thus making it possible that activity-related skeletal changes could be correlated with 'occupation'. All

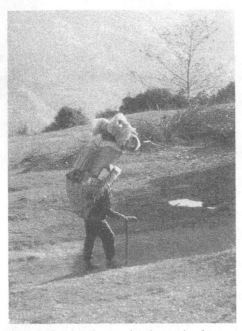

Fig. 6.10. Nepal: carrying heavy load on the back with a tumpline around the forehead on a trek.

the crew were male, and the majority were young adults or younger. Similar frequencies of spinal joint disease were found when compared with an older group of males from a late Medieval site in Norwich, England. It was suggested that activities undertaken by the crew of the *Mary Rose*, such as manhandling heavy guns, accelerated age-related changes in the spine; these people were probably a semi-permanent professional crew who had started their work as adolescents (Stirland and Waldron, 1997: 335). Studies of the differences between spinal joint disease frequency in two other skeletal samples in Britain have also been carried out, one of which had specific associated ethnographic accounts of activities carried out in the community (Sofaer Deverenski, 2000). The study of the site of Ensay on the Island of Harris, Outer Hebrides, Scotland (fifteenth–late nineteenth century AD) benefited from eighteenth-, nineteenth- and twentieth-century accounts of tasks, while it was assumed that the people from the rural site of Wharram Percy, North Yorkshire, England (tenth–sixteenth centuries AD) undertook general agricultural and related work. Features of joint degeneration were separately recorded in the spines of the individuals. Generally speaking the Ensay population had more joint disease overall. However, taking eburnation as the pathognomonic indicator of osteoarthritis in the apophyseal joints (Rogers and Waldron, 1995), 70 per cent of

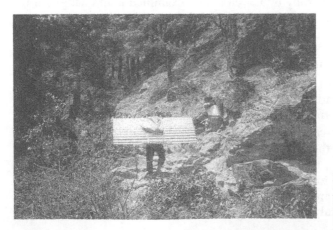

Fig. 6.11. Nepal: carrying a heavy load on the head (roofing for a building).

males and 71 per cent of females were affected, compared to 55 per cent of males and 39 per cent of females at Wharram Percy; there appeared to be little difference between the groups in distribution through the spines.

Another site with specific activities, assumed because of historical context, is that of the battlefield of Towton, North Yorkshire, England. There were thirty-seven burials, all male, and again the mean age at death was in the young adult category, and estimated to be 30 years (Boylston, 2001). Some 80 per cent of the spines examined had evidence of joint degeneration, mainly in the form of Schmorl's nodes and spinal osteophytes (Coughlan and Holst, 2001); 40 per cent of vertebrae had Schmorl's nodes, which is suggested to be the result of increased axial loading of the spine. Exploring the frequency of spinal joint disease as a means to identifying activity, however, has its problems because the spine may also be affected by the activities related to bipedalism – i.e. walking, running, etc. This was identified in a study of eighty-one skeletons from the thirteenth- and fourteenth-century site of St Andrew, Fishergate, York, by Knüsel et al. (1997). Three groups of differing status were identified from archaeological and historical data, but there was no significant difference in joint disease between the three. The conclusion reached was that spinal joint disease was not the ideal part of the skeleton to observe as a marker of activity-related stress.

ACTIVITY, OSTEOARTHRITIS AND MARKERS OF 'OCCUPATION'

It is clear from modern clinical data that people practising particular activities or occupations can suffer osteoarthritis (and other changes) at certain joints, although the links are not consistent (Jurmain, 1999). Study of, for example, osteoarthritic changes in skeletons from forensic contexts as an aid in identification has been noted, i.e. correlating osteoarthritis patterning (and changes in the robusticity of the bones) with the occupation of the individual who was the victim (Wienker and Wood, 1987). In archaeological contexts there has been a recent proliferation of work in this area as researchers try to 'put flesh on the bones' (e.g. Capasso et al., 1999), and the study of activity-related changes in the skeleton has been used to try to identify differences in lifestyle with subsistence change, e.g. the transition from hunter-gathering to agriculture. Waldron (1994), however, warns of the dangers of stretching the evidence too far and the lack of a consistent correlation of bone degeneration with specific occupations in modern studies; he summarizes the potential problems inherent in an archaeological study of lifestyle, occupation and osteoarthritis. If, today, one considers the multitude of activities people are engaged in during one week (or even one day) of their lives, for example, each of these could affect the body. However, what should be remembered is that 'the same kinds of activities will be performed over and over again particularly if they are necessary for survival' (Merbs, 1983: 1).

If a person practises a very heavy manual occupation which severely stresses the joints regularly, it is likely that a particular patterning may occur for that specific occupation (Fig. 6.12). Of course, many other factors (not least increasing age and obesity) can influence the development of osteoarthritis and these may determine whether osteoarthritis develops and is identifiable to a specific activity. To counteract the effects of age it may be useful to study younger individuals; if

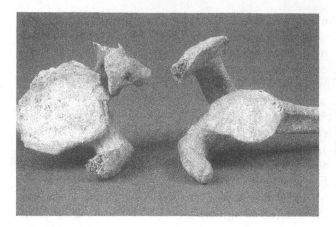

Fig. 6.12. Right glenoid cavity of scapula (with opposite as a comparison) showing enlargement of joint surface with osteophytes and porosity; perhaps this person used the right arm more than the left (early Medieval, fifth–seventh centuries AD, Pewsey, Wiltshire, England).

osteoarthritis is seen here in a particularly high prevalence and specific patterning, it may be possible to suggest an occupationally induced osteoarthritis for this group, because it is considered that for occupationally related changes to show, the person must start the activity young. What may be safer is to use multiple skeletal markers of activity such as enthesophytes (new bone formation at tendinous and ligament insertions as a result of increase in size of associated muscles), trauma patterns and changes in the size, shape and robusticity of bones, to try to suggest related activity. In addition, some 'non-metric traits' may be related to occupation (Saunders, 1989; Tyrrell, 2000), e.g. squatting facets, and research has suggested that differences in bone mineral content and density may be implicated as indicators of greater mechanical loading, particularly in the dominant arm (Faulkner *et al.*, 1993). Of particular relevance generally to occupationally induced changes in the skeleton was the law proposed in AD 1892 by a German anatomist Julius Wolff, known as 'Wolff's law of transformation', which stated that bone will adapt to functional pressure or force by increasing or decreasing its mass to resist the stress (Kennedy, 1989: 134); formation of bone, for example, will sustain and distribute the load, as we have seen in osteoarthritis. This means that if the body is involved with a repeated activity the skeleton will respond by becoming 'larger'. Enthesophytes will also develop at muscular attachments and degeneration of the joints will occur.

Biomechanical analyses (long bone cross-sectional geometrical analyses using the application of engineering principles) of the component bones of the skeleton have received much attention in recent years as a way of exploring the effects of activity or loading on the bones. There are a range of loading modes that can affect bone, and most of the time a number of different modes may be operating – e.g. tension, bending, compression, shear, torsion (Larsen, 1997: 196). Beam analysis is the method used to measure the geometric properties at cross sections taken perpendicular to the long axis of the bone, and these measures represent the amount and distribution of the bone at those points (Larsen, 1997: 199). Areas such as medullary and cortical area, and second moments of area (geometric properties that measure bending and torsional strength), are measured. Ruff (2000) provides a useful overview of the field and its use in biological anthropology. Plain film radiography, computed tomography and sectioning bones to measure cortical bone width and shape of the cross section have all played their part in biomechanical analyses, although non-invasive techniques are to be preferred. Archaeological examples of studies using this analytical technique include consideration of the change in shape of limb bones with the transition to agriculture, sex differences in cross-sectional geometry, and the effect of different terrain on the bones. For example, Bridges *et al.* (2000) measured humeri, radii, ulna, femora and tibiae of 372 individuals from West Central Illinois, United States, dating from the Middle Woodland (50 BC–AD 200) to the Mississippian period (AD 1050–1250); a subsample of 80 was scanned using computed tomography. Results showed humeral and femoral strength increased in females when native seed crops were being grown, females being implicated as key to growing and processing these crops. In the latest period, when maize use intensifies, female left-arm strength declines, which Bridges suggests could be the result of more efficient processing or because maize is an easier crop to process. From South Africa, a study of computed tomographic images of humeri and tibiae from eighteenth-century skeletons of low socio-economic status, a modern cadaver collection and a hunter-gatherer sample revealed that hunter-gatherers were a more mobile and active group. The humeral strength, however, of the eighteenth-century male skeletons was greater than for both of the other groups and was suggested as being indicative of their involvement in manual labouring (Ledger *et al.*, 2000). A more recent study of the effects of rowing on humeral strength in a number of skeletal samples with known subsistence activities showed that male ocean rowers had stronger humeri than river rowers or non-rowers, but that female non-rowers from the ocean rowing group had stronger humeri than non-rowing females (Weiss, 2003a). In the light of these results, Weiss suggests that assigning specific activities to a person on the basis of humeral strength is difficult because of the multi-task nature of arm use.

Studies in the **asymmetry of limb bone size** (length, width, circumference) as a possible indicator of the use of one limb more than the other for an activity/movement have also been undertaken using metrical analysis of bones and features on radiographs. Some 90 per cent of humans are right-side dominant when using their upper limb (Coren and Porac, 1977 in Ruff, 2000), and therefore it seems reasonable to assess whether this is present in past human groups, and if it is related to activity. For example, professional tennis players develop increased size of the dominant arm, including its bones (Jones *et al.*, 1977 in Larsen, 1997). The upper limb is usually used for analysis because lower limb asymmetry is smaller or more variable, and the arms are used for a multitude of tasks while the lower limbs are mainly used for locomotion (Ruff and Jones, 1981 in Ruff, 2000; Larsen, 1997: 213). Steele (2000) provides a useful summary of the subject of handedness and how it may be recognized in the skeleton, and some archaeological studies have explored the concept of handedness and activity. For example, antero-posterior radiographs of the second metacarpal of 120 individuals from the eighteenth-/nineteenth-century site at Christ Church, Spitalfields, London, were analysed (Mays, 2002). Measurements of bone length, bone width and medullary cavity width at the mid-shaft were taken, and the cross-sectional shape analysed with respect to sex and known or assumed occupation. Results showed that asymmetry varied with occupation but not strongly. Another study focused on the humeri of female and male lay people and a male monastic group from St Andrew, Fishergate, York, England (Mays, 1999). Measurements of the maximum length and, using radiographs, of the total bone width and medullary width at 35 per cent of the distance from the distal end were taken; the 35 per cent rule is appropriate, because there are no soft tissue attachments at this level, and the cortical walls are near parallel (Mays, 1999: 69). The results showed a difference in activity between the males and females and the male laypeople and the male monastic group. The humeral diaphyseal strength values were lower in the monastic males, suggesting that these people did not pursue heavy work; specifically what type of work that was is unknown. Biomechanical analyses of skeletal remains from archaeological sites do hold potential for more research, although it should be remembered that changes in size and shape of bones may be affected by many factors, including diet, biological sex, age, genetic factors, environment (terrain) and activity (Jurmain, 1999: 258). Jurmain adds that the type of loading, duration, amplitude, age at which loading began and stopped, bone element involved, and site within the element affected are all relevant for interpreting patterns.

The use of **enthesophytes** in the reconstruction of activity in the past has also received much attention. These musculo-skeletal markers of stress at tendon and ligament insertions indicate movement using specific muscles or groups of muscles (Fig. 6.13). For example, Eshed *et al.* (2004) considered musculo-skeletal stress markers in the upper limb bones of hunter-gatherer and Neolithic agricultural populations in the Levant. They found that the upper limbs were more heavily used in the Neolithic but that there were differences in expression in males and females for both periods. However, again there are many predisposing factors to the development of these markers, as described in Jurmain (1999); these include age, hormonal and genetic factors, dietary variables, disease such as DISH (see later) and activity. Weiss (2003b) in her study of muscle markers at seven sites in the upper limb bones suggests, for example, that age is the best overall predictor of aggregate muscle markers. However, the detailed anatomical and clinical basis for the development of enthesophytes has not been explored (Henderson, 2003). In terms of

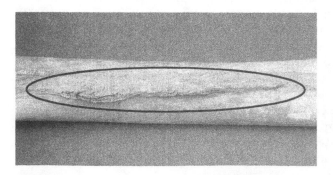

Fig. 6.13. New bone formation at the site of a muscle attachment on the femur, possibly a musculo-skeletal marker of stress.

clinical data and their application to archaeological populations, enthesophytes are not 'life threatening' and 'rarely produce identifiable symptoms' (Jurmain, 1999: 143); thus, data on enthesophytes from people with known activities are difficult to acquire. This may explain why many studies of enthesophytes in archaeological samples fail to relate the findings to clinical citations. Nevertheless, some useful studies have been published that discuss scoring criteria that are more transparent than has previously been the case (e.g. Hawkey and Merbs, 1995), and there has also been a focus on pattern of involvement of major muscle groups to reflect specific movements. The main problem to overcome, however, remains the fact that, if patterns of enthesophytes cannot be verified as indicating a specific activity, then the skeletal data alone are unconvincing (Jurmain, 1999: 159).

Historical data do exist about occupations in the past and how they may have affected health, but making a direct link to skeletal changes is extremely difficult. However, what we do know is that people did work in the past in a variety of occupations, for example, farming, craft industries, food processing and building; each one of these activities must potentially have impacted on the skeleton and caused changes we can recognize. Furthermore, males, females and different age groups probably had particular occupations, although we must not assume a direct stereotypical correlation (Panter-Brick, 2002). Whatever method of analysis is used to look at the link between occupation and skeletal changes, the process is not easy, and the use of comparative clinical data, ethnographic analogy and art and documentary sources, where available, is essential (Kennedy, 1989: 156).

The historical literature abounds with works on occupationally related diseases (see Kennedy, 1989 for a summary). Bernardino Ramazzini was the first author to write a treatise on diseases of workers, in Italy in AD 1700 (Louis, 1990). Called *A treatise on the diseases of tradesmen*, it described forty-two occupations, including miners, midwives and painters, and Ramazzini was awarded the title of 'father of industrial medicine'. From this time many people became involved in looking for relationships between occupation and changes in the body. The problem with many of the associated diseases described is that a large percentage do not involve the bone. There are certainly some fascinating occupationally related diseases in more recent literature (Cherniack, 1992); 'hatter's shakes' were the result of mercury poisoning in the hatter's trade when mercury was applied to rabbit skins in the manufacturing process, and 'potter's rot' occurred when workers in the pottery trade were exposed to silica, leading to silicosis. Furthermore, with the domestication of animals, human populations became subject to another set of diseases. For example, anthrax is contracted by humans mainly through contact with domesticated animals and their skins, and 'wool sorter's disease' was the name applied to anthrax in people working with wool in the nineteenth century (Meyer, 1964).

A number of archaeologically based studies have been published on the relationship between **occupation and arthritis**, some of which have already been described above (Spinal joint disease). They are of two types: in the first, the generalized distribution of osteoarthritis around the body in a skeletal population is often discussed with reference to occupation, while in the second the question of osteoarthritis prevalence and change in economy is addressed. Bearing in mind the premise that occupation is a difficult area to determine using skeletal remains, there have been interesting studies. Perhaps one of the most consulted examples of osteoarthritis and its relationship to activity is that of Merbs (1983). Osteoarthritis was recorded for both male and female skeletons in a Canadian Eskimo group. Males had more lower-limb osteoarthritis, and females had more changes in the temporomandibular joints and some of the vertebral joints. Osteoarthritis was seen more in the thoracic region in females and in the lumbar spine in males. By studying reports of accounts of meetings with the Sadlermiut Eskimos before their extinction, reports on discussions with the Aivilingmiut, who had lived with the Sadlermiut earlier, and the archaeological record, Merbs was able to reconstruct potential activities within this group of people (Merbs, 1983: 138–9). As he said, 'this is not as good as a first hand detailed ethnographic account, but it does allow a reconstruction of the most important elements of Sadlermiut behavior'. Merbs interpreted the osteoarthritic patterning seen in the material studied as being due to the male activities of harpoon throwing, kayak paddling and lifting and carrying heavy loads, and in the females as due to making clothes, carrying children and sledding. Similar work is reported by Lai and Lovell (1992) and Lovell and Dublenko (1999) who recorded joint disease and other skeletal changes (enthesophytes and increased bone robusticity) which may be consistent with habitual lifting, canoeing (paddling or rowing) in three males dated to the Fur Trade Period in Alberta, Canada. Transport of furs, provisions and officers of the Hudson's Bay Fur Trade Company was by canoe and boat on fast-flowing rivers; some journeys lasted seventeen or eighteen hours and it is possible that paddling and rowing induced the skeletal changes observed.

Other studies have used osteoarthritis as a means to answering questions about activity in contrasting economies, particularly in hunter-gathering and agricultural economies, and conclusions vary. Cohen and Armelagos (1984), in summing up the data for physical stress (including osteoarthritis and skeletal robusticity) in the studies in their book, suggest that there was a probable reduction in workload associated with the adoption of agriculture (1984: 590), but this did not necessarily imply less time spent on food production. Furthermore, many of the hunter-gatherer groups studied had greater longevity and this may have had an influencing effect on the development of osteoarthritis in these groups compared to the agricultural populations who lived shorter lives. Jurmain (1990) found a similar picture in his study of 167 skeletons from the south-eastern San Francisco Bay area of the United States, dating from AD 500 to pre-European contact. More osteoarthritis was seen than in comparative agricultural groups. Bridges (1991) also found this difference in the hunter-gatherer (6000–1000 BC) and agricultural (AD 1200–1500) groups she studied in north-east Alabama; the results, however, were not significant except for in a few joints (Fig. 6.14). Multiple aetiological factors affecting a population's predisposition to osteoarthritis are suggested as the reason behind inconsistencies in results of similar studies. Bridges (1991) suggests that examination of bone strength and osteoarthritis may help to explain activity patterns in past populations, as these changes may be responses to different kinds of forces. Her study in 1989 showed that the agricultural population had stronger bones than their hunter-gathering predecessors, suggesting an increased workload;

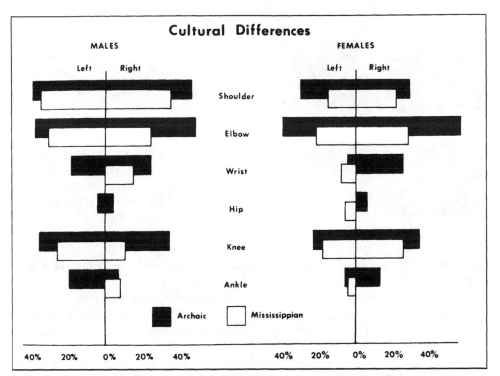

Fig. 6.14. Differences in osteoarthritis distribution in hunter-gatherer (Archaic) and agricultural (Mississippian) populations. *(With permission of Patricia Bridges)*

these findings are supported by osteoarthritis in the same populations, already discussed (Bridges, 1991). Goodman *et al.* (1984) also suggested significantly increased osteoarthritis in their Dickson Mound population with the transition to agriculture, and Walker and Hollimon (1989) noted increased mechanical stress with a shift to intensive exploitation of a marine environment from hunter-gathering by southern Californian Indians in the Santa Barbara Channel area.

Related to these studies of the change in frequency of osteoarthritis in joints in populations practising different economies, there have been other studies suggesting more specific activities. Molleson (1989) has described skeletal abnormalities of Mesolithic/Neolithic skeletons from Syria dated to around 8,000 years ago. Here, the abnormalities in the toe and ankle joints were suggested to be the result of extreme dorsiflexion of the joints of the foot in using a quernstone (Fig. 6.15), and robust arm bones, osteoarthritis of the lower spine, knees and big toes also contributed to this picture. Ubelaker (1979) noted similar changes on the metatarsals and first proximal foot phalanx in a prehistoric sample from Ecuador, and suggested that a habitual kneeling posture may be implicated for the changes. However, the observation of osteoarthritis as an indicator of occupation/activity is not clear cut, as we have noted above, and Jurmain (1999) provides an excellent overview of the clinical data. For example, Waldron and Cox (1989) found no

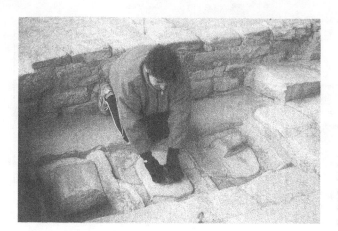

Fig. 6.15. The first author, at Mesa Verde, United States, on her knees simulating the actions of grinding grain on a mortar.

correlation between hand osteoarthritis and weaving in skeletons from the Christ Church, Spitalfields, London, site, as we have already seen.

Occupation has become of great interest to biological anthropologists worldwide because assessing a person's activity patterns in the past helps to complete one more part of the complex jigsaw puzzle of past human behaviour (see Capasso *et al.*, 1999 for the range of changes that might be occupationally induced). More specific studies of occupation should be discussed here briefly to show the range of potential in this area. The possible use of **traumatic lesions** (e.g. the clay-shoveller's fracture, Knüsel *et al.*, 1996; Fig. 6.16) and culturally induced **dental modifications** have already been described elsewhere in this book. What people specifically do for a living has been addressed by several authors. Kennedy (1986) considered the supposed correlation between **auditory exostoses** (bony growths in the ears, often recorded as a non-metric trait (Fig. 6.17)) and immersion in cold water in populations from different geographic regions. The hypothesis was that low frequencies would be expected in polar and subpolar areas (that is, avoidance of cold water because of the potential problem of hypothermia) compared to the

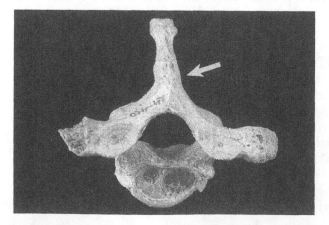

Fig. 6.16. Healed 'clay-shoveller's' fracture of spinous process in hunter-gatherer (Indian Knoll 24-410, Kentucky, United States)

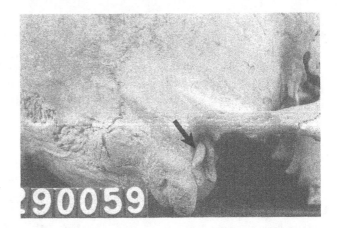

Fig. 6.17. New bone formation in the external auditory meatus (ear exostosis) of a hunter-gatherer (Indian Knoll, Kentucky, United States). *(National Museum of Natural History, Washington DC, United States, 290059)*

tropical latitudes, where people were accustomed to warmer water. Higher frequencies were expected in people who exploited either marine or freshwater resources through diving (Kennedy, 1986: 407); these hypotheses were substantiated and the previously suggested genetic predisposition for these abnormalities could not be sustained. More recent studies have upheld these findings, although some do not agree (e.g. see Hutchinson *et al.*, 1997). Standen *et al.* (1997) studied ear exostoses in 1,149 crania from forty-three sites in northern Chile dated from 7000 BC to AD 1450; a significant association was found between the condition and sex, and the condition and a coastal environment. An interesting study of ear exostoses in two skeletal samples from different social statuses dated to the first–third centuries AD from Rome, Italy, revealed no evidence in females but a higher frequency in the higher status males (Manzi *et al.*, 1991). This was suggested to indicate that those males frequented the thermal baths, which also included experiencing cold baths, which could have induced the exostoses observed. In fact, it is now suggested that many of the non-metric, epigenetic skeletal traits described previously in the literature (such as ear exostoses) may be culturally and not genetically induced (Saunders, 1989; Tyrrell, 2000). Stirland (1986, 2000) has considered the possible cause of non-fusion of the acromion of the scapula (**os acromiale**; Fig. 6.18) in skeletons from the *Mary Rose* which sank off the south coast of England in AD 1545. The acromion of the scapula usually unites at between 22 and 25 years

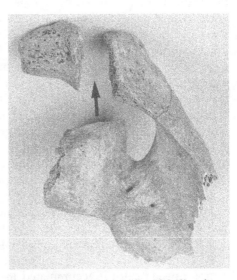

Fig. 6.18. Os acromiale (late Medieval, twelfth–sixteenth centuries AD, Chichester, Sussex, England).

but in 3–6 per cent of modern populations it does not. Of 207 scapulae from the *Mary Rose*, 26 had evidence of os acromiale (12.5 per cent); when it was possible to pair scapulae, of fifty-two pairs, ten individuals had the condition (19 per cent), six bilaterally (Stirland, 2000). There was also increased robusticity and size of the left humeri. Stirland associates this condition with the use of a bow and arrows in a defence mode on the Tudor warship, the action of drawing the bow and firing the arrows on a regular basis preventing fusion of the acromion. At this time Henry VIII, the owner of the *Mary Rose*, was considered a keen archer and encouraged the use of the longbow. Historical data indicate that boys were provided with a bow and arrows from as young an age as 7 years, and there were practice areas in all towns. The excavation of the *Mary Rose* also revealed 172 longbows and 3,969 arrows on board. The draw-weight of a longbow today is 20kg, but it is estimated at 75kg for the Medieval period. While os acromiale was not present in all scapulae, the evidence may represent a small group of very specialist archers. This condition was also found in three individuals from the North Yorkshire battlefield site at Towton, England (Knüsel, 2001); this was a frequency rate of 9.2 per cent of twenty-nine people whose scapulae were preserved to observe. Knüsel suggests that the condition may again have been related to activity such as archery but other 'occupations' could also be implicated. Of course, knowing the precise lifestyle of a person is useful for interpreting skeletal changes, and a study by Mann *et al.* (1991) is appropriate in this respect. Continued knee flexion, perhaps resulting from long-term paralysis, was inferred from the bony changes seen in the knees of three 'modern' skeletons. The medical histories of these individuals supported this interpretation, even though a specific conclusive cause could not be provided on the evidence.

To complete this survey, there are other 'occupationally' induced features in the skeleton that may ultimately aid our behavioural reconstructions in the future. Pollution both inside buildings and outside, in the general (including work) environment, may predispose people to develop specific conditions. For example, maxillary sinusitis has been used in archaeological studies as an indicator of industrial pollution as a consequence of work (Roberts *et al.*, 1998), the inhalation of residues of plants into the lungs may indicate subsistence economy (see Pabst and Hofer, 1998 on deposits in the Tyrolean Iceman's lungs), the presence of rickets may indicate the effects of working (or living) in a polluted environment without exposure to sunlight, and tuberculosis may suggest a person working with animals with the disease. Furthermore, congenital (Chapter 3) and neoplastic disease (Chapter 9) may be implicated as a response to pollutants in the environment as a result of industries such as mining, metalworking or textile manufacture. Indeed, the effects of prehistoric mining activities may still persist today to compromise health in some parts of the world (e.g. in Jordan, see Pyatt and Grattan, 2001). For example, Oakberg *et al.* (2000) analysed arsenic levels in individuals from the copper-smelting site of Shiqmim, Israel. They found in this pilot study that it was possible to identify people who had been working in that industry at that site.

At some periods in our prehistory and history **lead pollution** may also have compromised health if accumulated in high enough quantities. A classic example comes from the Roman period, when lead pipes brought water to inhabitants of towns, and lead was used for kitchen vessels and utensils; of course people would also have mined and worked the lead into usable items. Exposure to lead particles at such high levels could have compromised health (Roberts and Cox, 2003), and can affect a number of chemical processes in the body. For example, poor intellectual development, anaemia, kidney failure, gout and nerve paralysis may occur (Aufderheide and Rodríguez-Martín, 1998: 318). A study of human lead exposure in England from 5500 BP to the sixteenth century, based on lead concentrations in tooth enamel from archaeological sites, revealed that levels were high from the Roman period onwards (Budd *et al.*, 2003); at approximately 40 parts per million, this would be considered today as the effects of industrial pollution. However, lead isotope data refined the picture, suggested that exposure in the past was highly variable, and indicated that levels were actually similar to that reported for modern England (classed as 'natural' or 'non-technological' exposure), but increased levels were noted specifically for the Roman and later Medieval periods. This study controlled for the effects of post-mortem accumulations of lead from the soil, a factor that should always be taken into consideration in chemical analyses. Another study of mummified individuals also found high lead levels that, it was suggested, contributed to their demise. Three sailors on the John Franklin expedition to the Canadian Arctic in the nineteenth century were discovered and excavated in the 1980s (Beattie and Geiger, 1987 in Aufderheide, 2003). The lead levels in these men were about 133 parts per million, and the source of the lead was indicated to be from lead solder used on tins of food (Kowal *et al.*, 1989). Along with raised lead levels, we should also remember that lead lines might be visible on radiographs of long bones in affected individuals.

In 1998 Kennedy summarized the results of a symposium on markers of occupational status (MOS) and pointed the way forward. He highlighted the need for standards for making accurate identifications of MOS and determining aetiologies. He concludes by saying (1998: 309): 'Rather than continuing the venerable practice of first deciding that a bone modification is a marker of occupational stress, it is recommended that we initiate investigations with a sharper perception of how bone remodelling takes place and which kinds of modifications bone may assume within the configurations of habitual activity revealed in archaeological and historical sources.' How true this is. Jurmain (1999) also concludes in his book that osteologists often ignore clinical data if they do not support their skeletal findings, and that none of the osseous changes that have come to be associated with activity are simply the result of activity alone ('activity-alone myopia' (1999: 262)); all have many predisposing factors, as we have seen. Furthermore, ethnographic accounts may be useful in interpreting what activities might have been practised by a population, but in many cases the data, if used, are selected to fit what is being seen. The use of multiple indicators of activity may be a way to proceed (i.e. joint disease, enthesopathy, bone asymmetry and geometry, fractures, dental changes, certain non-metric traits, evidence of 'poisoning' such as lead, and other specific diseases such as tuberculosis). However, using many indicators does not rid us of the problem that we know little of the proportional contribution of each one in relation to activity (an analogous situation may be described with respect to using many methods of analysis for adult age estimations (see Chapter 2)). Jurmain (1999) suggests that studying young individuals, the use of bone geometry and exploring indicators of likely bone fatigue in early life may be the way forward. As he indicates, activities must begin early in life and be extreme to show on the skeleton. However, a number of different activities could produce the same changes, and therefore reconstructing 'movement' is perhaps the only safe interpretation with respect to activity that can be made using skeletal remains (as discussed also by Knüsel, 2000: 396). Clearly cultural context is also important for interpretation of skeletal changes, but again selectively choosing factors to fit what is seen in the skeletal data is unacceptable. Jurmain concludes by saying (1999: 267): 'Story-telling and scenario-building may have some (limited) utility. However, without clear empirical controls and application of rigorous means of verification, skeletal biologists can become lost in the same intellectual fog.' However, reconstructing 'occupation' or 'activity' is relevant for our interpretations of past human behaviour. Work today fills many waking hours, is a major part of adult life and can create stress; the type of work people do is also determined by many factors such as age, sex, ethnicity and status, and these variables are relevant when we come to try to explore work patterns in the past.

INFLAMMATORY JOINT DISEASE: SEPTIC ARTHRITIS

Several other specific joint diseases deserve discussion in this chapter. Septic or inflammatory arthritis is discussed in Chapter 7 under 'tuberculosis', but it can also be caused by organisms other than *Mycobacterium tuberculosis*. Arthritis caused by non-specific infection may have two aetiological pathways. The bacteria (usually *Streptococcus* or *Staphylococcus*; Resnick and Niwayama, 2003) spread via the blood to the joint cavity, but infection of a joint can also result from spread of an infection of the skin or from the bone to the joint (e.g. osteomyelitis). The joint is painful, hot and red; it is today considered a medical emergency (Shipley *et al.*, 2002: 555) and is treated with intravenous antibiotics and immobilization to prevent joint destruction, which can occur in a very short time (days). In a normal synovial joint the synovial fluid nourishes the cartilage, particularly with sugars. In septic arthritis the cartilage is starved of these sugars because of the competing needs of the bacteria. Septic arthritis usually affects one joint – the knee or the hip in two-thirds of cases (Ortner and Putschar, 1981: 399) – but other joints can potentially be involved. When compared to tuberculous arthritis, septic arthritis caused by other organisms (although usually an acute condition) is less destructive of the joint surfaces and is characterized by erosion of the bone around the edges of the articulating area and a reduced tendency to fusion. Whereas tuberculous arthritis primarily affects children, non-specific septic arthritis can affect all ages. Septic arthritis is an infrequent finding in archaeological material (Fig. 6.19), and distinguishing between a tuberculous and non-tuberculous aetiology is often problematic without other supporting evidence in the skeleton for tuberculosis, for example. Septic arthritis may also be complicated by non-septic osteoarthritis or other joint diseases, so that, in any one individual, a number of joint diseases may present themselves but are impossible to differentiate from one another.

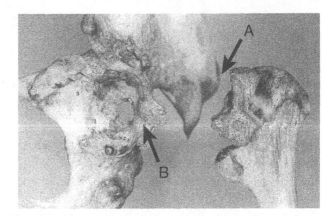

Fig. 6.19. Septic arthritis of the hip; loss of femoral head (A) and destruction of acetabulum of pelvis (B) (National Museum of Natural History, Washington DC, United States, 345394, Eskimo male, 20 years old, Yukon River, Alaska, ?Historic). *(With permission of Don Ortner)*

IMMUNE JOINT DISEASE
Rheumatoid arthritis (RA)

Compared to osteoarthritis, in the archaeological record rheumatoid arthritis is rarely seen. Although, in skeletal material, the palaeopathologist sees only the bony changes of rheumatoid arthritis, it is a disease affecting multiple systems of the body (Cotran *et al.*, 1989: 1349). It is a chronic inflammatory disease of connective tissue and has adult and juvenile (Still's disease) forms; it is one of the erosive joint diseases. Around 1 per cent of people in the world suffer the disease and females are affected two or three times more than males, especially in their third and fourth decades of life (Resnick and Niwayama, 1995a: 867). RA is classified as an autoimmune disease (i.e. an individual develops antibodies to their own body tissues), and around 80 per cent of people with the disease have circulating antibodies called the rheumatoid factor. The factors initiating an autoimmune response in RA are unknown, but what is certain is that people with RA experience more chronic symptoms in colder climates and with specific diets (e.g. including large proportions of red meat and red wine). High protein and saturated fat diets are also implicated (Buchanan and Laurent, 1990: 83). It is estimated that a familial predisposition accounts for 60 per cent of disease susceptibility (Shipley *et al.*, 2002: 538), familial meaning that more members of a family have a condition than would be expected by chance (*Dorland's Pocket Medical Dictionary*, 1995). RA affects multiple synovial joints symmetrically, especially the small joints of the hands and feet, wrist, elbow, knee, shoulder and cervical spine; less commonly affected are the ankle, hip and sacroiliac joints. The synovial membrane is affected first; this thickens and forms a layer of granulation tissue called pannus, which spreads over the cartilage of the joint, eventually destroying it. The bone underlying the cartilage and adjacent to it is also damaged. Ligaments and tendons associated with the joint are affected, often leading to partial dislocation (subluxation) of some joints, especially the metacarpophalangeal joints. Bone is eroded at the joint edges and later on the joint surfaces, and there is usually an associated osteoporosis. People with the disease are weak, often have anaemia and suffer weight loss and muscular weakness. Swollen, stiff, painful joints lead to reduced function and severe deformity in later years. Fusion of joints is less common than in other similar joint diseases.

RA has rarely been identified convincingly in the archaeological record and it is likely that the disease may be mistaken for other joint diseases. Its rarity has induced studies of joints from known RA sufferers to ensure diagnostic criteria are correct for identifying cases in the past (Rothschild *et al.*, 1990; Leisen *et al.*, 1991). Many of the examples described in Ortner and Putschar (1981), Short (1974) and Steinbock (1976) are only identified as possible cases. Short (1974) has argued that it is a very recent disease. However, many of the early medical writers (e.g. Hippocrates in the fifth century BC) do refer to a disease which could have been RA – 'a form of arthritis generally showing itself about the age of 35, first involving the hands and feet, which become cold and wasted, and next the elbows, knees and hips' (Short, 1974: 196). This type of non-specific description is not very useful in tracing the history of RA. The first good description was given by Sydenham in 1676 (Buchanan and Laurent, 1990), and Garrod in 1859 gave the condition its name (Duncan and Leisen 1993: 600). Paintings of people with RA also appear from the late and post-Medieval periods in Europe (Dequecker, 1977), e.g. the Flemish painters between 1400 and 1700 (Klepinger, 1979 in Duncan and Leisen, 1993). Of course, the skeletal evidence is the primary evidence for the disease.

If the cases highlighted already in the literature are accepted, then the disease appears to have been present in Egypt in 5500 BC (May, 1897 in Duncan and Leisen, 1993). Leden *et al.* (1988 in Ortner, 2003) also describe possible cases of RA in Sweden, but these individuals also have spinal osteoporosis which is believed to 'protect' against RA (Shipley *et al.*, 2002). Bennike (1985) describes two cases from Denmark dated to AD 200–400 (mature male) and 1800–800 BC (female adult). Ortner and Putschar (1981) and Ortner and Utermohle (1981) describe another two examples in an Alaskan male and female, the latter dated to AD 1200; Lewis (1998) documents a 2,000-year-old adolescent from Louisiana, United States, with juvenile rheumatoid arthritis; and Kilgore (1989) reports on a possible case in an elderly female from Kulubnarti, Sudanese Nubia, dated to between AD 700 and 1450. In Britain, examples dated from the seventh century AD up to the nineteenth century have been reported, although some of these cases have now been disputed (discussed in Kilgore, 1989). Waldron and Rogers (1994) claimed their eighteenth- to nineteenth-century female case to be 'the first evidence of rheumatoid arthritis in the United Kingdom' (1994: 165, and Fig. 6.20). This was also quickly followed by a report by Hacking *et al.* (1994) of a female skeleton from the later fifteenth-century layers of a cemetery associated with Abingdon Abbey, Oxfordshire, England. Changes characteristic of 'probable' (1994: 255) rheumatoid arthritis were recorded and included marginal erosions of the bones of the left wrist, and the intercarpal, carpo-metacarpal, metacarpo-phalangeal and interphalangeal joints of both hands. Erosive lesions of the acromial surfaces of the acromio-clavicular joints and the margins of the humeral heads were also observed. Radiographically the cortices of the bones were thin, suggesting osteoporosis. Farwell and Molleson (1993) also report on twenty-seven cases of erosive arthropathy in the Romano-British cemetery at Poundbury, Dorset, England, and ascribe possible specific diagnoses to them; fourteen cases

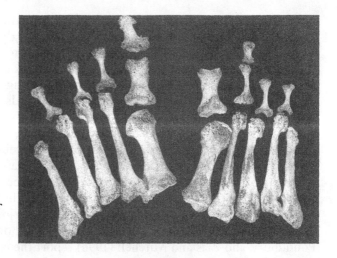

Fig. 6.20. Erosive lesions of the feet (metatarso-phalangeal joints) in rheumatoid arthritis (post-Medieval, eighteenth–nineteenth centuries AD, England). *(With permission of Tony Waldron and Juliet Rogers/John Wiley)*

are diagnosed as rheumatoid arthritic, out of 1,400 inhumations. Recent data from the Medieval site of Barton-on-Humber, England (Rogers, 2000: 174), indicates three individuals affected (0.2 per cent prevalence).

The rarity of the disease could be due to a number of factors. It may really be a recent disease, with the factors influencing its occurrence today absent in the more distant past. However, diagnostic confusion with other joint diseases, such as osteoarthritis, may be instrumental in the perceived picture. Other suggestions could be that the more severe and chronic bone changes do not appear to occur until later in life (did people live long enough to develop the disease?), or that the palaeopathologist just does not see the survival of enough of the small hand and foot bones from archaeological excavations and therefore does not see the evidence.

The three other joint diseases that must be considered in the differential diagnosis of RA are osteoarthritis, gout and psoriatic arthritis. In osteoarthritis there are usually no lytic lesions and the distribution pattern is often more asymmetrical. Gout has an asymmetric nature, 'overhanging edge' lesions (see below), and rarely has associated osteoporosis; it also predilects for the great toe joints. Finally, psoriatic arthritis (see below) is asymmetrical in occurrence, has 'pencil and cup' deformities at the joints, associated new bone formation and involvement of the sacroiliac joints, but rarely osteoporosis. Consideration of these very clear differences in character and distribution of lesions should make diagnosis straightforward; problems occur either when there are several different joint diseases present on the same joint, or when the skeleton is not complete and/or well preserved.

Psoriatic arthritis (PA)

The skin disease psoriasis occurs in 1 per cent of living populations, and around 5 per cent of sufferers develop joint changes (Rogers, 2000: 177). It has an association in 60 per cent of cases with the antigen HLA-B27 in the blood (Aufderheide and Rodríguez-Martín, 1998: 104), and people affected never have the rheumatoid factor in their blood. Although its cause is unknown, genetic, nutritional and infective factors may be instrumental in its development. The disease can affect any of the synovial joints, singly or multiply, and usually asymmetrically. Tendon and ligament attachments to bone may also be involved, with new bone formation or enthesophytes (Resnick and Niwayama, 1988: 1171). Males and females may be affected equally, and the age of onset is between 20 and 40 years (Rogers, 2000). The phalanges of the hands and feet become eroded at their joint surfaces and marginal to the joints, with development of 'pencil and cup' deformities in the distal interphalangeal joint, and the spine and sacroiliac joints can be affected, with ossification of vertebral ligaments. New bone formation on the shafts of the short bones of the hands and feet and around the joints is characteristic, and fusion of joints can occur. Few specific examples of psoriatic arthritis have appeared in the palaeopathological literature; perhaps some cases have been misdiagnosed as other erosive joint diseases or even leprosy (Rogers, 2000: 178). Farwell and Molleson (1993), however, list seven cases from Poundbury, and Zias and Mitchell (1996) report the condition in two males from the fifth-century AD site of the monastery of Martyrius in Israel.

Ankylosing spondylitis (AS)

Another of the autoimmune joint diseases is ankylosing spondylitis, or Marie–Strumpell's disease, named after the French and German doctors who first described the disease in the 1880s. It is a progressive inflammatory disease of unknown aetiology affecting the axial skeleton. Affected people have the HLA-B27 antigen in their blood (in up to 95 per cent of Caucasians with the condition (Shipley et al., 2002: 548)). People with AS are at risk from passing the gene to 50 per cent of their children; and then the children have a 30 per cent risk of developing AS (Shipley et al., 2002: 549). It affects males predominantly (5:1 male to female ratio (Rogers, 2000: 176)), with an age of onset of between 15 and 35 years. It is seen commonly in Caucasians and native American populations but rarely in Japanese or African groups; it is quoted to have an incidence of 0.1 per cent today (Resnick and Niwayama, 1988: 1105). The synovial and cartilaginous joints and entheses are affected and erosion and fusion of some of the joints, especially the sacroiliac joint, occurs; involvement of the sacroiliac joint is 'the hallmark of ankylosing spondylitis' (Resnick and Niwayama, 1988: 1112). The small joints of the spine fuse, and the vertebral bodies begin to fuse from the lumbar vertebrae upwards, not only via the joints, but also through ossification of the inter- and supraspinous ligaments (Fig. 6.21), formation of vertebral syndesmophytes (thin vertical outgrowths of bone) and ossification of parts of the outer fibrous layer of the intervertebral discs. As the spine fuses, the bodies remodel and their normal shape is lost; the ultimate appearance is smoothing and squaring of the vertebrae (Ortner, 2003: 572), or the 'bamboo spine'. Low back pain, limitation of chest expansion, immobility, weight loss and fever are some of the signs and symptoms. The hip, shoulder, knee, ankle, wrist, hand and foot joints are the most commonly affected peripheral joints of the body (Rogers et al., 1987) and appear to be affected in up to 50 per cent of people with the disease.

Cases of AS in the past have been described from Egypt, Nubia, Canada, the United States, Guatemala, France, Denmark and the UK, summarized in

Steinbock (1976) and Ortner (2003). It is possible that many cases of AS are not being diagnosed because of the problem of differentiating this condition from Forestier's disease (see below). However, several features can be used to distinguish the two conditions from each other, and from rheumatoid arthritis and psoriatic arthritis (Resnick and Niwayama, 2003). AS has significant erosions of the synovial and cartilaginous joints of the axial skeleton. PA involves the synovial joints of the appendicular skeleton and the cartilaginous joints of the axial skeleton, whereas both diseases promote erosion and repair of the entheses involved. Bony proliferation and fusion with no osteoporosis characterizes PA and AS, and in RA the cartilaginous joints may or may not be affected. If a complete skeleton is available for analysis, it should be possible to differentiate these erosive arthropathies.

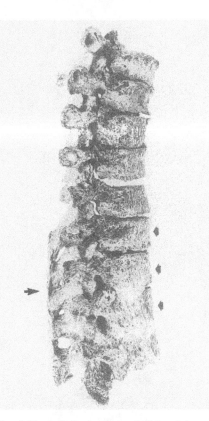

Fig. 6.21. Ankylosing spondylitis of the spine showing small syndesmophytes and ossification of the spinal ligaments (early Medieval, sixth–eighth centuries AD, Eccles, Kent, England).

Diffuse idiopathic skeletal hyperostosis (DISH)

Diffuse idiopathic skeletal hyperostosis (or Forestier's disease) also affects the spine, but it has very characteristic bony abnormalities elsewhere in the body that distinguish it from ankylosing spondylitis. Aufderheide and Rodríguez-Martín (1998: 97) rightly point out that 'it is not a true arthropathy' because it does not affect cartilage or synovium. It has been described in a Neanderthal skeleton from Iraq, dated between 40,000 and 73,000 years BP (Crubézy and Trinkhaus, 1992), the earliest known case. Although first described in 1950 (Forestier and Rotès-Querol) as a spinal disease, it has more recently become synonymous with extraspinal manifestations. Its specific cause is unknown, but it appears to be associated with obesity and Type 2 diabetes (Rogers and Waldron, 2001). Males are slightly more affected than females and the age of onset is usually over 50 years (Resnick and Niwayama, 1988: 1563). People affected are 'bone formers'. There is gradual and complete fusion of the spine (Fig. 6.22), particularly in the thoracic region, with retention of integrity of vertebral body surfaces, joint spaces and apophyseal joints. The anterior longitudinal ligament of the spine and paraspinal tissues ossify. The osteophytes produced are large and flow like

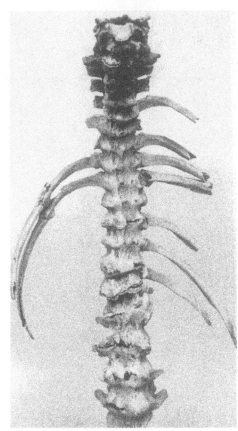

Fig. 6.22. Diffuse idiopathic skeletal hyperostosis involvement of the spine; note the flowing 'candlewax' new bone formation especially on the right side in the thoracic region, fusion of the spine, and some ribs (Roman, Droitwich, Hereford and Worcester, England).

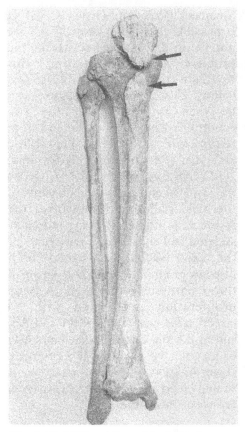

Fig. 6.23. Diffuse idiopathic skeletal hyperostosis: extra-spinal new bone formation at the knee joint (arrowed); same skeleton as Fig. 6.22.

'candlewax'; they are especially seen on the right side of the vertebral column at the level of the seventh to the eleventh thoracic vertebrae, and are probably prevented from developing on the left side because of the presence of the aorta (the major blood vessel of the body). Fusion of four contiguous vertebrae is necessary for a diagnosis. In addition, there are enthesopathies at tendon and ligament insertions (Fig. 6.23); it is not known whether these latter changes occur before or after spinal involvement but they are also necessary for a diagnosis. Cartilage also ossifies, especially in the neck and ribs. Pain, aching and stiffness are some of the symptoms of the disease.

DISH is found more in Northern European people (Julkunen *et al.*, 1971 in Rogers, 2000). Although not reported in high frequencies in the palaeopathological record to date, DISH is increasingly being seen in both monastic (Stroud and Kemp, 1993) and non-monastic cemetery groups (Waldron, 1993b). Its modern frequency is between 3 and 5 per cent, increasing to over 10 per cent in people over 65 years, whereas at Merton Priory in Surrey, England a frequency of 8.6 per cent was indicated in the forty-two skeletons examined, dated from the twelfth to sixteenth centuries AD (Waldron, 1985). It is suggested that a rich diet and lack of exercise predisposed people in the priory to obesity and late-onset diabetes. These high-status people may also have lived longer to develop the condition. However, Rogers (2000) notes that at Wells Cathedral in south-west England high status was more important than age in individuals diagnosed with DISH. Waldron (1993b) also reported on forty-seven skeletons with DISH excavated from the post-Medieval crypt at Christ Church, Spitalfields, London. The majority were male and of old age. Stroud and Kemp's study noted seven definite cases of DISH and a further eight individuals probably suffering from an early stage of the disease. All the skeletons were associated with Period Six of the site, that is the cemetery associated with the Gilbertine Priory of St Andrew, York, England. Janssen and Maat (1999) also report a 100 per cent frequency of DISH in twenty-seven canons from the Saint Servaas Basilica in Maastricht, the Netherlands, dated to 1070–1521. More recently Jankauskas (2003) documented the frequency of DISH in Iron Age to early modern period skeletons from Lithuania with defined social status, as indicated by grave structure and/or burial location. He found that it increased with age, was associated with males more frequently, and the frequency was highest in the high social status individuals (27.14 per cent) when compared to average or urban groups (11.86 per cent), and rural or poor groups (7.14 per cent). Nevertheless, it is suggested by Resnick and Niwayama (1988: 1600) that DISH 'may not represent a disease *per se* but rather a vulnerable state in which extensive ossification results from an exaggerated response of the body in some patients to stimuli that produce only modest new bone formation in others'.

Differentiating the bony abnormalities in DISH and AS is the first step to identifying the prevalence of both conditions in the past. DISH is usually found in older males and consists of characteristic thick, flowing spinal osteophytosis and enthesopathies extraspinally, but there is usually no fusion of the apophyseal joints or the sacroiliac joint. AS has thinner, vertically orientated spinal syndesmophytes, fusion of the apophyseal and sacroiliac joints and no extraspinal bone formation. Determining their specific aetiology in archaeological populations is more difficult than for modern groups, but the study of cultural factors at work in different populations with contrasting prevalence rates may shed light on the issue.

METABOLIC JOINT DISEASE: GOUTY ARTHRITIS

The final joint disease to be considered is much less common than many of the joint diseases already described. Gouty arthritis has a modern prevalence of between 1 and 3 per cent (Rogers, 2000: 173) and is increasing in frequency. For example, Rose (1975) documented a 10 per cent frequency in Maori males. It is characterized by a high level of blood uric acid (hyperuricaemia), caused by an excess of uric acid production or a reduced excretion by the kidneys. It affects males twenty times more frequently than females and occurs in older age groups (50 years +) (Resnick and Niwayama, 1988: 1619). There also appears to be a genetic predisposition in up to 20 per cent of cases (Aufderheide and Rodríguez-Martín, 1998: 108). Urate crystals appear in the synovial fluid of joints and lead to inflammation and erosion of cartilage and bone. The bone may be eroded on the joint surface, at its margins, or at a distance from the joint, producing overhanging bony lesions shaped like a hook. The joints affected are mainly those of the feet, hands, wrists, elbows and knees, with the first metatarsophalangeal joint (big toe) usually involved (90 per cent of cases); joints are affected asymmetrically. It is an extremely painful condition with swelling and redness of the joint affected. Urate crystals also accumulate in tissues associated with the joint, e.g. tendons and ligaments, and also away from the joints, e.g. in the fingertips and soles of the feet; these accumulations are called tophi. It is intermittent in its affectation, and it appears to be associated today with excessive alcohol intake and a rich high protein and fatty diet, diabetes and heart disease. The attribution to alcohol as a cause in the past is in part because during the distillation process a certain amount of lead was added in times long ago to improve the taste. The distillation process was also carried out in leaden vessels, a further source of the metallic poison. This lead, after prolonged and repeated ingestion, caused kidney failure and a consequent rise in blood uric acid concentration. It was not the alcoholic beverage *per se* but the lead which damaged the kidneys (Steinbock, 1976: 309).

Although the medical historical literature of gout goes back to the Hippocratic School and has been prolific ever since, the palaeopathological evidence is rare. The most celebrated example of gout is an Egyptian mummy of the Christian period in which actual deposits of urate crystals were identified (Elliot-Smith and Dawson, 1924). The osteoarchaeological evidence is no more than a few cases. Three male skeletons of the Romano-British period from Cirencester, England, dated to about AD 150, show the destructive features in several joints. Wells

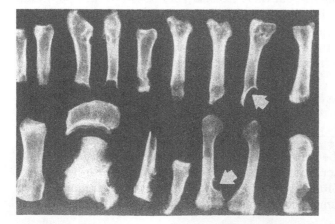

Fig. 6.24. Radiograph of erosive lesions in articular and para-articular surfaces (some arrowed) of the metatarsals, with sclerosis (Romano-British, fourth century AD, Cirencester, Gloucestershire, England).

(1982) considered these typical of gout (Fig. 6.24), although Rogers (2000: 173) is doubtful of the diagnosis of one skeleton. More recent data (Rogers, 2000) reports twelve individuals from St Peter's Church, Barton-on-Humber, Humberside, England, with gout dated from the tenth century AD to the post-Medieval period. In the mid-seventeenth century gout was treated with colichine, a purgative, with some effectiveness (Copeman, 1970 in Aufderheide and Rodríguez-Martín, 1998). Furthermore in Roman Gloucester, England, remains of this plant have been found, and this area of England (the Cotswolds) has always had a high frequency of gout (Wacher, 2000). Rothschild and Heathcote (1995) also found gout in 5.6 per cent of 250 skeletons from Guam, a Pacific Island, dated to AD 950–1450; along with Maori groups, Pacific Islanders have high frequencies of gout today.

This necessarily brief survey of some of the more commonly occurring and recognizable joint diseases visible in skeletal remains of past humans is but a small part of the total picture of the many hundreds of joint diseases known to modern medicine. No doubt more precision in diagnosis of specific aspects of these diseases in the past will be forthcoming since the diagnostic criteria are now better known. The further study of the skeletal manifestations of these diseases in living populations will aid in this goal. In addition, refinements in the correlation of osteoarthritis and activity are desperately needed to help place a perspective on lifestyle in past human groups. What people do for a living will affect their predisposition to any disease process and this information is, in effect, instrumental in the study of palaeopathology. In the absence of modern treatment, both drug and surgical, the symptoms of joint disease suffered by the elderly city dweller today are the same as those suffered by the elderly in the past. Unfortunately for the latter, they were denied the medical and surgical relief, such as joint replacement, and the creature comforts which we find so necessary in approaching old age.

CHAPTER 7

Infectious Disease

In demographic terms, infectious diseases . . . have likely claimed more lives than all wars, non-infectious diseases, and natural disasters taken together . . . as agents of natural selection, infectious diseases have played a major role in the evolution of the human species. (Inhorn and Brown, 1997: 31)

INTRODUCTION

In the past, the mortality, morbidity and misery wrought by micro-organisms must far have exceeded the consequences of warfare and famine. Today the degenerative diseases account for much illness in western society (e.g. see World Health Organization, 1997 which shows heart disease, cancer and strokes to be the biggest killers), and this is because people are living longer and have better access to health care (certainly in the western world). In the pre-antibiotic era, however, the infectious diseases occupied this position in the league table. Bacteria and viruses also accounted for most of the deaths in the past, although fungi and parasites also cause infections. It will be remembered that these deaths occurred at a much earlier age than today and this in part reduced the importance of the ubiquitous degenerative disease of the skeleton and cardiovascular system so familiar in the care of the elderly today. Infants and young children are particularly vulnerable to acute gastrointestinal and respiratory infection, and death from infections in these groups, even with modern care, is a high risk. It would have been much higher in antiquity without the availability of antibiotics and without the knowledge of correct rehydration procedures. It is likely, but without proof, that many of the young people represented by infant skeletal remains from archaeological contexts died as a result of acute fulminating infection before there was a chance for observable bone change to develop.

Until recently the western world felt that it had all but conquered the infectious diseases because of improvements in hygiene and sanitation, and the development of vaccination and antibiotics, but old infections are re-emerging and new infections are establishing themselves. For example, HIV (Human Immunodeficiency Virus infection) and AIDS (Acquired Immunodeficiency Syndrome), Rift Valley fever, Lyme disease and West Nile virus can be classed as new infections, although some have been around for more than a decade. West Nile virus, for example, appears to be favouring warmer climates, vulnerable human populations and unique bird and animal life in Latin America (Anasthaswamy, 2003). Re-emerging infections include tuberculosis, cholera and dengue fever. Barrett *et al.* (1998) document three periods in our history where infectious diseases increased or decreased. The first was the Neolithic revolution, when people started to farm and infectious disease increased. The second was at the time of industrialization in the mid-nineteenth century in both Europe and North America, when infections started to decline, probably as a result of an improvement in living conditions (although other parts of the world at this time did not benefit). The third is the current period of our history characterized by new infections, antibiotic resistance and re-emerging infections that were thought to have been controlled. Of course, the rise and fall of infectious diseases are affected by social inequalities today (Farmer, 1996), as they would have been in the past. In Britain, for example, from the 1850s onwards there were many social reforms to control infections and many infectious diseases declined from the second half of the nineteenth century. Today food poisoning, tuberculosis and HIV are the more commonly increasing infections, while childhood diseases such as mumps and scarlet fever have declined because of vaccination (Roberts and Cox, 2003). However, the public's declining confidence in vaccination is worrying (Motluk, 2002), and worldwide the development and distribution of vaccines is under threat (Rappuoli, 2002).

Factors responsible for the emergence and re-emergence of infections are many (see, for example, Morse, 1995; Farmer, 1996; Patz *et al.*, 1996; Barrett *et al.*, 1998). They include poverty, which leads to poor diet and depression of the immune system; this makes people more vulnerable to infections. Travel (Fig. 7.1) and migration put people into new environments with exposure to new pathogens to which they do not have any immunity, and they may also bring infections with them. For example, SARS (Severe Acute Respiratory Syndrome) made its appearance in China, Hong Kong and Singapore in 2003 but then spread by interpersonal contact to other countries. Climate change as seen in increasing temperatures allows pathogens to survive and be disseminated in otherwise foreign territory; this includes mosquito-borne diseases such as malaria and water-borne infections. Climate can also have an effect on the success of agriculture, and failure of crops could lead to malnutrition and predisposition to infectious disease. Human manipulation of the environment and technological and industrial

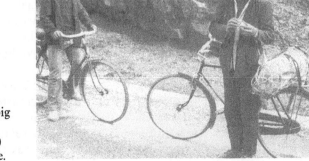

Fig. 7.1. China: taking a pig to market; movement of people (and their animals) potentially spreads disease.

development may create situations that favour the rise of infections. For example, dam building, agriculture and irrigation have led to Rift Valley fever and schistosomiasis in the area of development (Morse, 1995), and mass food processing can lead to contamination of meat and *Escheria coli* infection. Finally, micro-organisms can adapt and change because they are constantly evolving. Antibiotic resistance in the human population today is an illustration of this adaptation, and has affected the population's ability to overcome infectious disease. Other less commonly reported methods of transmitting infectious disease have also illustrated to us the hazards of living in the modern (and often terrifying) world: the transmission of hepatitis B from a suicide bomber to a victim via a bone fragment (MacKenzie, 2002), *E. coli* potentially passing to customers in restaurants from the dirty fingernails of chefs (Randerson, 2002), and of course the ever potential threat of biological warfare using infectious agents (Cohen, 2003). All serve to remind us of the still ever-present problem of infectious disease.

The fearful epidemics of plague, smallpox, malaria and other rapidly transmitted infections were responsible for large numbers of deaths in their years of visitation. The ever-present and much less spectacular bacteria and viruses would have accounted for the more or less constant and unremitting death rate of the non-epidemic periods. Most of these latter micro-organisms cause infection today just as in antiquity, but the advent of penicillin and synthetic antibiotics largely eliminated their fatal effect, even though antibiotic resistance later developed. The exception, of course, is still the virus, because, as yet, no universal antiviral agent comparable in efficacy to antibiotics has been discovered. In this context, however, the immunization of the young against such viral diseases as poliomyelitis, measles, mumps and rubella has reduced their incidence and has, therefore, reduced the impact of these diseases in the overall population profile of morbidity and mortality (although there are problems with vaccination programmes). In the current western generation, children physically disabled by poliomyelitis are a rarity, and the congenital defects resulting from maternal rubella are no longer a problem. The significance of vaccination against smallpox in the elimination of this disease is paramount in the history of disease control (Jenner, 1801) and, as a result of this and other public health procedures, the world is now free of this scourge of antiquity. But these are measures of prophylaxis. Once contracted, the misery, morbidity and, at times, mortality due to viral infection are unchanged. There can surely be no better illustration than the spreading global infection of HIV and its attendant clinical manifestation of AIDS (Grmek, 1989; Inhorn and Brown, 1990; Sattienspiel, 1990). Perhaps overall well-being and improved health status in developed countries today reduce the mortality risk of many viral infections, but in the less fortunate and subsistence-level communities of the world the morbidity and mortality of such commonplace viral infections as measles and influenza are considerable. Clearly, there are many factors responsible for lessening the effects of bacterial and viral infection during the passage of time and with increasing material prosperity. Doubtless the overworked and inadequately fed child living in the squalor of an early nineteenth-century industrial town was, relatively speaking, more susceptible to respiratory and gut infections than was the child of a Neolithic village. The general tendency has, however, been one of improving living and health standards since distant antiquity.

Infections are caused by bacteria, viruses, fungi and parasites. Whether a person is vulnerable to contracting an infection will be determined by intrinsic and extrinsic factors (Inhorn and Brown, 1997). Age, sex, genetic predisposition, nutritional factors, immune status, climate, trade and sanitation are just some of those factors that may help a person resist an infection or enhance their chances of contracting it. Infective lesions of greater or lesser degree are a very common finding in skeletons from archaeological sites. If we consider the infections from which we all suffer today, it is apparent that the vast majority only affect the soft tissues of the body. Even without active treatment, most of these infections resolve within a short time. Influenza, measles and bronchitis are but a few examples of this wide spectrum. More sinister, and often fatal in the absence of treatment, are appendicitis, meningitis and pneumonia. In all these examples, resolution of infection, or death of the individual, occurs fairly rapidly and long before the infective process will have spread to the bones. The infection, be it of soft tissue or bone, is associated with the pathological process of inflammation. Inflammation is a cellular reaction to the invading organism, be it virus, bacterium or larger parasite, and is manifest in the signs and symptoms of pain, swelling, tenderness and raised temperature. Inflammatory bone lesions are, therefore, manifestations of chronic, that is long-standing, infection in a person with a relatively healthy and strong immune system. However, many infectious diseases induce bone changes in only a small percentage of people (e.g. 3–5 per cent in tuberculosis), and males, females, different age and ethnic groups are affected in differing frequencies. For example, middle-ear infections are seen frequently in native Americans, Maoris and Melanesians (Polednak, 1989: 99). This is not to say that the micro-organisms causing the acute infections mentioned above do not cause bone inflammation under different circumstances, but that there is just not enough time for bone change to develop during the short course of these acute infections of soft tissues. By and large, the infective bone lesions of antiquity were created by bacterial and not viral infection, since the latter were more rapidly resolved or fatal, and did not lead to the chronic invasive process as did bacteria. There are certain characteristic infective lesions of bone that are caused by specific bacteria, so that the type of change noted in the bone can be ascribed to the particular bacterium, and the change is unlike that produced by other bacteria. These specific infections of tuberculosis, treponemal disease and leprosy will be considered later. The bone changes of infectious disease may be bone formation, bone destruction or a mixture of both. The bone formed will be woven in character at the start of the infective process, but will, with time, become incorporated with the underlying cortex and become mature lamellar bone. The distribution of these lesions, when compared to clinical cases of known infections, can help to identify more closely the infection from which the person was suffering. While most researchers in palaeopathology use macroscopic and radiological approaches to identifying infections, more recent work has emphasized the histological approach – i.e. taking thin sections of bone and observing infectious-related features under a microscope (e.g. see Schultz, 2001 for an overview).

NON-SPECIFIC INFECTIONS

The pathological changes of bone brought about by many bacteria are relatively non-specific; infection by one bacterium is indistinguishable from that of another. The bacteria commonly involved today in bone infection around the world are staphylococci, streptococci, pneumococci and, less commonly, the typhoid bacillus. Although unproven, it is likely that these were the cause of the non-specific infections of bone in antiquity, although fungi, parasites and viruses can affect the bone and marrow (Resnick and Niwayama, 1995b: 2326). In modern pathological bone specimens such individual bacteria may be isolated and identified. Clearly, however, the micro-organisms responsible for infections in antiquity do not persist in preserved skeletal remains, although specific parasites have been identified in mummified human tissues, and advances in techniques for identification of pathological processes suggest that molecular structures of bacteria do survive in some circumstances (Salo *et al.*, 1994). It is, however, impossible to distinguish the particular bacterial cause by the macroscopic examination of the non-specific bone changes from the past.

Each layer of bone may be involved in a bone infection. The terms periostitis, osteitis and osteomyelitis are applied to infection of the periosteum, cortex and medullary cavity respectively. Since bone is a single biological unit, such an arbitrary division of terms is perhaps artificial (Sandison, 1968) and some researchers use the single term osteomyelitis for all infective lesions of bone. However, a semantic discussion is inappropriate since both systems of description have their uses. Furthermore, differentiating between osteitis and osteomyelitis in clinical contexts using radiological analysis 'can be extremely difficult' (Resnick and Niwayama, 1995b: 2326), and 'radiography is usually unable to delineate the precise extent of the infection (suppurative periostitis, osteitis, or osteomyelitis)'. Furthermore, periostitis, if subtle in occurrence, will not be identified on a radiograph. In archaeologically derived skeletal material, identifying periostitis is usually straightforward, while identifying osteitis on the basis of thickening of the cortex is usually either by observation of the cross section of the bone or through radiographic techniques; osteomyelitis is often diagnosed on the basis of enlargement of the bone compared to its opposite (if a paired bone), the presence of a sinus (cloaca), an involucrum and a sequestrum. Radiological features will show destruction and formation of bone and areas of increased density. It should also be noted that, in archaeological material, if all layers are affected, it is usually impossible to be certain in which layer the infection started. Furthermore, these non-specific changes may be part of one of the specific infections discussed later. The following discussion will focus on osteomyelitis and periostitis.

Osteomyelitis

In osteomyelitis, the pathological process is one of bone destruction and pus formation, and simultaneous bone repair. In consequence, an individual bone frequently becomes enlarged in part or whole and is deformed from its healthy state. The bone destruction is manifest as pitting and irregularity of the bone surface and, possibly, cavity formation within the bone interior. This cavity, which is a pus-containing abscess, may gradually and progressively penetrate the compact bone wall and discharge pus into the surrounding body tissues. There is then to be found a clear and smooth passage between the surface of the bone and the internal abscess cavity. The longitudinal and transverse spread of bacteria and, hence, inflammatory process in bone is via microscopic channels known as Haversian and Volkmann's canals, which are found in all sites of compact bone. Thus the pathogenic micro-organisms are spread (from the initial focus) through the length and breadth of individual bones, producing satellite abscesses which may ultimately coalesce. More rarely the abscess may remain localized and contained within the bone interior and be undetected except by radiography or by bone section. Such a restricted cavity is known as a Brodie's abscess, and represents a site of active infection (Resnick and Niwayama, 1995b: 2327).

The bone-repairing process in osteomyelitis is seen as the development of new plaques of bone on the surface. The new bone applied to the original external cortical surface is produced by bone-forming cells (osteoblasts) in the innermost layer of the periosteum. Initially the new bone lacks an organized microstructure and is termed woven bone. Later, through the complementary action of bone absorptive cells (osteoclasts) and osteoblasts, the woven bone gradually assumes the microstructure of mature compact bone. In unresolved and progressive osteo-myelitis the original bone may become more or less ensheathed by a cast of new bone. In such an extreme circumstance the ensheathed old bone may die. Gradually and intermittently this bone, the so-called sequestrum, may extrude with the pus to the bone exterior. In consequence the enlarged, deformed and mechanically less efficient new bone, called the involucrum, may be the sole structural support of the specific skeletal part. All of these aspects of the pathological process of osteomyelitis are seen in Fig. 7.2 and its associated radiograph (Fig. 7.3) and Fig. 7.4.

Since these pathogenic, or disease-producing, bacteria are not normal inhabitants of bone, they must be transported to the affected bone from some other part of the body. In this process two main methods are involved. Probably the more common in pre-antibiotic antiquity was the transport of bacteria by the bloodstream from some primarily infected area, probably the throat, ear, sinuses or chest. Acute bacterial infections, usually by

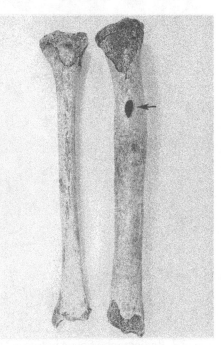

Fig. 7.2. Osteomyelitis of the right tibia (with opposite to compare), which is thickened and deformed (and longer). Sinus is arrowed into abscess in the interior of the bone (early Medieval, sixth–eighth centuries AD, Eccles, Kent, England).

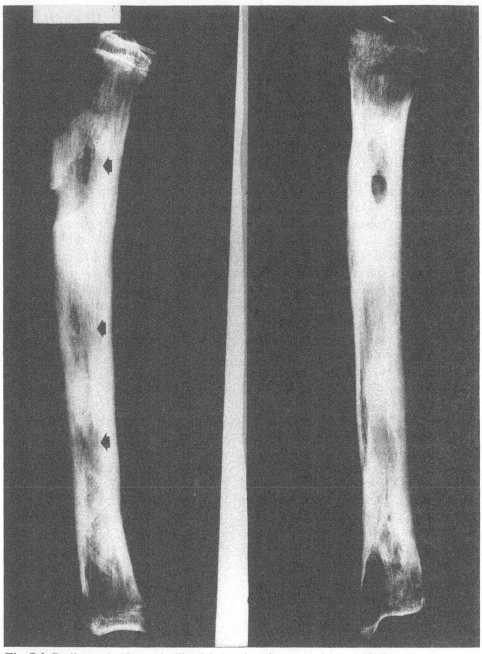

Fig. 7.3. Radiograph of bone in Fig. 7.2 showing abscess cavities within bone interior (arrowed).

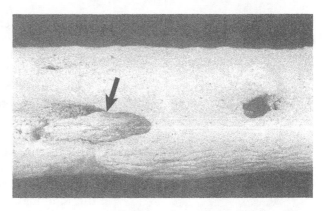

Fig. 7.4. Long bone with osteomyelitis showing extruding sequestrum on the left. *(NMNH 378243)*

streptococci, staphylococci, pneumococci or *Haemophylus influenzae*, of the tonsils, middle-ear cavity and bronchial tree are common clinical conditions today and must have been so, particularly in the young, in antiquity. *Staphylococcus aureus* is usually responsible for 90 per cent of cases of osteomyelitis today (Ortner, 2003). In the pre-antibiotic era these relatively insignificant infections of today would be followed by bacteraemia and the consequent haematogenous spread of the pathogens to more distant organs, including bone. For reasons unknown, in immature individuals, commonly only a single bone was involved in this secondary infective process. However, in adult individuals multiple bones were affected in approximately two-thirds of cases (Ortner and Putschar, 1981). Clearly, these were generalized infections only secondarily affecting bone, but commonly only a single bone was involved. No doubt the individual so afflicted was seriously ill with fever, pain and immobility in the affected area. However, in order for the bone changes observed in skeletal remains to take place, recovery from the generalized infection must have occurred. Septicaemia, or blood infection, is a very serious problem even today and carries a significant mortality risk. The infection was much more serious before the advent of antibiotics and survival in antiquity was probably uncommon. Maybe such cases of osteomyelitis in the archaeological record testify to the survival of the fittest.

As will be noted, osteomyelitis resulting from this mode of transmission is more common in some bones, notably the femur and tibia, than others; the reason for this is obscure. The initial site of secondary infection in a long bone is frequently at the metaphysis near the growing end in children, but the shaft is equally affected in adults. This zone of the bone has the most abundant blood vessel supply and is therefore most likely to receive the bacteria and sustain the inflammatory process. Less commonly, osteomyelitis may result from the direct injection of bacteria from the skin surface during a penetrating bone injury. The normal skin surface is a regular harbour of potentially pathogenic bacteria. In this case the bone infected is the bone injured and the injury will be evident. Infection may also spread from a severe and chronic skin lesion such as a leg ulcer, down through the deeper tissues, eventually infecting the bone surface itself (Fig. 7.5). In this case of direct spread, the site is usually one in which the underlying bone damage is fairly superficial. The third method of infection may be through

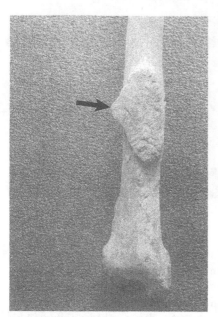

Fig. 7.5. Tibia with focal new bone formation, suggesting an overlying leg ulcer (late Medieval, twelfth–sixteenth centuries AD, Chichester, Sussex, England).

trauma or surgery. Both these latter methods of infection tend to be localized in extent compared to infection transmitted via the bloodstream (Ortner, 2003: 181).

Osteomyelitis tends to affect children between the ages of 3 and 12 years when bone growth is most active (Jaffe, 1972, in Aufderheide and Rodríguez-Martín, 1998), but people of all ages can potentially contract the infection. The knee, the distal third of the tibia and the proximal third of the femur are the most common sites for osteomyelitis, in that order, and account for 80 per cent of the cases in clinical contexts (Aufderheide and Rodríguez-Martín, 1998).

Periostitis

One non-specific inflammation of bone should be examined separately. Occurring in many populations through time and globally is bone surface inflammation, or periostitis, which is not part of a total osteomyelitic process of the bone. The inflammatory process is manifest as fine pitting, longitudinal striation and, eventually, plaque-like new bone formation on the original cortical surface (Fig. 7.6). Most common on tibiae, this is probably because it lies close to the skin surface and can be subject to recurrent minor injury. However, Resnick and Niwayama (1995c: 4435) note that there can be many causes of this non-specific bone change, but infection or trauma are usually implicated. Assessing what specifically caused periostitis in the past is problematic, but some researchers have made suggestions on the basis of histological observations (e.g. Schultz, 2001). Other reasons suggested for a predilection for the tibia include: a cooler surface temperature, which renders the tibia more susceptible to infection; that the surface of the tibia has a physiologically inactive surface, leading to bacterial colonization (Steinbock, 1976); and that blood tends to

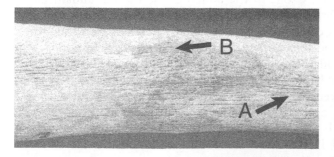

Fig. 7.6. Long bone showing striated new bone formation (A) and an area of porous woven bone (B).

stagnate in the lower legs, allowing bacteria to accumulate. Whatever the cause, it seems that bacteria probably lead to the changes seen in skeletal material and tibial infections are more commonly seen in settled communities practising agriculture. Alternatively, varicose veins, venous stasis and consequent ulceration of the lower leg may lead to chronic focally induced low-grade inflammation. Tibial periostitis has also been suggested by many to be one of the many indicators of stress visible in the skeletal record (Goodman *et al.*, 1988). Such trauma, stress or, in some few cases, varicose ulceration may have given rise to this superficial and insignificant inflammation of the lower legs. However, it was unlikely to produce the debilitating and even crippling symptoms of the more severe osteomyelitis.

Infective lesions are common findings in palaeopathology, especially periostitis. As with most diseases, the prevalence varies from place to place and from era to era. It was noted in an early Indian group from Texas that 18.3 per cent of adults possessed inflammatory bone lesions (Goldstein, 1957). In contrast, an analysis of 912 skeletons from South Dakota demonstrated a prevalence of infective disease of bone of 1.75 per cent (Gregg and Gregg, 1987). It has also been shown in an examination of early American populations that the frequency of bone-infective lesions rises with an increasing population density, for example at Dickson Mounds, Illinois. A decrease in longevity was also noted here (Lallo *et al.*, 1978). Comparisons between hunter-gatherers and agriculturists, certainly in North America, where nutritionally deficient maize was the main staple, have often shown an increase in infections with the transition to agriculture (see studies in Cohen and Armelagos, 1984) and through time (Steckel and Rose, 2002). However, this relationship is not globally consistent, nor is it always seen in North America (Larsen, 1997). Differences in non-specific infectious lesions between sex, age and status groups have also been documented. For example, Larsen (1998) examined skeletons from pre-agricultural, agricultural and European contact from the Georgia Bight, United States. He found an overall increase in periostitis with time but a greater prevalence in late Contact males than females. Ortner (1998) and Stini (1985) have documented the stronger and more effective female immune response in infectious disease, and Stinson (1985) has noted that males are less buffered against the effects of the environment than females. Furthermore, many bone diseases seem to affect males more than females (e.g. see table 6.2 in Ortner, 1998). All these factors have implications for discussions of male and female differences in infectious disease in past populations; if females have stronger immune responses, then either we may see no bone changes, or we could see chronic bone damage, the latter indicating survival through the acute stages of the disease into the chronic period when bone is affected. However, other, extrinsic, factors are also at work to cause differences. For example, Powell (1988, in Larsen, 1997) found no statistically significant differences in infection between elite and non-elite individuals, but did find some differences when considering individual bones affected. However, Lewis (2002a) in her analysis of urban and rural Medieval sites in England found that the high status children from Christ Church Spitalfields, London, had significantly less periostitis, osteitis and osteomyelitis. She suggests that this may be because these children were less exposed to causative factors.

Increased population density probably encourages the rapid and extensive spread of bacteria and viruses throughout communities. Associated with a rising population of increasing social and economic complexity, there is an extension of trade networks. The area of trading increases and the frequency of trade contacts increases. Such networks act as routes for the transmission of infectious diseases between communities. Thus the factors affecting the prevalence of infective disease in populations are multiple and varied. The immune status of the host, the virulence of the organisms, population density, malnutrition and ecological considerations are all significant, and the relationship between infection and malnutrition is well known.

A number of areas of the skeleton that may show evidence of non-specific infection have received attention mainly since 1990. Because they are seen in particular bones, their aetiology has been explored in more detail. They include infections of the facial sinuses, middle-ear and mastoid processes, the endocranial surface of the skull, and the ribs, which will be discussed below (for rib lesions see the section on tuberculosis).

Sinusitis

Although bone infection induced by blood-borne bacteria was a common disease in antiquity, the bacteria having probably spread from a primary focus of infection in the throat, ear, nasal sinuses or chest, the evidence for these infections in skeletal remains is sparsely reported. The nasal sinuses are air-filled cavities within the bones of the face and are therefore difficult to inspect, the more so since they are often full of soil on excavation. Probably, therefore, many examples of sinusitis from the past have been undetected, and the infection may not have been uncommon at all (but see Wells, 1964c, 1977). However, intact maxillary sinuses may be accessed by drilling a small hole at the back of the sinus and using an endoscope (Roberts et al., 1998). In dry bone, the condition is recognized as irregular pitting and new bone formation on the interior surface of the sinuses, and Boocock et al. (1995) have classified the changes (Fig. 7.7).

In a recent comparative study of skeletons from a Medieval rural population and a contemporaneous urban population, Roberts et al. (1998; and see Lewis et al. 1995) found evidence of maxillary sinusitis in 72 per cent of individuals from the urban site of St Helen-on-the-Walls, York, England, the highest frequency of all four sites examined (see Table 7.1). Overall, urban sites had more sinusitis than rural, but there was no consistent patterning of sex differences. Evidence for dental-disease-induced sinusitis was seen more frequently in the rural sites (Fig. 7.8). The cemetery of the site of St Helen-on-the-Walls served a poor parish in York, and it was suggested that the urban environment in which these people lived was such that pollutants in the atmosphere, both internally in the home (burning fuel for warmth and cooking), and externally in the parish, induced the high rates seen here. The higher male frequency could also be explained if one assumes the men worked in the neighbouring parish of Bedern, where contemporary historical data document polluting industries such as tanning and founding, which would have introduced particulate pollution. While high urban rates have been seen in Medieval England, Roberts and Lewis (2002) have also documented low rates in the urban London site of Christ Church, Spitalfields, in both children and adults (18 per cent and 3 per cent respectively of individuals). These frequencies may

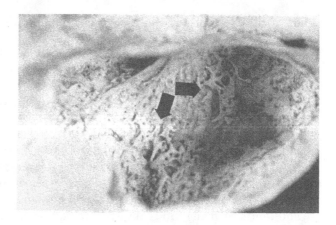

Fig. 7.7. New bone formation on the floor of the maxillary sinus (late Medieval, twelfth–sixteenth centuries AD, Chichester, Sussex, England).

well reflect that these high-status individuals were protected from the urban polluting environment. Indeed, McDade and Adair (2001) have highlighted the need to look at the finer detail and variables acting in urban and rural environments to explain differences in health in modern populations.

Other studies of sinusitis are rare, but Merrett and Pfeiffer (2000) note 50 per cent of 207 individuals with the condition in the ossuary at Uxbridge in Southern Ontario, Canada, attributing it to indoor pollution, and Panhuysen *et al.* (1997) record nearly 40 per cent of 126 individuals from Medieval Maastricht in the Netherlands with maxillary sinusitis, citing dental diseases as a major cause. More rare is the evidence for frontal sinusitis, as illustrated in a Bronze Age Spanish individual (Armentano *et al.*, 1999). Certainly from British contexts, maxillary sinusitis appears to increase through time with little evidence being reported in prehistory (Roberts and Cox, 2003), although one must consider, first, that, if intact sinuses present themselves for examination, the evidence may be invisible and, secondly, many researchers do not look for the evidence anyway. Certainly in the inhospitable climate of northern Europe today, the disease is common; allergies, indoor and outdoor environmental pollution, and house dust are just

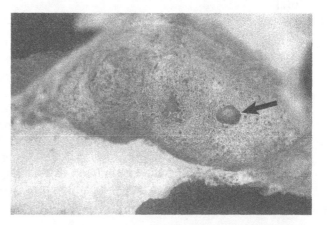

Fig. 7.8. Pitting of the floor of the maxillary sinus and an oro-antral fistula (connection between the mouth and the sinus) (early Medieval, eighth–tenth centuries AD, Raunds 5087, Northamptonshire, England).

some of the predisposing factors. For example, fuels such as wood, animal dung and coal can have considerable polluting effects (Ezzati and Kammen, 2001). The man or woman of the past, huddled around open hearths in the smoky, ill-ventilated houses of antiquity, would surely have been susceptible to this chronic and irritating infection (see Camuffo *et al.*, 2000 for a seventeenth-century Italian example of pollution). Such environments would favour the production and stagnation of pus within the sinuses and so create the chances of inflammation. In addition, today, and, as we have seen, in the past, the maxillary sinuses may become infected by dental disease and, more specifically, by the perforation into them of a dental abscess of the upper jaw (Lundberg, 1980). For example, Gregg and Gregg (1987) identified dental abscesses as the predominant cause of maxillary sinusitis in a series of Crow Creek Indians.

Pollutants of many kinds invade our indoor and outdoor space today, even though, certainly in the western world, there have been attempts to curb pollution. However, continuing pollution is noted for various reasons, and occupational health, respiratory and general medical journals are full of papers exploring the cause of respiratory problems. For example, studies have found a significant association between the occurrence of respiratory health problems in people exposed to wood smoke (e.g. Larson and Koenig, 1994; Riojas-Rodriguez *et al.*, 2001), and to particulate pollution from agriculture (McCurdy *et al.*, 1996). The documenting of maxillary sinusitis (and rib periostitis) as indicators of respiratory infection needs more attention in palaeopathology in the future.

Table 7.1 Frequency of maxillary sinusitis in four Medieval sites from England (individuals affected with at least one sinus to examine) (%)

Site	Overall frequency	Male	Female	Dental
Urban				
St Helen–on–the–Walls, York	72	76	69	9
Chichester, Sussex	55	55	55	7
Rural				
Wharram Percy, Yorkshire	51	44	60	27
Raunds Furnells, Northamptonshire	50	53	46	35

Note: Dental = evidence of dental-disease-induced sinusitis

Middle-ear and mastoid infection

In modern medical practice middle-ear infection, particularly in childhood, is a frequent occurrence (Daniel *et al.*, 1988). Untreated, the disease frequently settles following perforation of the eardrum and the discharge of pus from the abscess beneath. It must also have been common in the past. Indeed, studies of historical data for medicine from the Byzantine period (AD 324–1453), essentially a continuation of Hellenistic and Roman medicine, note the occurrence of ear disease and treatments (Lascaratos and Assimakopoulos, 1999). Perforation of the eardrum, otitis media, deafness and haemorrhage from the ear are included in the list of conditions, and herbal, animal and mineral remedies were recommended and applied via ear drops, poultices or special instruments. In the purely skeletal remains of the past, the delicate membranous eardrum does not survive and the evidence of perforation is therefore lost. However, during autopsy of the Egyptian mummy Pum II, perforation of the preserved eardrum was noted (Benítez, 1988). The pain endured by this man (dated to about 170 BC) was, no doubt, relieved by the perforation from the infected middle ear.

Although no observable bone change is associated with this acute infection of the middle-ear cavity, persistence of the infection with a chronically discharging ear induces inflammatory changes in the walls of the middle-ear cavity, and in the small bones (auditory ossicles) of the middle ear. Otitis media primarily affects children (Daniel et al., 1988; Aufderheide and Rodríguez-Martín, 1998), may be caused by a range of bacteria, and can be complicated by septicaemia, deafness and meningitis. It is estimated that 80 per cent of all children today will experience one or more episodes of acute otitis media, and children between the ages of 6 months and 24 months are most susceptible (Kemink et al., 1993: 866). A genetic predisposition, cleft palate and environmental factors such as climate, poverty and poor sanitation have been implicated as causes. Microscopic examination of ear ossicles has been carried out by Bruintjes (1990) on skeletons from a Medieval leprosy hospital cemetery. Erosive lesions suggesting chronic middle-ear infection were recorded in 51 per cent of ear ossicles (136 ear ossicles from 89 individuals were recorded; 69 had erosive lesions). For the general population such a frequency of middle-ear infection would, indeed, be very high and Bruintjes's findings are probably biased by the coincident infection of leprosy in the individuals examined. Dalby et al. (1993) found a lower frequency in Roman-British individuals of 1.5 per cent of 61 ear bones. Studies of ear bones from archaeological contexts need more attention, although survival for examination, through burial and excavation, remains a problem.

Infrequently, the middle-ear abscess bursts through into the surrounding bone and produces mastoiditis. Unresolved, this infection of the mastoid bone behind the ear ultimately bursts through the bone surface either to the exterior or to the interior of the skull. This opening in the bone surface should be visible, provided that bone preservation is good (Fig. 7.9). If the mastoid discharge was into the interior of the skull, the outcome was probably fatal, but if to the exterior then recovery was likely. In this disease, the infection may be recognized in archaeological material. However, this area of the skeleton is frequently damaged by burial and so the mastoid bone and its abnormal hole may be destroyed.

The disease is more common in children today than in adults and, because the air cells in the process develop at the same age as the high rate of mastoiditis, this condition can impair normal development (Aufderheide and Rodríguez-Martín, 1998: 253). However, from an examination of skeletons from Merovingian cemeteries in southern Germany dated to between AD 500 and 700, it was suggested that middle-ear infection was more common in older people and in the lower classes of society. On this finding, it was proposed that environmental

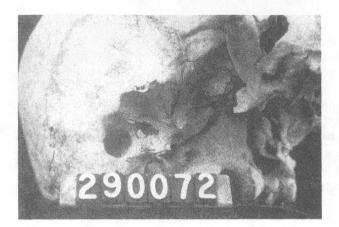

Fig. 7.9. Total destruction of the mastoid process, probably as a result of mastoiditis (hunter-gatherer from Indian Knoll, Kentucky, United States). *(National Museum of Natural History, Washington DC, United States, 290072)*

factors of poor diet and general health in infancy predisposed to the later development of the condition in the lower social groups (Schultz, 1979). Child skulls from the past are rarely well preserved because of the thinness, size and fragility of the bones, and this, too, makes diagnosis of the disease in antiquity difficult. Nevertheless, the diagnosis has been made on these criteria in several skeletons from Egypt, Europe and Britain (e.g. Wells, 1962).

However, the earliest recorded and most celebrated case is in the skull of Rhodesian Man from Broken Hill, Zambia. It is dated to the Upper Pleistocene, possibly about 40,000 years BP (Day, 1977), and clearly demonstrates a perforation of the left mastoid area. It is tempting to imagine this man suffering from intense earache and fever unrelieved by the benefits of modern medicine. Relief only came to him with the perforation of the mastoid bone and the discharge of pus. The long-term consequence was deafness, but this was preferable to the fatal alternative. However, doubt has been cast upon the diagnosis of mastoiditis in this early skull and the changes may, indeed, represent nothing more than post-mortem damage (Montgomery *et al.*, 1994). This is a further demonstration of the difficulty of palaeopathological diagnosis. Further evidence of mastoid infection may be found from radiography of the mastoid bone, because infection induces changes in the pattern and size of the air-containing spaces within the bone (Gregg and Gregg, 1987: 72–4; Dalby, 1994).

Endocranial changes

The presence of new bone formation on the endocranial surface of skulls from archaeological contexts has received attention in recent years, and some have suggested that it may represent inflammation of the meninges, or meningitis (Fig. 7.10). There is, however, debate as to whether a person could have survived in the past long enough for bone change to occur. This may, of course, have been influenced by the virulence of the organism, which may have been lower in past times (Roberts, 2000c). Meningitis is an 'acute inflammation of the meninges, the membranes covering the brain and spinal cord' (Patterson, 1993: 875). It is usually the result of a bacterial or viral infection (and can be a complication of infections such as tuberculosis), but may be caused by other

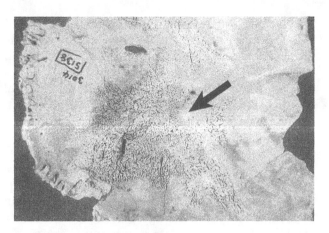

Fig. 7.10. New bone
formation on the endocranial
surface of skull (early
Medieval, eighth–tenth
centuries AD, Raunds 5138,
Northamptonshire, England).

non-infectious conditions such as a tumour. It is most commonly seen in winter and
spring (Patterson, 1993: 875). Of course, since the development of antibiotics, it has
been possible to treat bacterial-induced meningitis; this was not an option in the past,
however. In palaeopathological contexts Schultz (2001) notes that meningeal reactive
new bone can be divided histologically into new bone formed as a result of
haemorrhage (e.g. in a head injury) and as a result of inflammation (e.g. meningitis),
and from a mixture of the two. He also records an increase in meningeal conditions
from the Bronze Age to the late Medieval period in Central Europe and Anatolia,
relating this to changes in socio-economic and political conditions. However, most
researchers do not have access to such types of analyses and therefore can only record
the new bone presence (and character) or absence, and hypothesize about its cause. In
Britain, the earliest example of endocranial new bone formation comes from
Hambledon Hill, Dorset, dated to the Neolithic period (McKinley, 1996). However, in
a more extensive population study, Lewis (2002a) noted frequencies of 14 and 15 per
cent of individuals for children from two Medieval rural sites, and 12 per cent for an
urban site (Spitalfields). However, the urban children of Christ Church, Spitalfields,
London had only a 4 per cent frequency rate, correlating well with the low rate of
sinusitis observed and the infrequency of respiratory infection in general. More
recently, Lewis (2004) has cautioned the assigning of a specific cause to endocranial
new bone formation because of its multifactorial aetiology.

Soft-tissue infection

Unfortunately, direct evidence of infections of soft tissues alone is not found in the
dry bones of archaeology. Of course, one of the most devastating of soft-tissue
infections in the past, particularly in Medieval western Europe, where it killed
one-third of the population and devastated the socio-economic situation, was the
Black Death, a 'massive epidemic of plague' (Park, 1993: 612), which is caused by
Yersinia pestis. There have been three human pandemics, the Justinian plague
(sixth–eighth centuries AD), the Black Death (fourteenth–nineteenth centuries
AD) and the modern plague (nineteenth century AD to the present day), and it is
only recently that its genome sequence has been established (Parkhill *et al.*, 2001).

It is reliant for its transmission in humans on the rodent flea *Xenopsylla cheopsis*, which transfers the infection from rodent to human by biting the latter. The disease does not affect bone but has recently been identified using ancient DNA analysis of victims of plagues of the fourteenth, sixteenth and eighteenth centuries in Provence, France (Drancourt *et al.*, 1998; Raoult *et al.*, 2000). However, an alternative way of exploring the plague and other soft-tissue infections, without the use of ancient DNA analysis, is to consider whether there are differences between the demographic profiles of known plague and non-plague victims, or whether specific age and sex groups were more targeted by the bacteria. For example, Margerison and Knüsel (2002) and Gowland and Chamberlain (2005) have recently considered the profiles of the fourteenth-century plague cemetery of the Royal Mint in London. The latter found that Bayesian statistical analysis can be used to define and explain the age profile of a population affected by the plague. Additionally, historical data may testify to the use of a particular graveyard or pit for plague victims, as happened in both the cases in London and France.

A brief glimpse of these soft-tissue infections of antiquity usually comes from the detailed dissection and microscopic examination of mummies (see Aufderheide, 2003 for an overview). Pneumonia, which doubtless was a major cause of death in the past, has been diagnosed in Peruvian mummies from Chiribaya (AD 1000–1470), but this disease must have been more common in northern climates. An examination of an Aleutian mummy has demonstrated the lung changes of lobar pneumonia in which the normal aerated lung tissue becomes solid. The bacteria responsible have been partially identified and multiple abscesses secondary to septicaemia have been seen (Zimmerman *et al.*, 1971). By such meticulous post-mortem examination, the precise cause of death of this late seventeenth- or early eighteenth-century man was determined. A preserved Byzantine body has also produced evidence of appendicitis (Rowling, 1961), which may have been fatal, and a fungal infection (*Aspergillus*) has been identified in the lung of an Egyptian mummy by Horne (1995 in Aufderheide, 2003). The evidence of viral infection is more rare still even in mummified remains, and one example in the palaeopathological record classically rests upon the appearance of the skin of the mummy of Rameses V. The blistering lesions on the face, lower abdomen and thighs have been attributed to smallpox, but this diagnosis has not been supported by laboratory tests (Hopkins, 1980). A more recent study has identified smallpox in a sixteenth-century mummy (Fornaciari and Marchetti, 1986). Smallpox is no longer an active infection and survives only in laboratories (Crosby, 1993). It is caused by *Variola major* or *minor*, is transmitted by droplet infection and is therefore a population density disease, and it is focused primarily on the respiratory tract. It would obviously need highly populated urban areas for its success and it is unlikely it was a problem until urbanization occurred (Crosby, 1993). A skin infection of bacterial cause has also been identified in a mummy of the Tiahuanaco culture from Peru (Vreeland and Cockburn, 1980). This disease, called verruga, is confined to Peru and neighbouring countries and is characterized by multiple fungating skin lesions.

As already stated, viral infections are almost invariably fatal or resolved before inflammatory reaction in bones occurs. Direct evidence of viral infections is therefore absent in human skeletal remains, although some diseases may be indicative of viral infection – for example, Paget's Disease (Altman, 1993; Aufderheide and Rodríguez-Martín, 1998: 413). However, the potential for their identification may lie in the application of modern DNA extraction methods to human remains from archaeological and later contexts. There has already been some research in this area. In 1998 Marota *et al.* (1998) isolated hepatitis E virus RNA sequences from scrapings from the linen bandage applied to an ulcer on the left arm of a sixteenth-century female mummy from Naples, Italy. Furthermore, influenza virus RNA was isolated from lung tissues of two victims of the 1918 'Spanish' influenza pandemic (Reid *et al.*, 1999). Ribonucleic acid is a single strand molecule similar to the structure of DNA, a double-stranded molecule that contains the genetic code, which is essential for protein synthesis (Jurmain *et al.*, 1997: 43). This research shows the potential for identifying viral infections in the future in both archaeological and historical contexts, and assessing their role in the evolution of the human population. However, some examples of viral infections do exist in the skeletal record; a seventeenth-century example of osteomyelitis due to smallpox has been identified (Jackes, 1983). To date, this is unique, but controversial.

Another viral infection, this time of the central nervous system, is poliomyelitis, which is manifest clinically as the paralysis of one or more muscle groups. It is spread via the faecal-oral route (Wyatt, 1993), and may be accompanied by meningitis and fever. The disease is most common in early life, hence its alternative name of infantile paralysis. Paralysis of a limb at this early age results in muscle wasting and possible failure of growth of the bones in the affected limb. Therefore, marked inequality of bone growth in opposite limbs, a feature which will be apparent in skeletal remains, may suggest poliomyelitis. Other causes, both infective and traumatic, of bone growth arrest or muscle wasting must be considered (as noted by Brothwell and Browne, 2002), but poliomyelitis in recent times has been the most common cause of this phenomenon. Probable diagnoses of poliomyelitis in antiquity have been made on such features in a Neolithic skeleton from Cissbury, Sussex, England, a Bronze Age skeleton from Barton Bendish, Norfolk, England (Wells, 1964a), and a fifteenth-century male from Portugal (Umbelino *et al.*, 1996). The disease has also been diagnosed in Egyptian mummies, but the club foot of the Pharaoh Siptah, usually attributed to poliomyelitis, is more likely attributable to a congenital abnormality (Sandison, 1980a). Fig. 7.11 illustrates a male, aged 20–30 years at death, from Raunds, Northamptonshire, England, dated to the eighth to tenth century AD, in which there is failure of growth of the right femur, tibia, fibula and foot. Although possibly associated with tuberculosis, poliomyelitis is the most likely cause of this crippling abnormality. In summary, the skeletal and mummified evidence of non-specific bacterial and viral infection must represent only a very small part of the total spectrum of infectious disease to which people in antiquity were exposed.

In the present context of soft-tissue inflammatory disease, it is appropriate to consider the industrial contamination of the past. Clearly the problem is not infective, but the inhalation of dust particles does induce inflammation, as we have seen in sinusitis (above). Silicosis results from the inhalation of sand particles. It may represent the industrial contamination of a stone-worker's life,

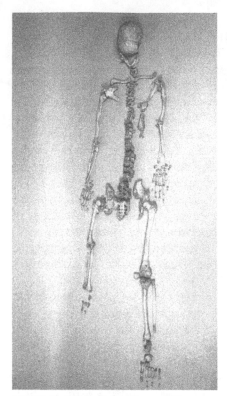

Fig. 7.11. Probable poliomyelitis showing failure of right leg to grow (early Medieval, eighth–tenth centuries AD, Raunds, Northamptonshire, England).

but in the Egyptian man or woman of long ago it may have been a consequence of living in a desert (Cockburn *et al.*, 1975). Only a quantitative assessment of silica content of lungs in a large number of mummies will separate those cases exposed by occupation to increased dust inhalation.

In ancient mummified human remains, carbon particles in the lungs can also be common findings. However, this element causes little in the way of physical incapacity when compared with silica. No doubt, when people enjoyed the comforts of companionship by the open fire, they exposed themselves not only to maxillary sinusitis but also to smoke inhalation and deposition of carbon particles in their lung tissue, a problem called anthracosis. Evidence for this is, of course, absent in skeletal remains of the past. The dissection of Aleutian mummies and the rehydration and microscopical examination of lung tissue has, however, demonstrated the changes of anthracosis (Zimmerman *et al.*, 1971), and a severe case in a young woman was also identified from Barrow, Alaska (Masters, 1984 and Thompson and Cowen, 1984 in Aufderheide, 2003). In the harsh, cold climate of northern Europe, deposition of carbon particles may have encouraged the chronic bronchitis so familiar to the modern medical practitioner. It should not be imagined, however, that the town residents of the past blithely accepted as inevitable the smoke of coal fires. There was agitation against this atmospheric pollution. So loathsome was it to Queen Eleanor that she felt obliged to leave Nottingham and its smoke in 1257 (Brimblecombe, 1976). It is perhaps only in the clean-air zones of the twentieth- or twenty-first century city that the results of at least 700 years of protest have been achieved, although many cities of the world are suffering increasing problems, and developing countries appear to be hardest hit.

SPECIFIC INFECTIONS

Specific infections are considered to be those where the exact causative organism is known, and there are three that have plagued populations through long periods of our history. They are tuberculosis, leprosy and treponemal disease. They may produce similar changes to the skeleton (for example, the lower legs in treponemal disease and leprosy, and the facial damage in leprosy and venereal syphilis). It is therefore important in palaeopathology to consider the distribution and nature of the presenting bone lesions. All three increased through time until the advent of chemotherapy in the twentieth century, but patterns of rise and decline in developing and developed countries today vary considerably and are very much related to poverty, poor living conditions and diet, and access to health care.

Tuberculosis

A queue of afflicted people awaiting the royal touch and the gold angel (or 'touch-piece') is one of the many aspects of the Medieval court (Crawfurd, 1911). Possibly originating in the reign of Edward the Confessor (AD 1003–66) (Mercer, 1964), this practice of the monarch touching individuals afflicted with King's Evil no doubt increased the royal claim to divine right. King's Evil was a term applied to scrofula, the tuberculous infection of the lymph nodes of the neck (Wiseman, 1696). The number of people 'touched' in the Medieval period may attest to the problem in France and England, but whether all the people actually had tuberculosis is debatable. Evans (1998) records that Charles II (1662–82) touched 92,102 people in his reign, and the seventeenth century saw its highest popularity. By the early nineteenth century the practice had waned.

A disease of considerable antiquity, tuberculosis increased steadily in prevalence in England, and by the seventeenth century it was responsible for 20 per cent of all deaths in London in non-plague years (Clarkson, 1975). The deaths were said to be due to consumption, a term which implies pulmonary tuberculosis or primary lung infection. However, by modern standards, diagnostic accuracy in the seventeenth century was probably poor. Many cases diagnosed as consumption may not have been tuberculous; these people may have been suffering from bronchitis or non-tuberculous pneumonia. The signs and symptoms of breathlessness, coughing up blood and other lung disease indicators would have made diagnosis a problem without the aid of modern diagnostic methods. However, the application of the term consumption does imply that tuberculosis at this time was a well-recognized and common disease. The London Bills of Mortality, written records of death, allow such figures to be known; doubtless other large centres of the English population suffered similar problems. No wonder then that Elizabeth I ordered that the weight of the gold touch-piece given to sufferers of King's Evil was to be reduced. With such an increase in tuberculous patients, England's exchequer stood to lose a great deal! It must be remembered in this context, of course, that many of the tuberculous men, women and children did not possess the manifestations of King's Evil. Cervical lymph node enlargement is merely one of the several presentations of tuberculous infection in humans.

Roberts and Buikstra (2003) have documented the increasing problem of tuberculosis, which now causes 3 million deaths per year and 8 million new cases. Among the many causative factors, the main ones responsible for its re-emergence are HIV/AIDS, poverty, antibiotic resistance, pleasure and business travel, and migration, often from war-torn areas of the world. Of course, for some, transmission of tuberculosis from animals presents a problem, along with poverty, and these two factors probably contributed most to its occurrence in past populations. Today, the presence of HIV and poverty weakens the immune system and makes people more susceptible to infections, while travel and migration may expose people to tuberculosis in a newly visited place. Additionally, people who are fleeing from conflict usually end up living in poverty, and access to health-care facilities may not be possible for the poor generally.

In 1882 the German bacteriologist Robert Koch discovered the bacillus responsible for tuberculosis. Since then the bacterium has been further investigated and classified, and there are now known to be several types of this bacillus. These types, together with others of similar characteristics, including the bacillus of leprosy, belong to the genus *Mycobacterium*. The relationship between the mycobacteria of tuberculosis and leprosy may be responsible for the historical differences between the two diseases (Grmek, 1983: 198–209; Manchester, 1991: 23–35); this will be considered later. The organisms *Mycobacterium tuberculosis, bovis, africanum, cannetti* and *microti* make up what is called the '*Mycobacterium tuberculosis* complex' and are closely related. *M. bovis* and *tuberculosis* cause tuberculosis in mammals, including humans, *M. africanum* in humans in some African countries, and *M. microti* in voles (Vincent and Gutierrez Perez, 1999). The *M. avium* complex is also described as causing tuberculosis in humans (Davidson, 1993), but also chronic bronchitis and pneumoconiosis (Wolinsky, 1992). Therefore, *M. tuberculosis* and *M. bovis* are the main organisms considered responsible for tuberculosis in humans for our purposes. These types may represent an evolutionary chain in the development of *Mycobacterium tuberculosis*, or the origin of the types may have been from a common mycobacterial ancestor millennia ago. However, recent work on the genomic structure of tubercle bacilli certainly indicates that *M. tuberculosis* did not evolve from *M. bovis* at the time of the domestication of animals, as was previously assumed (Brosch *et al.*, 2002).

Bovine tuberculosis is, as its name suggests, a disease of cattle but also of many other mammals, spreading secondarily to humans (O'Reilly and Daborn, 1995). It is probable, therefore, that a necessary condition for its transference from animal to human is the close association between the two (Fig. 7.12). Indeed it is found in North America that the prevalence of human tuberculous vertebral lesions increased as native American populations became more settled and dependent on agriculture (Roberts and Buikstra, 2003). Since domestication of animals is a feature of the Neolithic period in Europe the advent of bovine tuberculous infection in humans may be coincident with this phase of animal husbandry. It was about 10,000 years ago that people in different parts of the world began to settle in larger groups to produce their own food and domesticate animals and plants (Renfrew and Bahn, 1991). In the Near

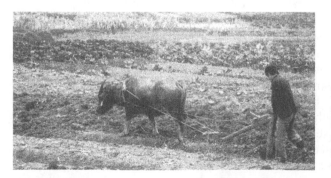

Fig. 7.12. China: ploughing; a close association between humans and their animals may have enabled tuberculosis to be transmitted.

East farming is evident by 8000 BC, with sheep and goats domesticated. By 6500 BC Northern Europe, the Mediterranean and India had adopted farming, and cattle had been domesticated in India. Plant domestication started in south-east Asia around 5000 BC and in sub-Saharan Africa by the third millennium BC. Domestication of plants and animals in the Americas started in South America by around 8000 BC, and in Central and North America by the seventh millennium BC and 1500 BC, respectively. Smith (1995) suggests seven primary areas of the world where domestication took place independently: the Near East 8000 BC, South China 6500 BC, North China 5800 BC, sub-Saharan Africa 2000 BC, South Central Andes in South America 2500 BC, Central Mexico 2700 BC and the eastern United States 2500 BC. Considering the areas of first domestication of animals and the establishment of settled communities, we would naturally expect the first evidence of tuberculosis to occur there in humans and other animals. Unfortunately the evolution and history of tuberculosis cannot yet be definitively written because several of these areas (notably China and sub-Saharan Africa) have not had any systematic analyses of skeletal remains for the evidence, so we do not know if there are any skeletal data to contribute to discussions. However, there is evidence in the Near East dated to $c.$ 3100 BC (Ortner, 1979) and the Americas from $c.$ AD 700 (Allison et al., 1981), although none of this evidence is as early as the dates for domestication cited above.

Of course tuberculosis can also be contracted by wild and feral animals, and therefore the argument that it was domesticated animals that introduced the bovine form of the infection to humans cannot necessarily be upheld. It is also apparent that mycobacterial species appeared first some 15,300–20,400 years ago, well before the domestication of animals (Kapur et al., 1994). Nevertheless, it should also be noted that domesticated cattle are believed to be the animals most infectious to humans (Grange, 1995). While archaeozoologists unfortunately have not produced very much evidence at all for tuberculosis in wild or domesticated animals from archaeological sites (plagued by problems of diagnosis (see O'Connor, 2000 for an overview)), we do have the human skeletal evidence for tuberculosis to confirm its presence in early settled agricultural communities. A rare example of tuberculosis in an animal was documented recently in a sixteenth-century Canadian Iroquoian context. Hypertrophic osteopathy in a dog as a result possibly of tuberculosis was diagnosed, and then confirmed using ancient DNA analysis (Bathurst and Barta, 2004). Furthermore, we also have evidence from historical texts that animals did get sick in the past, with Columnella (first century AD) describing tuberculosis specifically (Pease, 1940; Swabe, 1999). We must also not forget that other products of animals with tuberculosis may have been utilized in the past, such as dung for fuel and building rendering, and transmission to humans remains a problem in the developing world where tuberculosis in cattle is not controlled (Thoen and Steele, 1995). Furthermore, working with animals and their products, past and present, potentially exposes humans to tuberculosis – e.g. tanners, veterinary surgeons, butchers, zookeepers and farmers. However, the spread from infected animals to humans is largely by the drinking of infected milk and the eating of infected meat. Clearly, immediate and widespread animal infection and subsequent human infection with bovine tuberculosis could not have occurred with the advent of animal domestication; such a feature is not a biological reality. However, at present it is not known from archaeological evidence if the human form actually preceded the bovine form as a major infecting organism for humans.

Whatever its source, and whatever its evolutionary pathway, the tubercle bacillus capable of infecting humans has created chronic, endemic and widespread suffering in human populations throughout time. It is a truism that the introduction of a new infection into a human population produces a disease which is severe and often fulminating. This statement usually refers to a disease that is already endemic in a different group. To what extent this applies in tuberculosis, a disease totally new to humans, is of course not known. If the premise is correct, then the pathological changes of tuberculosis in very early eras must surely have been acute, of soft tissue only, and possibly fatal. The bone changes indicative of long-standing chronic disease would have been unlikely to develop until later generations of the population had developed some immunity and the infection was less virulent (Bates and Stead, 1993). Thus, the evidence from this time may not have survived in skeletal remains (see Wood *et al.*, 1992). However, research using ancient DNA analysis is now able to detect disease in skeletal and mummified remains showing no signs of tuberculosis (e.g. see Faerman *et al.*, 1999).

The human form of the infection is spread from human to fellow human. The infected person coughs and exhales bacilli, and their sputum and other excreta may contain bacilli which are capable of survival outside the body for some time (Fig. 7.13). The healthy person, particularly a child, coming into contact with these vehicles of infection may become tuberculous themselves. This then is a disease of closely gathered groups; in essence an urban disease. While originally it was suggested that the human-type bacillus was a micro-evolutionary development of the bovine type, and may have been the end of the tuberculous chain, Brosch *et al.*'s (2002) research rather overturns this hypothesis, as we have already noted.

The pathological changes of tuberculous infection occur in several areas and organs of the body, determined, to some extent, by the type of infecting bacillus and its portal of entry. For example, pulmonary tuberculosis is the common mode of infection by the human-type bacillus. The stomach and intestinal tract are the sites common to the bovine type. Bovine infection is more common in children than in

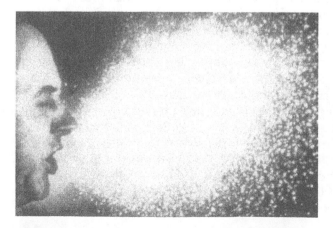

Fig. 7.13. Exhalation of droplets containing the bacilli of tuberculosis, and inhalation by others, allow the infection to spread between humans, but also between humans and their animals. *(With permission of Pia Bennike)*

adults, a fact possibly related to the consumption of milk in infancy. It should also be noted that bovine tuberculosis can be transmitted to humans via droplet infection.

The evidence for tuberculosis in antiquity mainly rests, as with most diseases, on the recognition of skeletal change, although ancient DNA analysis has, to date, focused mostly on diagnosis of TB (see Roberts and Buikstra, 2003). The evidence from mummified soft tissue is a significant but numerically small contribution to the picture of early disease (but see Aufderheide, 2003 for a summary in mummies). Tuberculosis may be primary, and is usually contracted in childhood in people who have never been exposed to tuberculosis before; the person either survives or dies. Post-primary or secondary tuberculosis occurs when a latent infection in a person is reactivated (perhaps because the immune system has become depressed), or the person is infected again with another large or repeated dose of tubercle bacilli. It is in the secondary form that skeletal changes occur. Apparently *M. bovis* tends to produce bone changes ten times more often than *M. tuberculosis* (Stead, 2000), but,

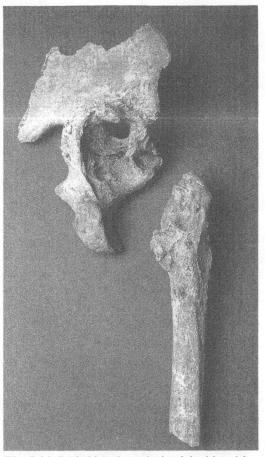

Fig. 7.14. Probable tuberculosis of the hip with extensive destruction of the femoral head and acetabulum with evidence of healing (late Medieval, twelfth–sixteenth centuries AD, St Oswald's Priory, Gloucester, Gloucestershire, England).

whatever the source of the infection, tuberculosis spreads to the bone from its original entry to the body via the bloodstream and lymphatic system. The skeletal features of tuberculosis are osteomyelitis which, largely because of the site in the body, is diagnostic. The areas of the hip joint and knee joint are the most commonly affected areas outside the spine, and spread of the infection through the blood to the joint, or spread of an adjacent lesion, leads to its establishment. This osteomyelitic process occurs at the ends of these long bones and frequently affects the joints themselves (Fig. 7.14) producing a septic arthritis, with characteristic destruction of the joint surfaces progressing ultimately to fibrous fixation (ankylosis) of the joint. However, a diagnosis of tuberculosis made on such evidence is usually tentative and may be confused with the other causes of osteomyelitis and arthritis. Unlike the

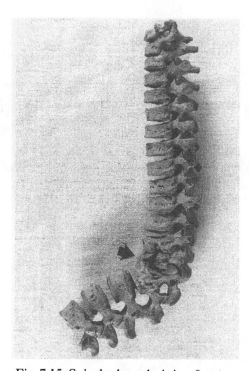

Fig. 7.15. Spinal tuberculosis in a 9-year-old child (National Museum of Natural History, Washington DC, United States, 327127, Pueblo Bonito, New Mexico, AD 950-1250). *(With permission of Don Ortner)*

degenerative arthritic diseases, the tuberculous involvement is usually of one joint only and the bone destructive process is more marked than the bone reparative process. In the context of palaeopathology, most diagnoses of tuberculosis are made on the presence of significant lesions of the spine.

Skeletal damage ocurred in 3–5 per cent of people in the 1940s and 1950s with tuberculosis (Resnick and Niwayama, 1995d: 2462). However, recent work has shown that this rate may be much higher, certainly for children (Bernard, 2003). Any bone of the body can be affected but involvement of the spine is present in 25–60 per cent of all cases of skeletal tuberculosis and it is not surprising therefore that this part of the skeleton is important in palaeopathological diagnosis, as noted above. The changes in the spine are usually found in the lower thoracic and upper lumbar vertebrae and between one and four vertebrae are involved. The involvement is often severe, with abscess formation within the body of the vertebrae, perforation of the abscess into the chest or abdomen, collapse of the affected vertebrae and the subsequent bony fixation of several pieces of the vertebral column. A characteristic feature of tuberculosis of the spine is the early involvement, by destruction, of the discs between the individual vertebrae and the relative absence of change in the neural arch, the most posterior part of the

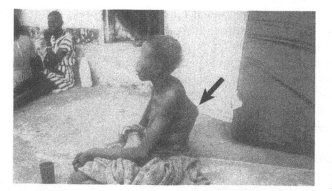

Fig. 7.16. Spinal tuberculosis in the living. *(With permission of Peter Davies)*

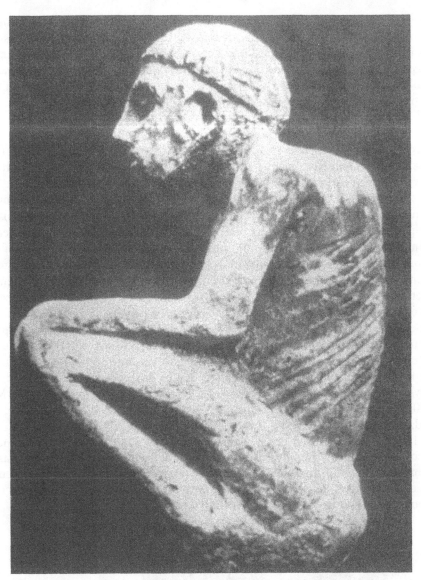

Fig. 7.17. Possible tuberculosis shown in the spine of this Egyptian clay statuette found in a clay bowl (height 20cm); supposed predynastic (4500–3000 BC); note also emaciated body (ribs) and sunken cheeks.

individual vertebra. Although they may be confused with other diseases causing spinal collapse, such as traumatic crush fractures and malignant disease (see Roberts and Buikstra, 2003: table 3.2), these spinal features of tuberculosis are known as Pott's disease (Figs 7.15 and 7.16). Sir Percival Pott, a surgeon at St Bartholomew's Hospital, London, described the condition in a monograph in 1779. The spinal collapse results in an angular deformity of the spine so frequently portrayed by authors and artists as the hunchback (Fig. 7.17). However, for reasons of diagnostic uncertainty, many of these portrayals may not be tuberculous. A person with osteoporosis of the spine may present a similar deformity. Spinal tuberculosis may also be complicated by an abscess in the psoas muscle anterior to the spine, and also by spread of the infection posteriorly to cause spinal cord compression. Weakness, numbness or paralysis of the lower limbs and unsteady gait, with loss of urinary control, may be sequelae of spinal tuberculosis (Luk, 1999).

Before we leave the changes of spinal tuberculosis, mention must be made of recent comments about the possibility of identifying this spinal infection in its early stages of development before spinal collapse and kyphosis. Baker (1999) described destructive lesions in the anterior vertebral bodies, which were suggested to be early evidence of tuberculosis. Subsequent work (Haas *et al.*, 2000) has successfully extracted ancient DNA of the *Mycobacterium tuberculosis* complex from skeletons with these lesions. However, as will be discussed below, this does not prove that the lesions are tuberculous. Furthermore, if one considers the normal development of the spine, in juvenile skeletons (where most of these lesions occur) these remnant holes of development are noted. As a person ages, the remnant features remodel and will disappear. Perhaps persistence of them into older adulthood could indicate a pathological cause, but, as yet, this evidence must be considered suspicious as a diagnostic criterion for early tuberculosis.

Because the spinal collapse of tuberculosis is identical in human-type and bovine-type tubercle bacillus infection, it is not known whether these early sufferers in antiquity contracted their infection through ingestion or inhalation, although ancient DNA analyses are now able to differentiate the two forms (e.g. Mays *et al.*, 2001). However, recent research (Kelley and Micozzi, 1984; Molto, 1990; Pfeiffer, 1991; Wakely *et al.*, 1991; Kelley *et al.*, 1994; Roberts *et al.*, 1994; Sledzik and Bellantoni, 1994; Roberts, 1999; Lambert, 2002; Santos and Roberts, 2001) has demonstrated criteria for the skeletal identification of pulmonary infective lesions. Although not definitive in aetiology, this work suggests that pulmonary infection by tuberculosis may cause an inflammatory response on the visceral surfaces of ribs (Fig. 7.18), but making a direct link is currently impossible, even using ancient DNA analysis (Mays *et al.*, 2002).

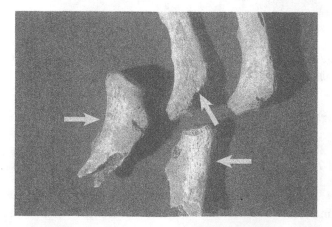

Fig. 7.18. New bone formation on the visceral surfaces of ribs (Romano-British, fourth century AD, Cirencester 189, Gloucestershire, England).

There are other non-specific indicators of tuberculosis that have been identified recently and that also deserve discussion (although they remain controversial), endocranial new bone formation as a response to tuberculous meningitis being one (see above and Hershkovitz *et al.*, 2002). Tuberculosis of the skin (*lupus vulgaris*) may also lead to destructive changes in underlying bone, usually in the facial area, and the pleura (membranes covering the lung tissue) may become calcified as a result of tuberculosis and other lung conditions (see examples in Roberts and Buikstra, 2003). These, however, are rare occurrences, archaeologically speaking, although they may be found together at one site, thus increasing the likelihood that tuberculosis may be present in the population (e.g. see Molnár and Marcsik's 2002 study of seventh–ninth-century Hungarian skeletons, where rib lesions, calcified pleura, endocranial new bone formation and spinal changes were found). The bone changes of secondary hypertrophic osteoarthropathy (HOA) as an indicator of tuberculosis have also been studied. New bone formation as a response to pulmonary conditions, including tuberculosis, can occur, mainly in the proximal and distal diaphyses of the tibiae, fibulae and radii with the femora, humeri, metacarpals, metatarsals, carpals, tarsals and phalanges being less affected (Resnick and Niwayama, 1995c). Some work identifying this condition in skeletons with known causes of death has been done (Rothschild and Rothschild, 1998; Santos, 2000), but very few cases have been identified archaeologically. More recent work, however, has used ancient DNA analysis of tuberculosis to correlate the infection with the changes of HOA (Mays and Taylor, 2002). While these non-specific indicators of tuberculosis must be considered in future studies of the infection, they should never be taken as definitively indicative of the disease. Nevertheless, Larsen (1997) suggests that, if a large number of skeletons from a site have, for example, rib changes, and there is definitive evidence of spinal tuberculosis, then correlating rib changes with tuberculosis may justified.

Early historical evidence for tuberculosis in the lymph glands of the neck dates back to 1550 BC in the Egyptian Ebers medical papyrus (Evans, 1998), and a medical text in China dated to 2700 BC suggests similar evidence (Keers, 1981). In India, the Rig Veda, a Sanskrit hymn dated to 1500 BC, describes phthisis, another term for tuberculosis of the lungs (Evans, 1998). More frequent references to tuberculosis appear in Classical antiquity from the fifth century BC, for example, in Hippocratic writings, and the later (ninth- and tenth-century) Arabian writers Rhazes and Avicenna also describe what appears to be tuberculosis. Naturally, as time went by and tuberculosis increased in frequency, references by writers, and drawings and paintings by artists, proliferated. Of course, historical data potentially provide us with much more evidence for tuberculosis than is seen in the skeletal record, although it can be more difficult to be sure that tuberculosis is being described or illustrated. The evidence from human remains for this devastating infection has recently been reviewed (Roberts and Buikstra, 2003) and the reader is referred to this source. What follows is a summary of the data from the Old and New Worlds. The earliest evidence of tuberculosis in human remains is from Italy, dated to the fourth millennium BC, and consists of a skeleton with the destructive and collapsed spinal lesions characteristic of Pott's disease (Formicola *et al.*, 1987). There is also a figurine (Fig. 7.17) of similar date from Egypt exhibiting spinal angulation and excessive weight loss which may represent advanced tuberculosis (Morse *et al.*, 1964). Perhaps more than any other form of evidence in the history of disease, such ancient figures are poignant reminders of the sufferings of our ancestors, although their interpretation as specific indicators of tuberculosis is debatable. Skeletal data suggest that tuberculosis became a major problem for humans in the later Medieval period in Europe and after AD 1000 in North and South America, although earlier evidence does exist. The earliest cases, as noted, come from Italy and are dated to the 5800±90 BP, or the Neolithic period (Canci *et al.*, 1996), while Egypt has produced evidence dated 4500 BC (Morse *et al.*, 1964). Neolithic cases from Spain and Poland complete the early evidence. In Britain the first evidence comes from the Iron Age site of Tarrant Hinton, Dorset, and is dated to 400–230 BC (Mays and Taylor, 2003). However, figures increase significantly from the twelfth century onwards in Britain and the rest of Europe. In the New World the earliest evidence of tuberculosis comes from South America, from Caserones in Chile, and is probably dated to around AD 700 (Allison *et al.*, 1981). It is suggested that here llamas may have been the source for the infection, and a higher frequency in males at some sites may support the argument that llama herding was a male occupation (notwithstanding the fact that both inhalation and ingestion routes would have been possible). There are few data from Central America except on its western side (probably as a result of trade from south to north America), and more data after AD 1000 in the south-eastern part of North America. Thereafter the infection continued to rise as population density increased in both the United States and Canada.

During succeeding periods the disease has become worldwide and even within living memory has been a scourge and a fear of humans. In the wake of the increasing phenomenon of HIV infection and AIDS, tuberculosis is once again increasing in incidence as a human disease (see summary in Roberts and Buikstra, 2003). The unfolding story is not yet told. The tuberculous victims of antiquity must have suffered the lingering ill-health, the gnawing and unassuaged bone pain of infective involvement and the extreme emaciation of advanced tuberculosis. No doubt also the human-type infection of the lungs produced the breathlessness, distressing cough and bloody sputum of pulmonary tuberculosis.

It is not surprising then that in the nineteenth and twentieth centuries the unfortunate sufferer of tuberculosis was confined to a sanatorium. Rest, fresh air, material welfare and segregation were perhaps the underlying principles of sanatoria before the advent of antibiotics (see MacDonald, 1997 for a personal

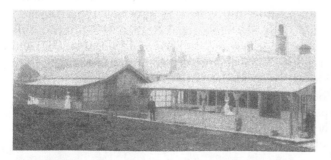

Fig. 7.19. Sanatorium in Keighley, West Yorkshire, England; note the verandas where patients were exposed to the elements. *(With permission of Ian Dewhirst)*

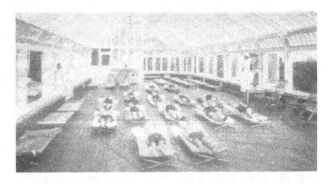

Fig. 7.20. Sun lounge at
Stannington children's
sanatorium near Morpeth,
Northumberland, England.
*(With permission of
Northumberland Health
Authority and the Secretary of
State for Health)*

account of being in a sanatorium and Roberts and Buikstra, 2003, for an overview of
the sanatorium movement (Figs 7.19 and 7.20)).

Leprosy

Throughout history few diseases have engendered such fear and provoked such
cruel and, at the same time, pious reaction as leprosy. Much of the Medieval
attitude to leprosy stems from the supposed biblical references to the disease,
references which today are considered largely incorrect. But what of the disease
itself? Today 'remarkable progress has been made in the control of leprosy in the
community and in the treatment of individuals in recent years' (McDougall,
2002: 17), and this is due to the use of multiple (antibiotic) drug therapy (MDT),
a therapy that is free to anybody suffering from leprosy. In 1991 the World Health
Assembly aimed to reduce the leprosy rate to 1 in 10,000 of a population by the
year 2000. Although twenty-four countries still had leprosy as a major public
health problem, by this time leprosy had been reduced by 86 per cent (World
Health Organization, 2000 in McDougall, 2002). The top eleven highest
prevalence countries now have a rate of 4.1 cases per 10,000 compared to a global
rate of 1.25, and these include India, Brazil, Nepal and Ethiopia. Indeed, India
claims about 60 per cent of the world total of leprosy cases, and reasons for its
maintenance in some populations include high prevalence rate, intense disease
transmission, civil strife and lack of infrastructure to diagnose and treat people
(McDougall, 2002: table 3). In early 1999 834,988 cases were registered, with
714,876 new cases between 1998 and 1999, plus an estimate of 1.5 to 2 million
people with undiagnosed leprosy between 1999 and 2001 (McDougall, 2002: table
2). Worldwide, in 2003 the World Health Organization reported 620,672 cases
detected during 2002 with the highest number in south-east Asia (520,632)
(Website 1).

Thus, the infection remains a significant problem for some parts of our world.
However, more disturbing are the many people with cured (and uncured) leprosy
who are disabled, and even handicapped, by their infection (Jal Mehta, pers.
comm.). While it appears easy to treat people with MDT, dealing with the disability
that is a feature of leprosy, often a consequence if the disease is detected late, is a
rising problem in countries that lack the infrastructure to cope. Furthermore, in
many parts of the world (including the western world) there is a general lack of

understanding of the meaning of leprosy, what causes it, how it is contracted and how it can be treated. For example, a study in Nigeria of people with leprosy found that males had problems with securing and maintaining a job, which of course led to loss of income, and divorce was usually instigated by males with leprous wives (rather than by wives of leprous men (Awofeso, 1995)). Another study in India found that quality of life declined progressively in leprous individuals because stigma was still associated with the infection and access to health care was difficult. Interestingly, women had a higher quality of life score, explained by females being more ready to accept the condition compared to males, and reflecting their secondary role in Indian society (Joseph and Sundar Rao, 1999). Leprosy therefore has the same impact and significance in many parts of the world today as it had in Medieval Europe; it has been likened to HIV and AIDS in terms of invoking a similar response from unaffected members of human societies (Jopling, 1991).

Leprosy is a chronic infectious disease caused by *Mycobacterium leprae*. Although leprosy is largely a disease of humans, it is not exclusively so; it has been identified in the chimpanzee, the Mangabey monkey, and the armadillo (Jopling and McDougall, 1988). However, there are differences in expression in experimentally induced leprosy in armadillos, which Meyers *et al.* (1985) have outlined. The infection in these animals is rapidly fatal in 1½ to 3 years and involvement of the nerves is not reported. Nevertheless, leprosy in wild armadillos in the southern United States (Texas and Louisiana) appears to be reasonably common, affecting nearly one-third of animals (Truman *et al.*, 1991), and they may be a risk factor for humans.

The mode of transmission of *Mycobacterium leprae* between people is still uncertain but may be both through skin contact with an infected person and, more likely, through exhaled droplets containing bacteria from an individual with a profuse nasal infection (Bryceson and Pfaltzgraaf, 1990). Interesting to note is that a nose blow of a leprous person can contain up to 20 million bacilli (Sreevatasan, 1993). Another possible route of transmission has been suggested, that of biting insects which transport the bacilli from the skin and blood of infected people to non-infected victims (Sreevatasan, 1993). In this review article, however, the conclusion was that insects were not major vectors in the transmission of leprosy from human to human. What is certain, however, is that the disease is not inherited and it is not transmitted venereally (although see Lewis, 2002b for some discussion), thus negating prominent Medieval thought. Leprosy is often acquired in childhood, and males are affected more than females. However, few cases of leprosy in young individuals have been found (but see Lewis 2002b; Ortner, 2002). After transmission there is an incubation period of some 2–5 years before the presentation of symptoms and physical signs of the disease (Jopling and McDougall, 1988). The bacterium multiplies only slowly, and therefore leprosy is a disease of slow progress; it has been known almost throughout time as the living death. In fact, '*Mundo mortuus sis, sed Deo vivas*' – be thou dead to the world but alive unto God – was the Medieval pronouncement to those diagnosed with leprosy. The infection is mainly of peripheral nerves and this, through the motor, sensory and autonomic modalities, is responsible for the majority of skeletal features in the disease and is therefore of profound significance in palaeopathology. The skin, the eyes, bone and the testes may also be involved in the disease process.

In addition to the skeletal and non-skeletal bodily changes, one must not forget that psychiatric disturbances have also been noted (Ranjit and Verghose, 1980). It is common for leprous patients to develop neurotic symptoms and psychotic reactions to their infection (both male and female alike), and the probable reason is the stigma attached to the disease. Furthermore, those people with physical deformity tended to be those with the most psychiatric problems, and the rate in this study was more common than in the 'normal' population (99 in 1,000 people with leprosy compared to 63 in 1,000). As Ranjit and Verghose (1980: 433) state: 'The psychology of crippling is a very important part of the psychology of leprosy.' While detecting the psychological aspects of leprosy in skeletal samples from the past is impossible, this type of clinical work can help us to understand the problems that the leprous sufferer may have experienced. Of course deformity has led to fear of the disease today (and in the past), but as Srinivasan and Dharmendra (1978: 197) state: 'If leprosy did not cause deformities and disabilities, it would not be a dreaded disease. It would have been considered as just another skin disease. The strong emotional bias . . . is mainly because the leprosy patients get deformed and disabled.'

After the long incubation period, the clinical manifestations of leprosy are variable in severity, bodily distribution and infectivity. The variation is, however, due not to differences in *Mycobacterium leprae*, but to differences in the immune status of each infected individual (Ridley and Jopling, 1966; see also Fig. 1.5). At one extreme the infected person exhibits low resistance, the disease is highly infective, and the physical signs involve multiple limbs, face and soft-tissue organs. This pole of the leprosy spectrum is termed lepromatous leprosy. At the other extreme of the spectrum, the manifestation of tuberculoid leprosy is relatively less infective, and the pathological lesions are of one or perhaps two limbs, with less severe soft-tissue reactions. In palaeopathology lepromatous leprosy is most commonly identified but the low rate of detection of tuberculoid leprosy may be because of non-recognition of the less severe bone changes. In lepromatous leprosy there may be bone damage to the nasal area and the palate, but in tuberculoid leprosy this is not seen. Likewise, in lepromatous leprosy the changes to the hands and feet are usually symmetrical, but these are unilateral in tuberculoid leprosy (Manchester, 2002).

Damage to the skeleton in leprosy involves the facial bones, hands, feet and tibiae and fibula. Some 5 per cent of people with leprosy are believed to develop bone changes (Resnick and Niwayama, 1995d). However, other conditions may lead to the same or similar changes. Observation of the distribution pattern of damage is key to diagnosis (Manchester, 2002). Documentation of the bone changes of leprosy in skeletal remains was first undertaken in the 1950s by Vilhelm Møller-Christensen (1953), a doctor from Denmark interested in archaeology and palaeopathology who excavated and analysed skeletons from Danish Medieval leprosy hospital sites (Bennike, 2002) (Fig. 7.21).

Involvement of the peripheral nerves results in their loss of function. There is consequent paralysis of muscle groups in the upper and lower limbs and resulting deformity (Figs 7.22 and 7.23). There is also loss of sensation, particularly of the hands and feet. The skin anaesthesia permits insensitive damage to the tissues, ulceration and secondary infection (Fig. 7.24). The bone changes in the hands and feet (Figs 7.25 and 7.26) and also the lower leg bones are the direct result of the

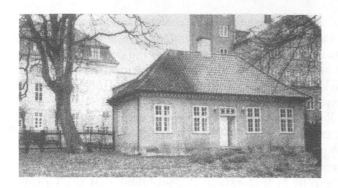

Fig. 7.21. Leprosy Museum, Copenhagen, Denmark, where the skeletons from Naestved are curated.

secondary infection and the deformity, and consist of inflammatory changes in the bones and joints (Møller-Christensen, 1961; Andersen *et al.*, 1994), joint fixation and deformity, and actual bone absorption, particularly of the toes and fingers (Andersen *et al.*, 1992). Interestingly, damage to the hands is less common than to the feet, and it is suggested that this may be because soft tissue lesions on the hands are noticed more often than those on the feet because of ease of access to observe them (Manchester, 2002). In archaeological contexts this is also the case. The more frequent damage to the plantar surface (sole) of the first and fifth metatarsophalangeal joint areas reflects the maximum skin pressure in the normal foot architecture. However, if the arch of the foot collapses (common in leprosy), then the pressure will be redirected to the mid-forefoot (Fig. 7.27). Today, in places where leprosy is common, protection of the feet by shoes, and hands by gloves/pot holders, is part of the educational process in dealing with leprosy (e.g. see Iyere, 1990; Soares and Desar, 1995).

The new bone formation of the tibia and fibula (periostitis) is a rather non-specific change that can be caused by many other conditions such as trauma, treponemal disease, scurvy and tuberculosis; recent work, nevertheless, has begun to use histological analysis to try to differentiate new bone formation as a result of leprosy from other causes (Schultz and Roberts, 2002). However, it has been suggested that this results from infection in the foot spreading upwards and affecting these bones, but it may be the result of trauma in leprous patients (although it has been seen in living leprous sufferers without bone changes in the

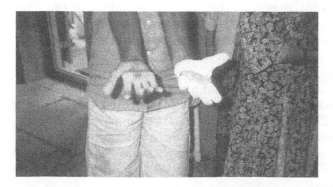

Fig. 7.22. Flexion deformity of hand (right) as a result of motor nerves being involved in leprosy; left hand is being treated with plaster of Paris splints to straighten the deformities (Pune, India).

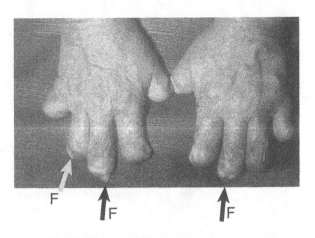

Fig. 7.23. Loss of mid and distal phalanges due to leprosy; note the retraction of the skin around the remaining metacarpals and the retained fingernails (F).

foot (Manchester, 2002)). Lewis (1995) documented 38 (76 per cent) leprous individuals from a Medieval leprosy hospital in Chichester, Sussex, England, with these changes to their lower leg bones, and 19 per cent (60) of the non-leprous individuals had the same changes. A small number of radii and ulnae were also affected, which may be the result of infection in the hand spreading to the forearm bones. While periostitis is not commonly described as a diagnostic criterion for leprosy in clinical contexts among those diagnosed with leprosy today, in archaeological contexts it does appear to be common. The former omission may be because the often subtle bone changes are not detected on radiographs and therefore are not described in clinical cases (Lewis, 1995: 82).

Direct infection of the soft tissues around the nose and mouth by *Mycobacterium leprae* results in the characteristic changes in the bones of the face (Møller-Christensen, 1978; Andersen and Manchester, 1992; Fig. 7.28). The face becomes nodular, the bridge of the nose collapses and is associated with a persistent nasal discharge, the eyes become infected and, in the extreme, blindness supervenes. Invasion of the larynx produces the hoarse, coarse voice characteristic of advanced leprosy. The bone changes in the face of people with

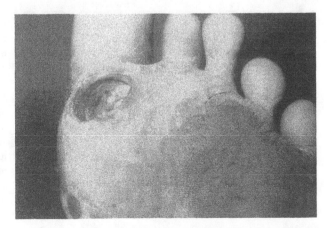

Fig. 7.24. Ulceration of the foot in leprosy as a result of loss of involvement of the sensory nerves and loss of sensation.

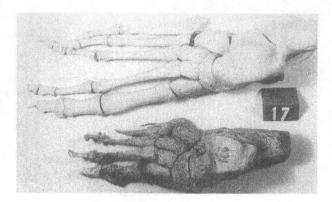

Fig. 7.25. Loss of some of the foot phalanges and 'pencilling' of the metatarsals in leprosy (late Medieval, twelfth–sixteenth centuries AD, Naestved, Denmark); normal foot (top) for comparison.

leprosy include inflammatory pitting of both surfaces of the palate with possible perforation (inflammation), loss of alveolar bone of the upper jaw in the area of the incisor teeth and subsequent loss of teeth, absorption of the anterior nasal spine, remodelling of the nasal aperture, and inflammation of the nasal conchae and septum. The changes were called 'facies leprosa' by Møller-Christensen (1978) and, more recently, the 'rhinomaxillary syndrome' by Anderson and Manchester (1992). While these changes are deemed pathognomonic for leprosy, other disease processes may lead to similar changes: they include treponemal disease and tuberculosis (see Manchester, 1994 and Cook, 2002 for a discussion).

No wonder that the chronically disfigured and possibly blind man or woman with deformity or loss of fingers and toes provoked such reaction and fear. The diagnosis and misdiagnosis of the disease in antiquity has been, and still is, a subject of debate. The extent to which the non-leprous diseases of the nervous system, the skin and eyes were attributed to the 'biblical scourge' is questionable (see below). Elucidation of the problem comes from the evidence of documents and, more particularly, from the evidence of osteoarchaeology. Some 68 per cent of the skeletons from the Medieval leprosarium at Naestved, Denmark, exhibited the changes of leprosy (Møller-Christensen, 1978). It is fortunate indeed from a

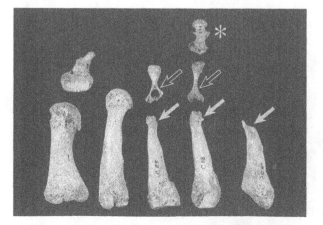

Fig. 7.26. Detail of bone changes in leprous individual's metatarsals and phalanges (late Medieval, twelfth–sixteenth centuries AD, Chichester, Sussex, England); note the loss of the distal ends of the metatarsals (closed arrows), autonomic nerve involvement leading to concentric atrophy of the phalanges (open arrows), and fusion of mid and distal phalanges (*). *(With permission of Don Ortner)*

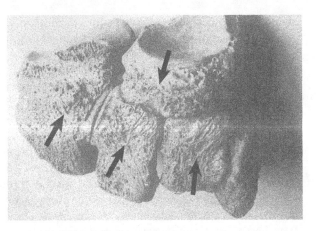

Fig. 7.27. Dorsal surfaces of the tarsals of the foot from a leprous individual showing new bone formation at ligament insertions due to strain following 'drop' foot.

historical viewpoint that leprosy leads to characteristic bone changes and that these changes can be recognized from skeletons of long ago. Subsequent to Møller-Christensen's seminal work on leprosy, further refinement of the diagnostic criteria for leprosy and examination of the specific pathological processes that lead to the bone changes so familiar to the palaeopathologist have been undertaken (Andersen, 1969; Andersen and Manchester, 1987, 1988; Andersen *et al.*, 1992). More recently biomolecular analysis has been utilized in confirming diagnoses for leprous cases in palaeopathology (e.g. Taylor *et al.*, 2000; Spigelman and Donoghue, 2002).

The changes and clinical manifestations of leprosy were present in antiquity just as today, and there is no reason to suppose that the disease has changed its features throughout history. The sufferings of the lepromatous leprous individuals in a twenty-first-century African or Indian leprous community are more or less those of Medieval communities, but the social reaction (to a certain extent) and medical treatment have changed. What a piteous spectacle on the Medieval scene: poor ostracized men, women or children, deformed, and smelling of the discharging ulcers, who were forced to give notice of their presence with a wooden clapper and then had to beg with hoarse voice for their material needs. The pattern of

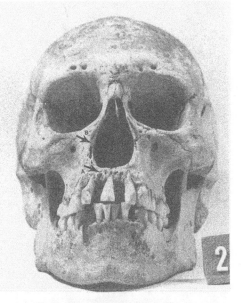

Fig. 7.28. Facies leprosa in leprosy: A: alveolar bone resorption of maxilla and loss of teeth; B: remodelling of nasal aperture (late Medieval, twelfth–sixteenth centuries AD, Naestved, Denmark).

social abhorrence and the persistent reaction to leprosy (Jopling, 1991) is unique among diseases in its intensity, inventiveness and ubiquity.

However, leprosy appears to have been a late arrival in the history of bacterial disease. Pending the discovery of early skeletons, the earliest history of leprosy relies upon literary sources. The earliest reference to leprosy in humans is in the Sushruta Samhita, an Indian document from the period around 600 BC. The description of loss of sensation, falling off of the fingers, deformity and ulceration of the limbs, and sinking of the nose, are almost diagnostic of advanced lepromatous leprosy (Dharmendra, 1947). A similar description is also identified in a Chinese bamboo book of the third century BC (Skinsnes, 1980; Skinsnes and Chang, 1985). Thus, lepromatous leprosy was established in India and the Far East at an early period, and the clear and accurate contemporary description implies that the authors possessed an acute clinical acumen. It is quite possible that the disease may have had a significant prevalence in those parts of the world at that time.

Until the sixteenth century, Medieval paintings represented leprosy as spots, tumours and pustules distributed over the entire body (Gron, 1973). There can be little doubt that artists of this period recognized the gross deformities of the limbs and face, but it was the early Renaissance artists who first portrayed the limb and facial deformities in leprosy (Hollander, 1913). Notwithstanding this early artistic stricture, there is a sculpture of 1250–1350 from Burton Lazars leprosarium in Leicestershire, England, which illustrates the facial features of advanced lepromatous leprosy (Marcombe and Manchester, 1990). A very similar figure is seen on a carving from the high altar of a church in Krakow, Poland, and a figurine illustrating both the facial and the peripheral limb features of the disease has also been identified (Fig. 7.29) in the Abbaye de Cadouin, France (Manchester and Knüsel, 1994). It is likely that the sculptor of this most poignant figure had a first-hand and intimate knowledge of a sufferer of advanced lepromatous leprosy. Carvings of less certain diagnosis are known from European and Middle Eastern sources (Grmek, 1992).

Whence the bacterium came to infect humans remains unknown. However, it has been found that bacteria similar to mycobacteria can survive on very simple hydrocarbon chemicals which are found in fossil fuels on the ground surface (Chakrabarty and Dastidar, 1989). Could it be therefore that this source resulted in

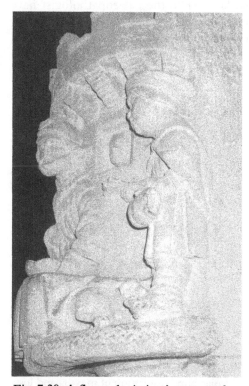

Fig. 7.29. A figure depicting leprosy and holding a clapper in the Abbaye de Cadouin, France.

the implantation of potentially pathogenic bacteria into broken human skin, thus establishing disease? Dols (1979) considers that there is no persuasive evidence that leprosy occurred in ancient Egypt, Mesopotamia or Persia before the time of Alexander the Great. The literary and osteological evidence for the Mediterranean and European areas is of a later period. Largely based upon the evidence currently available, it has been suggested that leprosy was brought to the Mediterranean from the Indo-Gangetic basin by the returning armies of Alexander the Great (356–323 BC). Its earlier existence in the Far East is, as yet, without supporting skeletal evidence. The Alexandrian Indian campaign occurred in the years 327–326 BC, and the soldiers or the camp followers may have contracted leprosy during this expedition. The movement of people, either in 'trade', military or religious expedition, is an efficient vehicle of disease transference (Kaplan, 1988; Wilson, 1995). It may be of significance therefore that the earliest skeletal evidence of leprosy known at present is from the Dakhleh Oasis in Egypt (Dzierzykray-Rogalski, 1980). The four skulls showing features of leprosy are of the Ptolemaic period and are dated to 250 BC, a relatively short time after the Alexandrian campaign. It is of interest also that the skulls are of 'European' type and not the Negroid type typical of that area. Dzierzykray-Rogalski suggests that these people were members of a high stratum of society who, because of their disease, may have been segregated from the more urban centres of the Empire. If this supposition is correct then, bearing in mind the possible time taken to develop such socio-medical attitudes, leprosy in the Ptolemaic Empire may have been a recognized disease for many years. This is consistent with its entry into the Mediterranean area with the Alexandrian army. Molto, more recently (2002), has identified a further two early/mid-fourth-century AD male burials with leprosy, and isotopic data indicates they lived elsewhere before they died at Dakhleh Oasis. This is further supporting evidence for a possible origin in the African area.

Following this, evidence of the disease in human remains is not recognized until the Egyptian coptic mummies of the fourth to seventh centuries AD from El Bigha near Aswan (Møller-Christensen and Hughes, 1966). The earliest evidence of leprosy in western Europe is of the fourth century AD. For example, a diagnosis of leprosy has been made from the bones of the legs and feet of a Romano-British skeleton from Poundbury (Reader, 1974, and see Roberts, 2002 for a summary of the British skeletal evidence); a skeleton of similar date with unequivocal signs of leprosy has been identified in Sweden (Arcini, 1990), and in France two skeletons dated to AD 500 have been diagnosed with leprosy (Blondiaux et al., 2002). Since the western European evidence post-dates the Roman expansion into Europe, it is possible that the disease was transported from the Mediterranean by the Roman Imperial campaigns into northern Europe. The Roman combatant soldier is of course very unlikely to have had leprosy, but camp followers, the group of 'hangers-on' who have accompanied armies since time immemorial, may well have been leprous. The mercantile routes were also, no doubt, a ready road for dissemination of disease. Although less infectious, less mutilating and less obvious than lepromatous leprosy, the tuberculoid and borderline forms, if they existed, should not be forgotten in the transmission of leprosy at this time. From succeeding centuries the evidence of leprosy in Britain becomes more abundant (Roberts, 2002). Elsewhere in continental Europe Blondiaux (1989) has identified leprous skeletons of a similar early date, and Pálfi (1991) has diagnosed leprosy in a skeleton dated to the tenth century from Hungary.

Much reliance for the early history of the disease in the Near East has, until recently, been placed on the biblical references to leprosy. There are no fewer than sixteen separate references to leprosy in both the Old and the New Testaments. However, it has been demonstrated by several researchers (Andersen, 1969; Hulse, 1972, 1976) that biblical references to the disease are probably false and result from a mistranslation of the word *tsara'ath* in the Hebrew version. What is apparent is that the word *tsara'ath* does not denote any specific disease but rather describes the state of ritual uncleanliness. Such a description implies that the individual was not fit to enter a holy place. It has nothing to do with the infection that we now call leprosy. Because it is now known that leprosy was present in the Near East by the second century BC, discussions on New Testament leprosy are probably irrelevant. The disease was probably known throughout the eastern Mediterranean area at that time. Indeed, the earliest skeletal material diagnostic of leprosy in the Holy Land is from a mass grave of the ninth century AD (Monastery of St John the Baptist) in the Judaean Desert (Zias, 2002). Regrettably the biblical association remains with the name Lazar, a name suggestive of 'leper' and 'leper' hospital. From the meagre clinical description (Luke 16: 20) it is not possible to state whether Lazarus the beggar was leprous or not. He certainly did not suffer from *tsara'ath* because he was not segregated from society. Further confused Medieval thinking has linked the name of this Lazarus with Mary and Martha. Many of England's leprosy hospitals have been dedicated to these three, and as late as the nineteenth century the name Maudlin, the abbreviated and conjoined Mary and Martha, had historical associations with leprosy (Richards, 1977). It is perhaps tragic that much of the prejudice against leprosy throughout history has been due to an error of translation. Furthermore, the leprosy in the literature of the Graeco-Roman period is referred to by the terms *elephas* and *elephantiasis*, and in the Medieval period by the term *lepra*. Investigating the written sources of antiquity for the early history of leprosy is clearly very difficult. The attribution of the loosely applied names of the past to the specific disease recognized today is a major pitfall in the investigation of diseases in antiquity.

The spread of leprosy throughout Europe in the Medieval period was probably due to expanding trade, the opening of mercantile routes and the increasing movement of people. The developing Medieval period saw a gradual increase in leprosy in urban centres, although it is essentially a rural disease (Aufderheide and Rodríguez-Martín, 1998). The osteoarchaeological record becomes more abundant and by the twelfth and thirteenth centuries legal and socio-medical measures aimed at the control of leprosy had become established (Roberts, 1986a). Leprosy hospitals as a means of isolating those with leprosy in Medieval Europe is of course a subject in itself that has been discussed by many. Once diagnosed, the Medieval leprous were supposedly segregated via a symbolic funeral into leprosy hospitals and retained there so they could not mingle with the non-leprous of their community. However, it is clear that the rules were not strict, which meant that people with leprosy had the opportunity to wander at will and go to markets, allowing their infection to be transmitted to others. Furthermore, not all people with leprosy would be segregated. This may have been because the clinical signs of the infection were not visible (and that they had a high resistant – i.e. tuberculoid – form of the disease), they may have evaded detection or their community could have accepted them as 'normal' citizens. Clearly, people with leprosy have been buried in non-leprosy hospital cemeteries, as shown by recent work in Britain (Roberts, 2002). Nevertheless, leprosy hospitals were sited on the edge of towns and were founded usually by benefactors who then supported the needs of those in the hospital. Leprosy hospitals saw their height of 'popularity', in Britain at least, during the twelfth and thirteenth centuries (Roberts, 1986a; Fig. 7.30), with a decline from the fourteenth century onwards. Whether this reflected a decline in the infection is much debated. The situation in North America is somewhat different in that the evidence for early leprosy is non-existent. This is perhaps expected, since, by the fifteenth century and the Columbus expedition to America, leprosy in Europe was declining and it is very unlikely that somebody with lepromatous leprosy would have joined the expedition. Recent excavations in Guam (a Pacific island in Indonesia) of graves pre-dating European contact with North America have revealed skeletons with features characteristic of lepromatous leprosy (Trembly, 1995). Almost certainly, the route of arrival for the disease in Guam was from the Asian mainland. The isolation of North America until long after this period, at least according to currently available evidence, remains a mystery.

The decline and elimination of leprosy in northern Europe illustrates the complex and interrelated bacter-iological, social and environmental factors implicated in infectious disease change. These factors differ from country to country and even within individual countries themselves, which may explain the survival of leprosy in one community and its simultaneous disappearance from another. The persistence of the leprosy hospital may not be a true guide to the persistence of leprosy within a society. There is no doubt that by the late Medieval period in England people with leprosy were considerably more rare than his or her supposed place of refuge. The leprosy hospital, like the sanatorium in a later period of history, maintained its name and dedication but changed its function. It is well known that by the mid-twentieth century many sanatoria contained few, if any, tuberculous patients but instead accepted patients with other pulmonary diseases. So it may have been with leprosy hospitals in the late Medieval period. To all intents

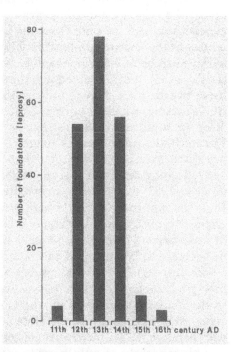

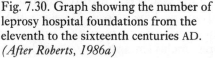

Fig. 7.30. Graph showing the number of leprosy hospital foundations from the eleventh to the sixteenth centuries AD. *(After Roberts, 1986a)*

and purposes, leprosy was a non-existent disease in England by the sixteenth century, and in the fifteenth century was a rarity (Richards, 1977).

Similar changes took place in southern Scandinavia, and yet in northern Scandinavia and in Iceland leprosy persisted even until the twentieth century. What identifiable factors operated in northern Scandinavia in the twentieth century and in mid- and southern Europe in the late Medieval period? It is appropriate to narrow the horizon and consider England alone as representative, because the history of the disease, its hospitals and general population movements are fairly well known. In spite of the vigour with which it was often enforced, segregation of the leprous possibly contributed little to the decline of the disease. Leprosy is a highly infectious disease, but the ability of the bacterium to produce clinical disease in patients is poor in comparison with other infectious diseases, and there are, in fact, recorded instances of healthy individuals taking residence in leprosy hospitals and remaining clinically free of the disease themselves for many years. This illustrates the variation in individual susceptibility to infection, a phenomenon common to most infectious diseases. Effective medical treatment of leprosy in the Medieval period was non-existent. Nevertheless, leprosy declined from its fearsome prevalence in the twelfth and thirteenth centuries to its virtual absence in the sixteenth century.

Although other reasons for leprosy's decline have been explored (e.g. Duncan, 1994), what is apparent during the period of decline of leprosy in the later Medieval period in England is the concurrent increase in tuberculosis. To some extent the evidence for this increase at this time is assumed and is a projected expectation back in time from the known very high prevalence in the urban centres of the seventeenth century. The reaction of the body at a microscopic level to *Mycobacterium tuberculosis* and to *Mycobacterium leprae* is essentially the same (Lurie, 1955). It is also noted that there is a degree of cross-immunity induced by these two bacteria. It is found, for example, in modern investigations that the BCG vaccine, which is normally used for protection against tuberculosis, does offer some protection against leprosy ranging from 20 per cent to 80 per cent. Furthermore, some authors suggest that around 75 per cent of people may be protected from one mycobacterial species by exposure to another (Clark *et al.*, 1987; Jopling and McDougall, 1988; Fine, 1984, 1995). It was suggested by Grmek (1983) that there is an evolutionary chain of mycobacterial development from the non-pathogenic through and including the human pathogens. In this chain *Mycobacterium tuberculosis* is regarded as an earlier entity than *Mycobacterium leprae*. If this phase of bacterial evolution has resulted in a decrease in bacterial virulence (and the relatively low pathogenicity of *Mycobacterium leprae* and variable human susceptibility may suggest this), then, because of biological competition, tuberculosis will take precedence over leprosy. Exposure to tuberculosis, regardless of whether it results in overt disease or rapid self-conquest of infection, may therefore induce a degree of immunity to leprosy, and will therefore reduce the chances of contracting leprosy (Manchester, 1991).

This is clearly of only passing interest to the individual with relentlessly advancing tuberculosis. However, the human type of tuberculosis has its primary focus of infection in the lungs and it is a common response today (and, presumably, in antiquity also) that this process becomes arrested early without advancement of the disease. Henceforth the individual is immune to tuberculosis and, by the above reasoning, in part to leprosy also. Therefore an increasing community exposure to tuberculosis may result in a decreasing community incidence of leprosy. Clearly, those individuals dying with tuberculosis will not prevent leprosy gaining or maintaining a foothold in a community, but the background of people immune by exposure to tuberculosis will fulfil this role. Exposure to tuberculosis is likely to be more widespread through human-type bacilli, and a prerequisite for this is close human-to-human contact. This is achieved by urbanization. The revival of urban living in Europe gathered momentum from the tenth century and the number of new town foundations reached a peak in the late thirteenth century (Pounds, 1974). The early fourteenth century onwards witnessed a falling-off in the number of new foundations. What should be significant, however, is not merely the number of urban centres developing within a territory, centres defined by social organization rather than number of inhabitants, but the actual population size and density within these centres. During the later Medieval period the population of England doubled (Dyer, 1989), although the fourteenth century saw famine and the Black Death impact on population numbers (Roberts and Cox, 2003). At the end of the thirteenth century, the period of maximum demographic growth, very few urban centres in Europe had populations in excess of 50,000 and these were mostly in Italy. Perhaps no more than 15 or 20 towns had populations greater than 25,000, and again most of these were in Italy. The number of towns containing smaller populations was greater, with the majority containing 2,000–10,000 inhabitants (Pounds, 1974). As for England, in 1199 Peter of Blois reported that London had a population of 40,000, a figure incorrect for that period but possibly correct for the mid-fourteenth century (Green, 1971). The development of urban centres was somewhat later in northern Scandinavia, and it is observed that the decline of leprosy there was also later than in England. Thus, certainly for England, a decline in population in the fourteenth century may explain, to a certain extent, the decline in available people to contract leprosy. Interestingly, however, research on the frequency of leprosy and tuberculosis in 'modern' Africa suggests that a decline in leprosy is associated with the increase in cities and tuberculosis, and there is a negative association between leprosy and urbanization; as leprosy is a rural disease, this seems to make sense.

The osteoarchaeological record may be supportive of this hypothesis. Leprosy is attested in several hundred skeletons in Europe as a whole (Møller-Christensen, 1967). Tuberculosis is not uncommon in both the skeletal and the literary record. However, the presence of both tuberculosis and leprous lesions in the same skeleton is rare, although a skeleton with evidence of both has been described from the Medieval cemetery at Naestved in Denmark (Weiss and Møller-Christensen, 1971a). The tuberculous changes are suggestive of human-type infection of the lungs. The rarity of this combination of diseases is support for the mutually exclusive nature of leprosy and tuberculosis and, by inference, for the above hypothesis. However, in modern populations, pulmonary tuberculosis is a major cause of death in leprosy hospitals. Although tuberculosis frequently occurs in leprous patients, leprosy rarely develops in tuberculous patients (Jopling, 1982). It seems that, although tuberculosis confers some immunity to the development of leprosy, the converse does not apply (Chaussinand, 1953). However, very recent research has cast some doubt on this theory of leprosy decreasing while tuberculosis increases. Wilbur *et al.* (2002) analysed leprosy and tuberculosis data from two eras (1938–80 and 1991–8) from Texas, United States. They found that, as leprosy increased and declined, then so did tuberculosis. While admitting that lack of diagnostic accuracy, medical intervention and under-reporting may have affected the results of the study, Wilbur *et al.* offer 'possible though not conclusive evidence against a model of cross-immunity' (2002: 255). Leitman *et al.* (1997) are of the opinion that Chaussinand's hypothesis of competitive exclusion of leprosy by tuberculosis cannot be tested experimentally, but their research indicates that, in any case, it would take centuries for tuberculosis to eradicate leprosy. Interestingly, exposure to leprosy provides 'little protection, if any' against tuberculosis (Chaussinand, 1953). Leitman *et al.*'s (1997: 1926) final word on the matter states that 'if conditions were such that the basic reproductive rate of leprosy was relatively low, then, as Chaussinand proposed, tuberculosis could have played a major role in the disappearance of leprosy from western Europe'. Clearly, there is still research to do regarding the decline of leprosy. However, in Britain, where leprosy and tuberculosis were major diseases in the later Medieval period, the stratigraphic data available from cemetery sites are not robust enough to be able to look at the rise and decline of these two infections through the mid-eleventh to sixteenth centuries AD, and see if tuberculosis does increase while leprosy declines (Roberts, 2002).

Whatever the manifold reasons for the decline of leprosy, Europe is now largely spared this most emotive and mutilating of the mycobacterial diseases. The scourge is now a problem of the tropical and semitropical areas of the world. When prejudice, fear and geographic and economic barriers have been overcome, leprosy may also disappear from these zones and become a disease of purely antiquarian interest.

Treponemal disease

For many years the human diseases caused by bacteria of the genus *Treponema* have been the subject of controversy. These diseases are pinta, yaws, endemic syphilis (treponarid/bejel) and venereal syphilis. The controversy centres on whether these are different disease entities caused by different species of bacteria within the genus, or whether they are merely different clinical manifestations of infection by one species, *Treponema pallidum*. If they are truly separate diseases, then collectively they may be referred to as the treponematoses. If they are but different clinical manifestations, then the disease entity is the treponematosis and the syndromes have to be explained by other intrinsic (e.g. age, sex) and extrinsic (e.g. diet, living conditions) factors. Upon this distinction depends the most emotive controversy, regarding the evolution and history of venereal syphilis. Although to many it may seem an argument of bacteriological nicety, this controversy is of more worldly significance. No finger of rectitude is pointed at pinta, yaws and endemic syphilis, but in the past, and even today, certain moral judgements surround the problem of venereal syphilis. Much time and thought have been devoted to the question of global venereal syphilis and its New World or Old World origin (Baker and Armelagos, 1988; Dutour *et al.*, 1994).

Before discussing the evolution and spread of the treponemal diseases, it is appropriate to consider *Treponema* and its identity. Pinta, yaws and syphilis (both endemic and venereal) have been customarily attributed to the bacterial species *Treponema carateum*, *Treponema pertenue*, *Treponema pallidum endemicum* and *Treponema* subspecies *pallidum* respectively, and it is the specificity that is under scrutiny. These four 'species' were, until recently, indistinguishable in appearance and physical laboratory characteristics (Dooley and Binford, 1976). For example, certain immunological changes in the blood of infected individuals were indistinguishable in the three bacterial infections. These facts, together with some epidemiological aspects of the diseases themselves, have led to the conclusion that there is only one species of *Treponema* involved in these infections, and that has been labelled *Treponema pallidum* (Hudson, 1958). However, analysis of the DNA of the bacteria causing treponemal disease has shown a difference between venereal syphilis and the non-venereal types (Centurion-Lara *et al.*, 1998 in Ortner, 2003), although it is suggested (Ortner, 2003) that this will not affect the clinical manifestation of the syndromes. Other research using ancient DNA analysis isolated the DNA of *Treponema pallidum* subspecies *pallidum* as the causative agent of bone changes in a 200-year-old individual from Easter Island (Kolman *et al.*, 1999). This method of analysis holds promise for the future identification of treponemal disease in human remains from archaeological sites, although problems have been highlighted (Bouman and Brown, 2005). Counter-arguments to the 'one-species' theory, and based on the different clinical features, and on the different geographic distribution of the individual diseases today, have led to the conclusion that the bacteria are, in fact, separate species (Hackett, 1963). The problem is not solved and no doubt awaits further refinements of bacteriological techniques.

However, if the laboratory questions are as yet unanswered, the clinical effects of infection have been known for many years. The basic pathological changes, both gross and microscopic, of the infectious diseases of pinta, yaws, endemic syphilis and venereal syphilis are identical. Differences between them are purely quantitative and of degree, and are not qualitative. There is, however, valid reason for regarding pinta as a somewhat different problem, despite the identical reaction of inflammation. In this disease the pathological change is of the skin only, unlike the other diseases. It is therefore not manifest in skeletal material. It has not been found possible to inoculate animals with this infection under experimental conditions, as is possible with the other infections of the group. The clinical severity in terms of morbidity and mortality does seem to progress from pinta, the least significant, through yaws and endemic syphilis to venereal syphilis, at which point, for the present anyway, the story stops. However, evolution, if this is what is in the evidence, is not a finite phenomenon and there is no reason to suppose that an end point has been reached in the treponemal diseases any more than in the other infections.

Yaws, endemic syphilis and venereal syphilis are all associated with inflammatory changes in most tissues from the body surface to the bones, although the bones affected usually have little overlying soft tissue (Ortner, 2003). A considerable amount of information concerning the bone changes of venereal syphilis has been derived from studies of untreated people in Norway (Gjestland, 1955) and the United States (Jones, 1993). Recent work has also reviewed the proposed mechanisms by which the bones are affected in treponemal disease (direct extension from soft tissue lesions in the secondary stages of the disease, and local trauma to bones close to the skin), with the suggestion that spread of the infection to bone may be from adjacent lymphatic nodes and vessels (Buckley and Dias, 2002). Venereal syphilis, being the most severe, is also characterized by involvement of the arterial circulation and the nervous system in the final stages. All are purely human diseases. All are transmissible from infected person to non-infected person without the intervention of an intermediate animal host. Only venereal syphilis was thought transmissible from infected mother to unborn child (congenital syphilis), but there is also evidence of yaws being congenital (Heoprich, 1989; Ortner, 2003). All are characterized by recognizable clinical stages of development. The early stage is at the site of entry of the bacteria and is a relatively mild inflammatory lesion. A later stage marks the generalized spread of bacteria within the body characterized by skin and soft-tissue changes. In the later stage there is inflammatory change in the bones, which is mainly of a destructive nature but which also demonstrates considerable regeneration and repair. It is with the evidence of this stage that the palaeopathologist is concerned and Hackett (1976b) documents the skeletal changes well. It is from this stage alone that the skeletal evidence for the antiquity of treponemal disease comes.

It must be remembered that, albeit uncommonly, an individual can overcome the disease in an early stage and recover. Thereafter they will remain immune to further attacks of this disease. Because infection by one of the group will confer immunity to the other diseases, that is, there is cross-immunity, a recovered individual will thereafter be immune also to the other treponemal diseases. This is possibly of significance for the evolution of endemic and venereal syphilis.

As already stated, the diseases differ quantitatively and in the prevalence of bone involvement (Rothschild and Heathcote, 1993; Hershkovitz et al., 1994; Rothschild and Rothschild, 1994). Pinta need not, of course, be considered further in the present context. The bone changes of yaws, endemic syphilis and venereal syphilis are of osteomyelitis, induced in part by an inflammatory reaction specific to *Treponema* (Canci et al., 1994). This reaction, which results in gross bone destruction, is called a gumma. However, unlike some of the cases of non-specific osteomyelitis discussed earlier, the osteomyelitis of the treponemal diseases is accompanied by extensive bone regeneration and exhibits specific microscopic characteristics (Schultz, 1994, 2001). In consequence, in the later stages of the bone infection, the bone affected assumes a much altered shape. The frequency of bone involvement in these diseases is suggested to be between 5 and 15 per cent of all cases of yaws (Steinbock, 1976), up to 20 per cent of all cases of venereal syphilis, with endemic syphilis lying between the two.

In **yaws** the tibia is the most commonly affected bone (Dooley and Binford, 1976), and only to a lesser extent are the other bones of the skeleton involved. Moreover, the joints may become eroded (erosive joint disease). The skull is infrequently involved but, when it is, the destruction is generally more severe than in venereal syphilis, particularly in the oral and nasal areas (Manchester, 1994). The usual result is a few irregular crater-like depressions of the skull surface. Occasionally the destructive element may be extensive. This may result in the condition of gangosa, in which the whole nasal area and upper jaw may be destroyed, associated with extensive destruction of the soft tissues of the face, a severe and mutilating stage surpassing even the mutilations of leprosy. More common, however, is the tibial osteomyelitis which, due to the deposition of new bone, gives rise to the sabre shin, so called because of its shape. As yaws is contracted in childhood, active lesions are seen then, but these may heal if the child reaches adulthood (Ortner, 2003: 275).

As with yaws, skull involvement in **endemic syphilis** is uncommon, but may result in extensive destruction of the nasal area and upper jaw. Also in common with yaws, the tibia is the most commonly affected bone, resulting in the sabre shape (Anderson *et al.*, 1986; Hershkovitz *et al.*, 1994). The difference between yaws and endemic syphilis lies in the earlier stages of each disease and in their individual geographic environment. Both diseases are common and endemic in hot climates, but yaws has a predilection for the humid tropics whereas endemic syphilis is prevalent in the arid zones lying north and south of the yaws territory (Froment, 1994). In fact, to avoid confusion of terms in syphilis, endemic syphilis has been renamed treponarid (Hackett, 1963) but the new term is not yet used universally. Pinta is a disease usually acquired during the third decade, whereas yaws and endemic syphilis are infections primarily of children, but of course children become adults and the lesions can persist.

The emotive discussions on treponemal diseases, often with undertones of morality, largely surround **venereal syphilis**, an infection that, between 1995 and 2000, saw an increase of 145 per cent in England, Wales and Northern Ireland (Goldmeier and Guallar, 2003). The names given to the disease perhaps betray the interest in the condition and suggest an element of blame in its origin: Mal de Naples, Arboyne pimple, Scottish sibbens, Swedish saltfluss, Morbus gallicus and Spanish pox are but a few. In view of the arguments regarding its New World or Old World origin, it is surprising that a name implicating North America does not seem to have been used.

Despite the similarities that yaws and endemic syphilis possess, venereal syphilis displays several differences. The mode of transmission from person to person is perhaps the most obvious difference; yaws, endemic syphilis and also pinta are transmitted by bodily contact which is not of the intimacy of sexual intercourse. They are, as mentioned, diseases with an onset in childhood. Venereal syphilis is acquired in adulthood through the act of sexual intercourse with a person infected with *Treponema pallidum*. Pathologically the most striking and significant difference is in the severe, incapacitating and frequently fatal circulatory and central nervous system involvement of venereal syphilis, features not manifest in pinta, yaws or endemic syphilis. The most advanced stage of venereal syphilis has given rise to the apt term 'general paralysis of the insane'. The affected individual with stumbling faltering gait, given to bouts of irrational madness, has good reason to regret his or her previous indiscretion. Relief from worldly suffering may come dramatically from the rupture of a grossly dilated major artery and the consequent catastrophic haemorrhage. It is noteworthy, however, that up to 20 per cent or so of venereal syphilitic individuals may possess bone changes (Resnick and Niwayama, 1995d). Since the only truly reliable evidence of venereal syphilis in antiquity is derived from osteoarchaeological study, it is quite probable that the prevalence of venereal syphilis in the distant past may be underestimated by as much as 90 per cent. This may in some measure explain the apparent rarity of the disease in past society. The bone changes develop between 2 and 10 years after the infection (Ortner, 2003: 279). As in yaws and endemic syphilis, the tibia is the long bone most frequently affected in venereal syphilis (Clairet and Dagorn, 1994), presenting as a deformed osteomyelitic bone, but multiple bone involvement throughout the skeleton is frequently noted. Venereal syphilis may also result in destructive change of joints, characteristically the knee. The joint itself may be the seat of infection or, at a later stage of the disease, may become damaged by the loss of sensation due to nervous system involvement. This so-called Charcot joint adds further to the unstable gait of the relentlessly advancing syphilitic disease. In contrast to the other two diseases, however, the skull is commonly affected in venereal syphilis and it is upon this change that a palaeopathological diagnosis is mainly reached. The plate bones of the cranial vault exhibit a characteristic 'worm-eaten' appearance that has been given the name *caries sicca* (Figs 7.31 and 7.32). Most commonly the parietal and frontal bones of the vault are affected, the pathological process being one of gross destruction and irregular repair. The inflammation commences within the internal substance of the skull bones

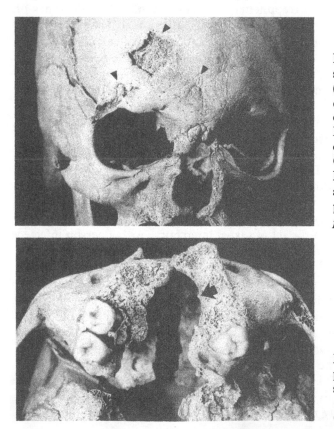

Fig. 7.31. Involvement of the skull in venereal syphilis (*caries sicca*); note the arrowed destructive lesions, with some evidence of healing (late Medieval, twelfth–sixteenth centuries AD, Blackfriars, Gloucester, Gloucestershire, England). This skeleton is archaeologically dated to the pre-Columbian period. *(With permission of Don Ortner)*

Fig. 7.32. Destruction of the palate, with healing, in the same individual as Fig. 7.31. *(With permission of Don Ortner)*

themselves and gradually spreads both outwards and inwards. Eventually perforation of the skull may result (Hackett, 1981). Although changes do occur at the nasal area and palate, these are not so marked as in yaws and endemic syphilis.

There is yet another difference that adds a further dimension to the treponemal diseases. This is the ability of the *Treponema pallidum* of venereal syphilis to pass from an infected mother across the placenta to an unborn child. This unwelcome infection of a totally innocent victim gives rise to **congenital syphilis**. It may suggest a difference between the species of *Treponema*, but the absence of congenital infection in endemic syphilis is rather puzzling, except of course that this latter is largely a disease of the young who are not as yet involved in reproduction. It is probable that transplacental passage of the bacterium occurs in pregnancy during the secondary stage of venereal syphilis, during which phase there is haematogenous spread of *Treponema*. It is considered (Grmek, 1994) that pregnancy will not occur during this secondary stage in endemic syphilis because of the young age of the infected female. The clinical features of congenital syphilis are in some respects similar to those of acquired venereal syphilis. The osteomyelitis of the tibia produces the sabre shin so characteristic of the treponemal infections, but the combination of multiple bone involvement (Panuel, 1994), the notched, so-called Hutchinson's, incisors, and mulberry and Moon's molars comprises the cardinal features of this disease. Hillson *et al.* (1998), however, have recently noted that Hutchinson's incisors and moon molars are likely pathognomonic of congenital syphilis, but mulberry molars display changes that could be caused by other conditions. The rarity of congenital syphilis in palaeopathological contexts is largely due to the fact that the disease carries a 50 per cent mortality in the very young. The skeleton of a newborn case of congenital syphilis recovered from an archaeological excavation will rarely, if ever, be recognized for what it is (although see Mansilla and Pijoan, 1995). As always, it is seen that palaeopathological diagnosis is dependent upon age at death, preservation and recognition.

For many years the search for the origin and evolution of the treponemal diseases centred on venereal syphilis and its relation to the trans-Atlantic expeditions of Christopher Columbus (Baker and Armelagos, 1988). In general, Europeans chose to relate the European onset of the disease to the return of the Columbus expedition, which, it was said, infected Europe with the treponemes from America. The Americans, in their turn, chose to regard the disease as of Old World, but not necessarily European, origin. Although the argument has not ended, and some still believe the answer to the treponemal question lies in the years following 1493 (Møller-Christensen, 1969b), it is probable that the recent, but pre-antibiotic, global distribution of pinta, yaws, endemic syphilis and venereal syphilis holds the key to the origin of these most elusive diseases of antiquity (Hudson, 1968).

Fig. 7.33 indicates the worldwide distribution of the treponemal diseases at about 1900 – that is, before effective antibiotic therapy. It is noted that pinta occupies the area of Central America only, yaws the belt around the equator in many countries, and endemic syphilis the arid regions north and south of the yaws territory. Venereal syphilis is widespread, and to some extent without geographic frontiers, but with a predilection for the crowded urban centres of civilization. It is considered (Hackett, 1963) that pinta was the primitive human precursor and, at about 15,000 BC, was

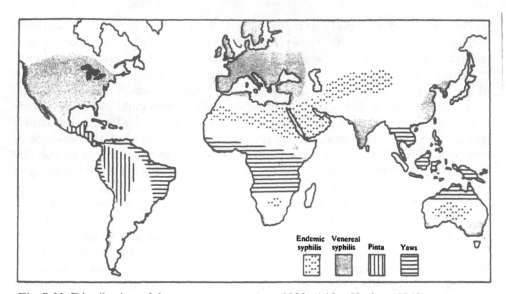

Fig. 7.33. Distribution of the treponematoses, AD 1900. *(After Hackett, 1963)*

widespread following the migrations of people out of Central Africa. It was carried to the Americas across the Bering land bridge and, for some reason not understood at present, there it remained, even after its disappearance elsewhere. Thus, a Central African cradle origin is accepted, as is the primeval status of pinta. Contrary to this opinion of the primogeniture of *Treponema carateum*, Grmek (1994) notes that a species that is isolated in a territory at the edge of the geographic area in which its group has expanded should not be considered primitive. This is precisely the case with pinta in the modern world, isolated as it is to Mesoamerica. On this basis, Grmek considers that yaws, not pinta, is the most ancient clinical manifestation of treponemal infection in humans. Thereafter opinions vary. Some (Hudson, 1958, 1965) regard pinta, yaws, endemic syphilis and venereal syphilis as different clinical manifestations of but one disease, treponematosis.

The proposition holds that the migration of people carried the treponeme to different climatic areas and that this climatic variation resulted in the apparently different diseases. The change was not, however, of the bacterium but rather of people's social adaptation to their new environment. The absence of clothes in the humid tropics allowed the easy transference of yaws by skin-to-skin contact. The more huddled, closely knit villages of the arid Near East encouraged the treponeme to become endemic, particularly in the increased child population. Such a change is due to many factors, not least an increased population size unit, a more settled existence and, as a cause or a consequence, the more year-round assured food supply. With increased urbanization of the temperate zones, the relaxation of sexual attitudes, increased climatic necessity for clothes and an increased element of unsettled and maritally unattached individuals, the treponeme was encouraged to find new routes of transmission. In such circumstances transmission by the intimacy of sexual intercourse replaced the more casual skin contact of yaws and endemic syphilis. Venereal syphilis entered the scene and, like many infections, its spread was facilitated by urbanization, prostitution and military and religious pilgrimage (Hudson, 1963). Prostitution, the familiar reservoir of venereal infection, has no place in village society.

It has been found that there is a back and forth transition from one treponemal disease to another even within a single group of people when changing from one environment to another. This support for Hudson's theory has led to his statement that every social group has the kind of treponematosis that is appropriate to its geographical and climatic home and its stage of cultural development (Hudson, 1965). It is also noted that there can be differing presentations within separate peoples living in the same geographic environment. For example, in the yaws regions, groups such as Europeans with higher standards of living rarely develop yaws but do develop venereal syphilis (Cockburn, 1961). The relationship between geographic area, climate environment and treponemal infection is therefore by no means straightforward.

The second major theory of treponemal evolution regards the causative bacteria of pinta, yaws and syphilis as separate species of the genus *Treponema* (Hackett, 1963; Brothwell, 1970), ascribing their origin to the mutation of the primeval *Treponema carateum* under the influence of climate variation. Mutation is a phenomenon that must be common in the rapidly multiplying world of bacteria. By the Darwinian process of natural selection, certain mutants may be better adapted to the new climate. Their reproduction at the expense of the parent species will thus ensure the new clinical presentation of disease. The two theories, which, in practice, are not so widely different, centre around the taxonomy of *Treponema*.

Notwithstanding these theories, there remains to be explained the startling, almost meteoric, rise to importance of venereal syphilis in sixteenth-century Europe (e.g. see Arrizabalaga *et al.*, 1997). Lending support to the Columbian theory, documentary records attest the near-epidemic status of the disease around 1500. Clearly, a decade or so after the return of Columbus's force, be it syphilitic or not, is insufficient time to unleash a European pandemic. This is not an epidemiological reality with a chronic disease such as venereal syphilis. It is possible, however, that Columbus brought back from the Americas a more virulent strain of *Treponema pallidum* and that this was responsible for converting a long-standing and comparatively mild disease in Europe into one of fulminating character. It has been further proposed (Hackett, 1967) that venereal syphilis in Europe prior to the Columbian expeditions was not identified specifically from several other diseases, including leprosy. Possible support for this is noted in the Medieval belief in the venereal mode of transmission of leprosy. However, skeletal evidence from Medieval leprosy cemeteries does not support this proposition (see Crane-Kramer, 2002, on the lack of evidence of skeletons with venereal syphilis in late Medieval European cemeteries). Holcomb (1940), in discussing the possible Medieval diagnostic confusion of leprosy, cites syphilis as one of the confusing diseases. He refers to the writings of observers as early as the fourteenth and fifteenth centuries, among them Paracelsus and Guy de Chauliac. These workers refer to diseases that may now be interpreted as venereal syphilis. There is, however, no general agreement on these interpretations, which rely so much on the observations, acumen and accuracy of recording of the early physicians.

Doubtless, discussions of these theories will continue for many years, but what of the skeletal evidence? Clearly, palaeopathological evidence of pinta is not found. In order to place in true perspective the corporeal evidence of treponemal infection from antiquity, it must be restated that less than about 20 per cent of infected individuals display bone changes of their infection. Taking into account such aspects as the often-assumed earlier age at death in antiquity, it is likely that, in studying the skeletal evidence from the past, one is seeing merely the tip of the iceberg. The earliest evidence of yaws comes from the Mariana Islands and is dated to about AD 850 (Stewart and Spoehr, 1967). The diagnosis has been made on the classic cranial and long-bone features of the disease. Evidence of yaws from later periods has come from pre-European-contact Australia, pre-contact Tonga, Easter Island, Borneo and Puerto Rico (Steinbock, 1976), and Guam (Rothschild and Heathcote, 1993).

The separation of venereal from endemic syphilis in early skeletal specimens depends upon the geographic origin of the specimen just as much as the bone lesions. An example of endemic syphilis showing skull and long-bone changes in an Australian Aboriginal skeleton of pre-European-contact date has been described (Sandison, 1980b). A further case has been described in a skull from Tasmania, and it is suggested that the disease accompanied the original inhabitants on their migration from Australia into Tasmania some 10,000 years ago (Hackett, 1974). A European example has also been noted from this period (Anderson et al., 1986).

For reasons already discussed, which were perhaps not always scientifically motivated, concentration of thought has been on venereal syphilis almost at the expense of the other treponemal diseases. The early evidence of syphilis in the Old World is sparse but increasing. Examples from Siberia dated as early as 1000 BC have been diagnosed as possible syphilis (Steinbock, 1976). However, an extensive examination of several thousand early Egyptian and European skeletons has failed to reveal evidence of syphilis prior to AD 1500 (Møller-Christensen, 1969b). A single female skull with typical caries sicca was discovered in the burial ground of Christ Church, Spitalfields, London, and dated prior to 1537 (Morant, 1931). Unfortunately the terminus post quem is 1197 and further dating precision cannot be made. Evidence of the early presence of syphilis in England has also come from the cemetery of St Helen-on-the-Walls, York. A skull from this cemetery displays caries sicca. The burials are mainly dated to the fifteenth and sixteenth centuries (Dawes and Magilton, 1980) and this particular skull has been radiocarbon dated to before AD 1492. With increased cemetery excavations and skeletal examination using improved diagnostic techniques and dating precision, further examples of pre-Columbian treponemal disease have been identified in the Old World (Stirland, 1991a, 1994 (England); Power, 1992 (Ireland); Gladykowska-Rzeczycka, 1994 (Poland); Henneberg and Henneberg, 1994 (Italy); Roberts, 1994 and Mays et al. (2003) (England), Mitchell, 2003 (Israel), Steyn and Henneberg, 1995 (sub-Saharan Africa)). A diagnosis of congenital syphilis, and thus venereal syphilis, has also been proposed for fetal remains from Hyères, France (Pálfi et al., 1992). Higher precision dating and a Bayesian approach to the interpretation of radio carbon dates are key to exploring the history of venereal syphilis, and recent research shows the use of Bayesian analysis to offset the effect of a marine diet on dating acuracy (Bayliss et al., 2004).

Evidence of early treponemal disease in the Old World may be inferred from the documentary records of treatment, but this is, of course, circumstantial evidence only. It appears that, in the twelfth and thirteenth centuries, the Crusading forces in the Levant were using 'Saracen ointment' to treat a disease that they diagnosed as leprosy. This ointment contained mercury and, for whatever disease it was efficacious, it was certainly useless in the treatment of leprosy. For many years, mercurial compounds were used in the treatment of syphilis. The suggestion is therefore that the Crusaders were using their mercurial ointments to treat syphilis. Such evidence is tentative when compared to the irrefutable evidence of palaeopathology.

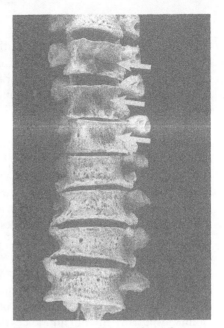

Fig. 7.34. Bone destruction of vertebrae possibly due to an aortic aneurysm. *(Terry Collection 1190, National Museum of Natural History, Washington DC, United States)*

In contrast to the sparse evidence from the Old World prior to AD 1500, North and Central America afford indisputable evidence of pre-Columbian syphilis (Baker and Armelagos, 1988; Larsen, 1997 for a summary). For example, cases of the disease have been diagnosed from Pecos Pueblo, New Mexico, Arizona, Alabama and Ohio (El-Najjar, 1979) and North Carolina (Reichs, 1989). This also includes evidence for pre-Columbian congenital syphilis in Mexico (Pineda *et al.*, 1998). However, skeletal evidence of the cardiovascular sequelae of late-stage venereal syphilis is rare indeed, from the northern plains of North America, although a single skeleton exhibiting erosion of the posterior surface of the manubrium and the anterior surfaces of the second and third thoracic vertebrae is indicative of an aneurysm of the aorta, an arterial dilatation probably responsible for the death of the individual (Walker, 1983). Furthermore, in England, an archaeological site has revealed a skeleton with lesions consistent with an aortic aneurysm in the spine (Brothwell and Browne, 1994), although there was no supporting evidence of skeletal changes consistent with venereal syphilis (see Fig. 7.34 for an example of bone changes of aortic aneurysm).

Ideas concerning the bacteriology and the history of the treponemal diseases will no doubt be modified from time to time. With increasing archaeological excavation and with firmly established diagnostic criteria, the evidence for early treponemal disease will accumulate. The evolutionary models already discussed, based in part on theory and in part on the observed skeletal evidence, suggest that human infection due to bacteria of the genus *Treponema* existed in both pre-Columbian Europe and pre-Columbian America. Infective diseases are not solely microbiological entities but are a composite reflection of individual immunity and social, environmental and biological interaction.

Brucellosis and the mycoses

Brucellosis, caused by bacteria of the genus *Brucella*, is a zoonotic infection that relies on humans working with animals to enable contamination of the skin and droplet infection, the latter being rare (Aufderheide and Rodríguez-Martín, 1998: 192), and/or consumption of animal products. It is a chronic disease of the lungs and other organs (Ortner, 2003: 216), with recurring bouts of fever ('undulant fever'). It may come to humans from pigs (*B. suis*), from goats and sheep (*B. melitensis*) or from cattle/horses (*B. abortus*) – (Wilkinson, 1993). All are widespread around the world where these domesticated animals are utilized. Fever caused by *B. melitensis* is, in effect, a septicaemia and it may last days or months, and can relapse; symptoms include muscular pain, sweating, chills and weakness. *B. abortus* apparently is less likely to cause disease in humans (Wilkinson, 1993). Males are more affected than females and most modern sufferers are over 30 years of age (Aegerter and Kirkpatrick, 1975 in Aufderheide and Rodríguez-Martín, 1998).

Around 10 per cent of people with the infection will develop bone changes (Aufderheide and Rodríguez-Martín, 1998), although higher rates have been reported. The bone changes of brucellosis are a result of spread of the infection via the bloodstream, starting in the bone marrow. They include degeneration of the joints, especially the hip and knee, the sacroiliac joint and the interphalangeal joints of the hands, and involvement of the spine, or brucellar spondylitis/anterior vertebral epiphysitis (Capasso, 1999). Most cases affect the lower thoracic and lumbar spine, and the spinal ligaments, intervertebral discs and vertebral bodies are involved (although the spinal changes do not occur in children). The antero-superior vertebral area is destroyed in the area of the annulus fibrosus of the disc (Capasso, 1999). Unlike in tuberculosis, there is reactive new bone formation and no spinal collapse. Radiographically, a hemi-ring of greater density around the lower part of the destroyed area, due to an increase in size of individual trabeculae and their numbers, is considered pathognomonic for brucellosis. If the infection progresses, then more extensive destructive lesions of the vertebral bodies may be expected.

Few examples of brucellosis have been reported in the palaeopathological literature to date but are summarized in Ortner (2003). Capasso (1999) identified 16 individuals out of 151 from Herculaneum, Italy (AD 79) with characteristic brucellosis changes in the spine. Of 29 affected vertebrae, 9 were of the fourth lumbar. His interpretation of these skeletal data, and an understanding of the historical data on the Roman use of animals in the Mediterranean, indicated that goats were probably the most likely source of the disease here. Interestingly, 11 of the individuals had associated new bone formation on the visceral surfaces of their ribs, possibly as a reaction to pleurisy (one of the localizations of *Brucella* in the early stages of the disease (Capasso, 1999: 284)). Etxeberria (1994) also notes two cases from later Medieval Spain and one from the Chalcolithic.

The mycoses, or fungal infections, may also affect the skeleton (systemic mycoses from soil inhabiting fungi), but they are rare and infrequently affect the bones; lesions are also randomly distributed, and skeletal distribution is similar for most (Ortner, 2003: 325). The bone lesions are destructive and may affect multiple elements. Today there are around 200 fungi that have been identified as being pathogenic to humans (Ainsworth, 1993), and inhalation of the fungus, or infection via traumatized skin, are the most common routes of transmission (Aufderheide and Rodríguez-Martín, 1998: 212). Spread of the fungal infection to the skeleton is via the bloodstream or lymphatic system. The different mycoses tend to be located in specific geographic regions. If one assumes that this distribution has remained constant throughout time, then geographic location will be key to diagnosis. For example, North American blastomycosis is found especially in North Carolina and the Mississippi and Ohio valleys (Ortner, 2003: 326), paracoccidiomycosis is a Central and South American variant, while coccidiomycosis is found only in the western hemisphere (Ortner, 2003: 326), and warm dry regions (Ainsworth, 1993: 733). Like brucellosis, the fungal infections have rarely been reported in the palaeopathological literature. However, Allison *et al.* (1979) note histological evidence for paracoccidiomycosis in a Chilean mummy, and Kelley and Eisenberg (1987), along with tuberculosis, identified blastomycosis at two sites in the United States at Mobridge, South Dakota, and Averbuch, Tennessee, dated to the late seventeenth/early nineteenth centuries AD, and AD 1275 to the end of the fourteenth century AD, respectively.

PARASITIC INFECTION

In many parts of the world today, particularly those bordering the tropics, infection by the larger parasites is a cause of considerable morbidity. By and large it is the **endoparasites**, which live within the host's body, that tend to give rise to chronic disease and are therefore responsible, in part, for the chronic ill-health that characterizes some of the poorer nations of the world, at least in the recent past. A similar situation must have existed in the more distant past also. Since many of these parasites do not solely attack humans but have animal host stages in their life-cycle, a prerequisite for human infection is close animal-to-human contact (humans are 'an accidental host'). Many parasites have infected humans only when, in the evolutionary process, the latter have become omnivorous, eating meat as well as vegetable foods. Several parasites, either as adults or at some stage in the life-cycle, live within the flesh of animals. It is by eating such flesh that humans become infected. This may, in part, explain the food taboos of certain religious groups. For example, the Jewish avoidance of pork may be due to their knowledge in the distant past of infection of pigs by *Taenia solium* (one of the tapeworms), and its transference to humans by the eating of infected pork. This knowledge was obviously not gained by scientific observation but was the result of years of conscious experience. Parasitic infection of people is likely to have become more widespread with animal domestication, and its increase may therefore have run parallel with tuberculosis.

In palaeopathological terms, the evidence for these parasitic infections is sparse, but techniques of investigation are improving and ancient DNA analysis may help in the future. Some parasites can be seen by the naked eye but others need a microscope, and the range of parasitic infections in antiquity is becoming known (Sandison, 1981). The parasites themselves are, like our own flesh and blood, soft tissues. Just like our own soft tissues, these parasites putrefy and disappear after burial of the host. Occasionally, however, parasitic remains are discovered in mummified human remains. Perhaps the earliest observation of this kind was made by Ruffer (1910). He found eggs of the parasite *Schistosoma haematobium* in the kidneys of two mummies of XX Dynasty date. This condition, known at one time as bilharziasis, induces bleeding into the urinary tract and, even today, is a source of considerable morbidity in parts of Africa and the Mediterranean. In more recent mummy investigations, evidence of many more parasites has been found (see Aufderheide, 2003).

Unfortunately, the osteoarchaeological evidence of parasitic infection consists of very few examples. A tapeworm of the genus *Echinococcus* lives in the intestines of sheep, dogs, foxes and rodents. The parasite eggs are passed in the faeces of these animals and if, due to food or water contamination, they are ingested by humans the eggs enter the life-cycle phases of the worm. The larvae of the eggs penetrate the gut wall, spread via the blood (Aufderheide and Rodríguez-Martín, 1998: 241) and develop into multiple cystic structures called hydatid cysts which inhabit various organs of the body, principally the liver and, to a lesser extent, the lungs. By good fortune, at least for the palaeopathologist if not for the affected individual, these cysts calcified in a Medieval Danish woman with leprosy and were discovered on excavation (Fig. 7.35). Seventy-two identified cysts and many fragments of similar cysts were found in the area of the abdominal cavity (Weiss and Møller-Christensen, 1971b). A solitary cyst measuring 47 × 35 mm was also found in the chest cavity of a Romano-British woman; this hydatid cyst was presumably in the lung (Wells, 1976b). A solitary egg-shaped lesion was also found in the area of the abdomen of a skeleton from Medieval Winchester. The lesion was shown on radiography to have a smooth inner lining characteristic of a calcified hydatid cyst

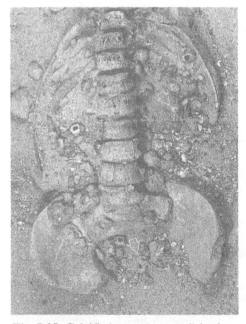

Fig. 7.35. Calcified cysts (arrowed) in the abdominal cavity of a female burial (late Medieval, twelfth–sixteenth centuries AD, Denmark).

(Price, 1975). Bone lesions affect 1–2 per cent of people with hydatid disease (Aufderheide and Rodríguez-Martín, 1998: 242), and destruction of cancellous bone by the rupture of the cysts, especially in the lower spine, is the usual change observed. Long bones and the pelvis may also be affected but not commonly. The presence of infection caused by *Echinoccocus* species must, of course, be an indication of the close association between humans and their domesticated animals – for example, the herding of sheep with dogs. People have for a long time lived in fairly close association with dogs. Animals may have been used for hunting or may, as in recent times, have been kept as pets and companions. The potential for this parasitic transfer from dog to human has been ever present. The squalid and unhygienic lifestyle of the Medieval town possibly increased human population prevalence. It is then surprising that more evidence of such cysts is not forthcoming. These cysts are, however, thin walled and fragile and may not have survived their environment of deposition over several hundred years of burial. Their presence should nevertheless be looked for during the archaeological excavation of human skeletal remains.

Of course, another parasitic infection, malaria, caused by the protozoan *Plasmodium* species and transmitted by the mosquito *Anopheles* species, may (indirectly) reveal itself in the skeleton through the occurrence of the bone changes of sickle-cell and thalassaemia, as an adaptive response (see Chapter 8). However, recent research has managed to extract and amplify the ancient DNA of the parasite from the skeleton of a twentieth-century individual from the Hamann-Todd Collection, Ohio, whose cause of death was defined as malaria (Taylor *et al.*, 1997), thus indicating that now direct evidence can be retrieved from bone as a result of developments in analytical methods. A more recent report by Sallares and Gomzi (2001) managed to extract the DNA of *Plasmodium falciparum* from skeletons from a Roman site dated to the fifth century in Italy.

Knowledge of the parasitic infections of humans in antiquity is becoming more extensive in another way, arising from a perhaps unexpected source. The excavation of settlement sites is producing material from latrines and rubbish pits, and certain environments will preserve evidence. Examination of this material is revealing the presence of parasitic eggs which were presumably passed in the faeces of humans and animals of antiquity (Reinhard, 1990; Reinhard *et al.*, 1992). Fortunately the eggs of these worms of the distant past have specific and characteristic forms. Microscopic examination of latrine deposits not only confirms the infection of earlier people but allows a specific diagnosis to be made. Eggs of *Trichuris trichiura* (whipworm) and *Ascaris lumbricoides* (roundworm), both helminth infections, have been found in the Medieval cesspits of York, England (Jones, 1985). With such knowledge, the clinical symptoms and consequences of infection can be deduced. Abdominal discomfort, diarrhoea and constant blood loss associated with tapeworm infection must have accounted for much morbidity in past populations. Maybe the chronic iron deficiency anaemia causing cribra orbitalia and porotic hyperostosis, to be considered in the next chapter, is in part due to such infection. These microscopic findings of environmental archaeology are reliable, if circumstantial, evidence of parasitic infection of humans.

Of much wider distribution and of much less clinical significance are the infestations of humans by **ectoparasites**. These organisms do not enter the body but live on the skin surface and hair. For survival they suck the blood of the host. Ectoparasites such as the flea, head and body lice, and ticks usually cause no more serious problem than a rash and the social embarrassment of itching. Occasionally, however, these arthropods may be the vectors of serious disease. Harbouring smaller organisms, notably the different species of *Rickettsia*, within their intestinal tract, the human ectoparasites may transfer these agents of disease directly to the bloodstream of humans.

The infectious disease of typhus is a serious, sometimes fatal, sequel to life in insanitary conditions. Also known as camp fever, typhus was well known to campaigning troops in recent wars. No doubt it was common too in earlier times, particularly among the besieged and the besiegers in prolonged Medieval warfare.

However, there is no skeletal or mummified evidence of this acute infectious disease, but there are preserved ectoparasites in mummified remains. Of a small series of North American Indian mummies examined, 44 per cent had head lice (El-Najjar and Mulinski, 1980). Zias and Mumcuoglu (1991) also found head lice preserved in hair combs in Israel, and Capasso (1998) reports head lice at Herculaneum, Italy, in a young female. The eggs of the head lice *Pediculus humanus* var. *capitis* are also common findings in the mummies of Peru (Vreeland and Cockburn, 1980).

Although the palaeopathological evidence of ectoparasites is scant, when found their prevalence in a burial group is high. It is deduced therefore that ectoparasitic infection was commonplace in antiquity. Presumably, the diseases such as typhus, dependent upon their parasitism, were also common. It is unfortunate that knowledge concerning the range and prevalence of parasitic infection in the distant past is incomplete because of the limited nature of preservation. Such evidence as there is suggests that the problem was as widespread and varied, if not more so, as it is today. The improvements in food care, hygiene and animal husbandry during the passage of time have, by and large, restricted the problems today to the less developed areas of the world.

INFECTIOUS DISEASE IN PALAEOPATHOLOGY AND BIOMOLECULAR ANALYSIS

While research in the palaeopathology of infectious diseases that has utilized ancient biomolecular analysis has been noted in the relevant sections of this chapter, further comment is appropriate at this stage. It is true to say that it is the infectious diseases that have received the most attention from biomolecular analysis. Tuberculosis has been the target for most studies (e.g. Gernaey *et al.*, 2001 on ancient DNA and mycolic acids), but leprosy (Taylor *et al.*, 2000), treponemal disease (Kolman *et al.*, 1999), plague (Drancourt *et al.*, 1998), malaria (Sallares and Gomzi, 2001) and the 1918 Spanish flu (Reid *et al.*, 1999) have also received attention, as have hepatitis E in an Italian mummy (Marota *et al.*, 1998), bacterial DNA in the colon of a Chilean mummy (Ubaldi *et al.*, 1998) and in the skin and muscle of the 'Iceman' found on the Austrian/Italian border (Rollo *et al.*, 2000), and *Escheria coli* in the Lindow Man bog body (Fricker *et al.*, 1997). Clearly these analyses help to confirm a diagnosis in human remains, identify an infection when no changes in the bodily tissues are apparent (for example, if the person died before bone changes occurred), and diagnose diseases that do not affect bones, such as plague. Furthermore, identifying the specific organism causing a disease is now potentially possible, although correlating bone changes directly with a positive result for ancient microbial DNA is not. While these are significant advances for our understanding of the evolution and palaeoepidemiology of infectious disease, the necessary costs involved, the need for technical expertise, the destructive nature of the analysis and the problems of non-survival of DNA (and possible contamination with external microbial DNA) can limit us. Moreover, most people working in palaeopathology utilize, and will continue to use, macroscopic and radiographic methods of diagnosis.

CHAPTER 8

Metabolic and Endocrine Disease

In view of the prevalence of malnutrition in the world today, it is unlikely that it did not occur in the past, despite the vast increase in world population. (Brothwell and Brothwell, 1969: 175)

INTRODUCTION

Unfortunately, classification in clinical medicine is not all-embracing. There exist diseases of palaeopathological significance which do not lend themselves to the foregoing classes used in the present volume. These diseases may loosely be considered as the abnormalities of deficiency or excess, not only of dietary constituents, but also of hormones, those chemicals manufactured by the endocrine glands of the body for the maintenance of its health.

METABOLIC DISEASE

Past societies are often assumed to have trodden that fine knife-edge between subsistence and starvation. As has been noted in connection with population expansion, the improved techniques and refinement of agricultural methods shifted some groups away from starvation, albeit temporarily, even if there was a greater risk of dietary deficiencies through reliance on a less varied and poorer-quality diet (Cohen and Armelagos, 1984). Starvation is still a familiar sight today in the less developed areas of the world, particularly where the rainfall level is critical. Of course, the recent developments in growing genetically modified (GM) food may help or hinder the problem of feeding the world's population in the future (Coghlan, 2002). Certainly there may be potential in developing genetically modified foods to combat diseases due to deficiencies in some crops – for example, anaemia as a result of low iron levels in rice (Holmes, 1999); higher crop yields may also be enabled (Le Page, 2002). No doubt in the past an increasing community size still stretched the food resource. It is not just the total lack of food, or the overall starvation problem, which is of relevance. A lack of quality, particularly in respect of essential vitamins and chemical trace elements, is just as important. Evidence of chronic food shortage, by living on the wrong side of the 'knife-edge', may be deduced from the study of skeletal and dental remains. Many factors may be involved in the production of such skeletal and dental abnormalities, but a direct causal relationship with poor diet cannot be inferred as it is likely that multifactorial causes may be implicated.

The metabolic diseases can also be described as 'indicators of stress', a term used increasingly in the anthropological literature over the past 20 years. The abnormalities observed in skeletal and dental remains represent the individual's adaptive response to stressors working on the body during his or her growing years. That response will be determined by a number of factors, for example the individual's immune status and genetic predisposition, environmental constraints and cultural systems (e.g. see Schell, 1997). In effect, the environment will provide 'resources necessary for survival and the stressors that may alter the health of the population' (Larsen, 1997: 6). However, stressors will affect individuals disproportionately (Schell, 1997), and detecting why some people are more stressed than others can be complex in both modern and archaeological contexts. Clearly a skeleton with no indicators of stress may either suggest a healthy person or it may represent somebody who never recovered from the insults to the body, i.e. they were continually stressed (Wood et al., 1992). Selye (1950) suggests that stress is a non-specific response to stimuli, i.e. the body can be stressed by multiple stressors but it displays a very characteristic form and composition when it adapts. Factors in a person's environment may buffer the impact of stress but others may enhance it, and some populations may overcome some stressors but some may not. Although it is seen as physiological stress, some authors have considered psychological stress as being instrumental in predisposing to disease (Bush, 1991). It is known, for example, that emotional stress can lead to the formation of enamel hypoplastic lines on the teeth (see Chapter 4) and Harris lines of arrested growth in the long bones (see below). Although it may be possible to identify factors in a population's environment, culture or biology that may cause physiological stress, it is virtually impossible to read into their psychology. Although we know that psychological factors and health are strongly correlated (Taylor, 1995), and that stress may vary throughout any one year, decade or more, and cause psychologically induced stress (e.g. see De Garine, 1993 on seasonal stress in Africa), detecting psychologically induced stress as a cause of skeletal and dental indicators of stress in the past is problematic. Stress may affect function and reduce cognition and ability to work (Larsen, 1997: 6), and this in turn could affect the production of essential resources such as food. A consequence of this could be dietary deficiency disease, and a decline in fertility, ultimately affecting reproduction in, and maintenance of, a population.

Normal growth of the body (and skeleton) follows two main periods of activity, the first being up to about the age of one year, and again in adolescence (Larsen, 1997: 8). One should remember that the period of weaning, around three to four years, is a crucial time when passive immunity to disease is lost from the breast milk, and the child is then inherently more susceptible to health problems. Intrinsic and extrinsic factors, such as genetic inheritance and nutrition respectively, can affect normal growth. However, infectious disease may also affect growth, and there is a strong relationship between infection and nutritional status. Generally speaking, stature has been increasing through time, and much of this reflects improved nutrition and less infection due to improvements in living conditions, certainly in developed countries. However, growth can be intermittently affected if there are famines, crop failures or other crises in a population. A problem with growth, compared to earlier hunter-gatherer populations, has been recorded at a number of archaeological sites with evidence of agriculture (see Cohen and Armelagos, 1984 for some studies). The stature of an individual or population therefore is taken to reflect the level of childhood health, although a genetic predisposition to be short or tall can be present for some populations – e.g. Central African Pygmy people who have a male average stature of 4ft 9in and female stature of 4ft 6in (Bogin, 2000). Nevertheless, environment also has its part to play here, as many pygmies are undernourished.

Goodman *et al.* (1988) provide a useful summary of the recognized stress indicators shown in prehistoric, historic and contemporary populations. A number of these indicators have already been discussed, and two are particularly relevant here, mortality and stature. Mortality rates provide an indication of how healthy and adaptive (or not) a population was by their age at death profile, always assuming that their ages have been determined accurately (see Chapter 2). High infant mortality, for example, suggests that an acute infectious disease may have precipitated deaths in this age group. In addition, integrating mortality data with identified stressors may highlight earlier death in individuals who were stressed (Huss-Ashmore *et al.*, 1982; Duray, 1996). Final attained stature, when compared to that expected of the group, may also differ, and decreased stature may indicate poor nutrition during growth. Nevertheless, humans can adapt well to stress and growth may not be affected (see Ribot and Roberts, 1996 for a study of the relationship between indicators of stress and growth in Medieval England). For the purposes of this chapter those indicators that show a clear relationship with nutritional inadequacy will be considered; these are anaemia, osteoporosis and Harris lines, plus the specific vitamin deficiencies of scurvy and rickets. Dental enamel hypoplasia and periostitis are discussed in Chapters 4 and 7 respectively.

Diet and its relationship to disease

The quality of food a person eats will affect health in two ways. First, if the diet is not adequate and the person is malnourished, then his or her immune system and thus the ability to withstand disease are diminished. Secondly, if the diet is lacking in one specific constituent, then the person may develop a dietary deficiency disease. Furthermore, whether a person eats a marine or a terrestrial diet may affect whether he or she develops certain diseases, and a poor diet will affect normal skeletal and dental development. Study of past diet can be undertaken in a number of ways and includes the analysis of plant and animal remains from archaeological sites, including their containment within coprolites (ancient faeces), and the study of artefacts associated with growing and processing food. These must be classed as indirect evidence because we cannot be sure that they represent specifically the diet consumed by our population. However, direct evidence for diet can be gleaned in other ways. If studies of mummified remains are possible, then analysis of the contents of the intestines may help shed light on the last meal the person ate before death, bearing in mind that this may have been a 'special' rather than a normal meal. Analysis of pollen and larger plant remains, along with small bones from the consumption of meat or fish in intestinal contents, can be very helpful in highlighting actual food consumption. For example, Rollo *et al.* (2002) analysed the contents of the intestines of the Tyrolean iceman (Ötzi) using ancient DNA analysis, and it was possible to conclude that his last meal consisted of red deer and possibly cereals, preceded by a meal based on ibex and cereals. However, there are two main ways of exploring what type of diet a person was eating and whether there were any vital constituents missing; this is better termed a 'consumption profile' (Larsen, 1997: 270).

First, evidence of dietary deficiency diseases in the skeleton may be considered indirectly, or the evidence for 'indicators of stress' such as the analysis and interpretation of enamel hypoplastic defects on the teeth. Secondly, chemical analysis of the stable carbon and nitrogen isotope values in the protein of teeth and bone can be undertaken, along with assessment of the stable isotopes of carbon, oxygen and strontium from the mineral component of bones and teeth (Katzenberg, 2000); work in this field began in the 1970s. While trace element analysis of bone and teeth for details of palaeodiet also had its inauguration in the 1970s (Sandford and Weaver, 2000), subsequent work has illustrated the problems of diagenesis and uptake of elements from external sources during burial (Pate and Hutton, 1988; Lambert *et al.*, 1989; Price, 1989; Price *et al.*, 1992). Therefore, it is to isotope analysis that biological anthropologists turn for dietary information. Stable carbon has two isotopes: ^{12}Carbon and ^{13}Carbon. C_4 plants come from hot and dry climates and C_3 plants come from temperate areas. Relevant to isotopic analysis, the C_4 plant maize, a tropical grass, has relatively more ^{13}Carbon (heavier isotope) relative to ^{12}Carbon than most other plants from temperate regions (Katzenberg, 2000), while temperate C_3 plants have relatively less ^{13}Carbon. Marine plants have ^{13}Carbon values between the values of C_3 and C_4 plants, while marine fish and mammals have ^{13}Carbon values 'less negative . . . than animals feeding on C_3 based foods and more negative values than animals feeding on C_4 foods' (Larsen, 1997: 272). Nitrogen isotope levels will also vary. There are two, ^{14}N and ^{15}N, and nitrogen isotopes are useful for distinguishing marine from terrestrial diets. ^{15}N levels for terrestrial plants are lower than for marine plants (Larsen, 1997: 283), and higher levels are seen in hot areas compared to lower values in cooler areas.

North American research has used stable isotopic analysis extensively to explore the adoption of maize agriculture (e.g. Buikstra and Milner, 1991; Katzenberg *et al.*, 1995), indicating spatial differences. Furthermore, maize consumption and social status have been considered and are summarized in Larsen (1997). In England, Privat *et al.* (2002), in their study of carbon and nitrogen isotope values of individuals buried at the Anglo-Saxon cemetery at Berinsfield, Oxfordshire, found differences in diet between different social groups, but they found no differences between males and females. Nevertheless, differences between the sexes in maize consumption have been identified (e.g. males eating more maize than females in Central America (see White *et al.*, 1993)). The consumption of marine versus terrestrial diets has also been considered, particularly in Europe. For example, in Portugal Lubell *et al.* (1994) found more plant and animal domesticates being consumed in the Neolithic compared to the Mesolithic, while Lillie and Richards

(2000) found in both the Mesolithic and the early Neolithic Ukraine that hunting, fishing and gathering produced the protein component of the diet, and there was an increase in fish consumption into the Neolithic. More recent work (Lillie *et al.*, 2003) indicates that prior to the Mesolithic (Epipalaeolithic, or 10,400–9,200 cal. BC) animal protein and freshwater resources such as fish were the main components of the diet. In Greece, Papathanasiou (2003) used the analysis of stable isotopes of carbon and nitrogen to examine Neolithic individuals from coastal and inland sites. She found that marine foods were a minor component of the diet, even at the coastal sites. In a study in Belgium of a Medieval monastic community, Polet and Katzenberg (2003) also found that diet consisted mainly of terrestrial foods but also included some marine products. Clearly, these studies (and many others) have shed light on the components of the diet for a range of populations in time and space.

Stable nitrogen isotope analysis can also inform us about the weaning of infants in the past because levels will change at this point and later. These differences are because the nursing infant is at a different trophic level compared to the mother (the former is higher). Pre-weaned infants have a higher isotope value than weaned and older individuals (Larsen, 1997: 284). There is a general reduction in ^{15}N through childhood which indicates that the replacement of breastfeeding with other foods is gradual rather than abrupt (also see Wright and Schwarcz, 1998 and a study of individuals from Guatemala dating to 700 BC–AD 1500). Dupras *et al.* (2001) also made a study of infants from the Roman site of Dakhleh Oasis, Egypt (*c.* 250 AD), and found that the start of the weaning process was at the age of 6 months and it was completed by 3 years of age. However, at Wharram Percy, Yorkshire, England, Richards *et al.* (2002) found that weaning had occurred by 2 years of age or before. Further research at this site reflected a decrease in the consumption of isotopically enriched breast milk and the introduction of less enriched weaning foods (Fuller *et al.*, 2003). With the use of dentine sections, it was possible to study the temporal relationship of breastfeeding, weaning and dietary patterns in individuals. Some studies have also shown a correlation between enamel defects of the teeth and the age of weaning, as determined by nitrogen isotopic analyses, while others have noted a relationship between a decline in ^{15}N isotopes, weaning, loss of passive immunity and mortality (Herring *et al.*, 1998 in Katzenberg, 2000).

To date, little attention has been paid to correlating the evidence for metabolic disease with direct evidence for diet using stable isotope analysis, but no doubt this will be a focus for the future. Consequently, by considering the dietary consumption profile of individuals from archaeological sites, this may shed more light on the meaning of the metabolic diseases to be considered below. However, Katzenberg and Lovell (1999) warn that isotope signals may be affected by samples taken from pathological bone, which therefore should not be used (although usually teeth are sampled).

Anaemia

The study of the skeletal changes of anaemia attracted a great deal of attention in the twentieth century and is continuing to do so. These data have been applied to questions such as: what happened to a population's health when they started to

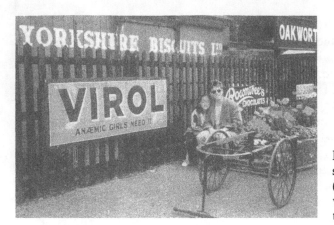

Fig. 8.1. Oakworth railway station, West Yorkshire (restored, Victorian period) with sign showing a treatment for anaemia.

practise agriculture, and was it more unhealthy to live in an urbanized or a rural community? There are a number of anaemias of different causes but this section will deal mainly with the most common form of anaemia today, that caused by **iron deficiency**. Even today 30 per cent of the world's population (500 million people) have been estimated to be iron deficient (Murphy *et al.*, 2002: 412; Fig. 8.1).

Anaemia results from a variety of disease processes, and can be defined as a reduction in concentration of haemoglobin and/or red blood cells below normal for the age and sex of the person, or a reduction in the volume of packed cells in the blood. Iron is needed for the development of haemoglobin in newly formed red blood cells in bone marrow, but in anaemia a person's red blood cells become pale and small, and they have a much shorter life span, up to half the normal life of 120 days. Iron is usually stored in the liver and the spleen when old blood cells are broken down. Around 90 per cent of the iron in old red blood cells is needed to form new cells and, as iron deficiency develops, these stores are depleted while the body attempts to absorb increased amounts of iron. As well as being needed for haemoglobin formation in red blood cells, which then transfer oxygen to the body cells from the lungs, iron is also necessary for the transmission of nerve impulses for collagen (protein) synthesis, and contributes to the strength of the immune system.

There are two forms of iron, non-haem, which is mainly derived from cereals and is poorly absorbed by the intestines, and haem iron, which comes from red meats and is more easily absorbed (Murphy, Wainscoat and Colvin, 2002: 412). For example, only 1.4 per cent of iron from spinach is taken in by the body, while 20 per cent of iron from red meat can be absorbed (Scrimshaw, 2000: 252). Compounds called phytates in staple cereal crops such as maize, nuts and legumes inhibit iron absorption (whereas vitamin C aids absorption). Cereals are themselves poor sources of iron (Stuart-Macadam, 1992), and it is notable that iron is added today to most of the cereals we eat at breakfast (Fig. 8.2). Thus, the transition from hunter-gathering to an agriculturally based economy relying on these crops for an adequate varied diet (Fig. 8.3) may have led to iron deficiency in the past. Increases in anaemia have been reported at many archaeological sites at the transition to agriculture (e.g. see Cohen and Armelagos, 1984; Steckel and Rose, 2002). In British contexts too there seems to

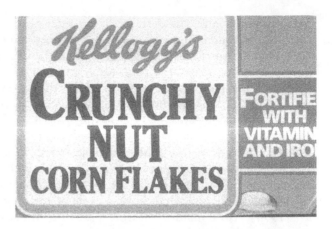

Fig. 8.2. Cereal packet showing the addition of essential dietary constituents.

be an increase in anaemia through time (Roberts and Cox, 2003), although absolute frequency rates are difficult to determine. While it is not possible to assess whether there was an increase in anaemia with the transition to agriculture in the Neolithic period, because of the lack of pre-agricultural skeletal remains available for study in Britain, it seems that an increase in anaemia may represent intensification of agriculture, but also other factors. For example, today iron-deficiency anaemia appears to increase closer to the equator and at lower elevations (Stuart-Macadam, 1998: 53). The picture is not that clear cut, however, because many factors can predispose to the development of anaemia (Kent, 1987). A diet low in iron, poor hygiene and increased infection with the development of settled agricultural communities could all contribute together or individually to anaemia. In fact Walker (1986) categorically states that, in his study of 400 crania from a Californian fish-dependent group of people living in

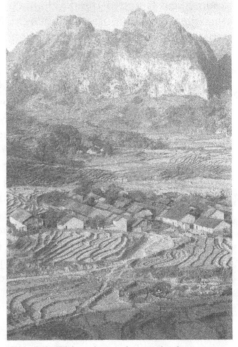

Fig. 8.3. China: intensive agriculture, which could generate a less balanced and varied diet.

the prehistoric and historic periods, this iron-rich diet did not prevent the occurrence of anaemia. However, some fish do have a low iron content; for example, white fish has 0.5mg/100g compared to 7.0mg/100g in kidney and liver and 1.9mg/100g in beef (Her Majesty's Stationery Office, 1985). These results, of course, support the suggestion that diet is only one of the causes of anaemia.

Apart from an iron-deficient diet, excessive blood loss through injury, menstruation and chronic disease such as cancer and parasitic infection of the gut, which inhibit iron absorption, probably all had a large part to play in the past. It is known from the survival of parasites in archaeological deposits that humans were subject to gut infections (Reinhard, 1988); their prevalence, both geographically and through time, is, however, unknown. Last, but certainly not least, is the impact of infection on a population; most nutritional deficiencies are aggravated by infection, and poor living conditions and sanitation would predispose people to infections. Work on the Medieval skeletons from a Danish leprosy hospital at Naestved indicated that two-thirds of the group with bone changes of leprosy had skeletal indications of anaemia. At that time Møller-Christensen (1953) believed the lesions in the orbits indicative of anaemia to be the result of leprosy. Carlson *et al.* (1974) also consider the role parasitic infection had in influencing the occurrence of anaemic changes in skeletons from prehistoric Nubia, and Stuart-Macadam (1992) summarizes the evidence for infectious disease as a major aetiological factor in the development of iron-deficiency anaemia. It is believed that the process of infection leads the body to withhold iron from the pathogens, which need it to survive and reproduce in the body; this makes the body iron-deficient. If this theory holds true, then changes in settlement pattern and increasing population density with the transition to agriculture would have led to an increase in infectious diseases (Fig. 8.4); the study of infectious disease in some populations seems to support this theory (Cohen and Armelagos, 1984), although others do not. There are studies (e.g. Møller-Christensen, 1953; Mensforth *et al.*, 1978) where anaemic bone changes and infection have also been observed in the same skeleton. If iron-deficiency anaemia is induced by the body as an adaptive response to infection, both the skeletal changes of anaemia and infection may reflect different aetiological factors. As Stuart-Macadam (1992: 159–60) suggests, these causes could be a function of many factors such as climate, geography, hygiene (Figs 8.5 and 8.6), diet, time period and economy.

Fatigue, pallor, headaches, shortness of breath, fainting, palpitations and increased heart rate characterize the disease, with more severe forms creating growth and cognitive development problems (Ryan, 1997), gastrointestinal disturbances, cardiac failure and abnormalities in the skeleton. Spoon-shaped

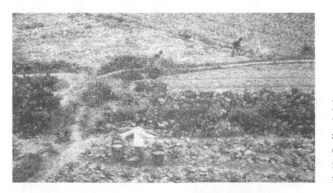

Fig. 8.4. China: watering vegetables with 'night soil' in an area with little naturally occurring water. Parasitic infections are prevalent from this farming practice.

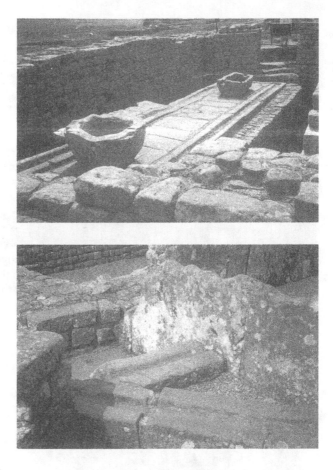

Fig. 8.5. The Romans in Britain developed mechanisms to improve hygiene and dispose of sewage and waste water (toilets at Housesteads Roman fort, Hadrian's Wall, Northumberland, England).

Fig. 8.6. Drainage channels for waste water (Housesteads Roman fort, Hadrian's Wall, Northumberland, England).

(koilonychia) brittle nails can also occur. This latter feature has been identified in a bronze fourth-century AD arm from Gloucestershire, England (Hart, 1980). The bone changes probably only develop in childhood (Stuart-Macadam, 1985), although adults do display the lesions. On the basis of studies of radiographs of patients with anaemia, specific criteria for identification of this condition in archaeological groups have been produced (Stuart-Macadam, 1987). Although anaemia occurs in all areas of the world in the past and today, the bone changes vary in extent and severity. Thinning of the outer table of the skull, due to vertically orientated trabeculae in the diploë causing pressure on the table (the 'hair-on-end' appearance radiographically), and thickening of the diploë between the two skull tables are two of the main criteria highlighted (Figs 8.7 and 8.8). These changes are the result of the body being stimulated to produce more red blood cells in the marrow to compensate for lack of iron. This stimulation comes from the hormone erythropoetin produced by the kidneys. Apart from the (external) skull lesions, particularly seen on the parietal and occipital bones (porotic hyperostosis) (Fig. 8.9), the orbital roofs are affected (Fig. 8.10) in the form of 'holes' in the bone surface (cribra orbitalia). The skeletal changes of anaemia

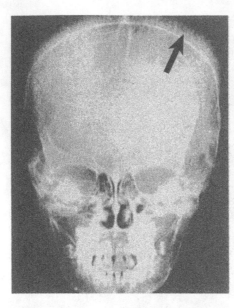

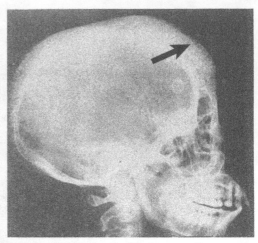

Fig. 8.7. Radiograph of 'hair-on-end' appearance in porotic hyperostosis of anaemia. *(Calvin Wells Photographic Collection)*

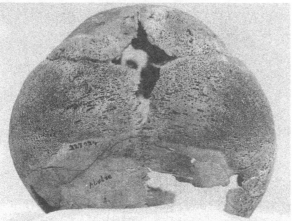

Fig. 8.8. Cranial porotic hyperostosis in anaemia (National Museum of Natural History, Washington DC, United States, 327074, 1–2-year-old child, Pueblo Bonito, New Mexico, United States). *(With permission of Don Ortner)*

appear to come in two forms: the orbital lesions alone, and both orbital and vault lesions together – the bones are often symmetrically affected and vault lesions do not tend to occur without the orbits being involved. It has been suggested that the vault lesions indicate a more severe form of the anaemia (Stuart-Macadam, 1989a) but that, because of the similarity of orbital and vault lesions radiographically, both are caused by the same aetiological factor. In archaeological populations in Britain the vault lesions are rarely seen, with cribra orbitalia being much more common, and an increase in porosity of the vault surface is often observed (Fig. 8.11), sometimes with no attendant cribra orbitalia. This, of course, may purely be a variation in the normal appearance of the skull for that particular population. Similar lesions in the skull vault may also be seen in vitamin C and D deficiency (scurvy and rickets respectively), inflammation of the skull and some tumours.

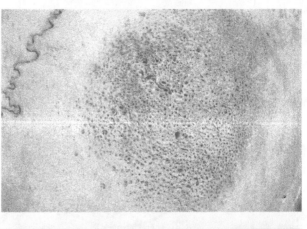

Fig. 8.9. Detail of lesions of porotic hyperostosis in the parietal bone.

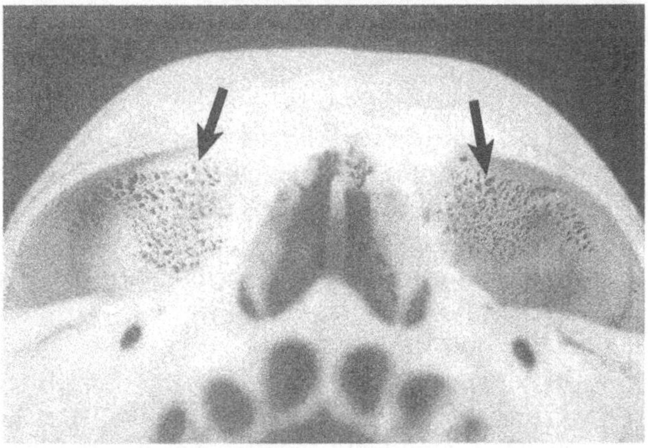

Fig. 8.10. Cribra orbitalia of both orbits. *(National Museum of Natural History, Washington DC, United States, 266456, Pachacamac, Peru, South America)*

Attempts differentially to diagnose these conditions using histological analysis have been undertaken (Schultz, 2001; Wapler *et al.*, 2004). Standards for recording of the lesions of anaemia have also been described by many most recently by Buikstra and Ubelaker (1994) and Stuart-Macadam (1991). However, it is clear that standardization of recording of the lesions so that data are comparable between population studies is far from perfect (Jacobi and Danforth, 2002).

In a study by Stuart-Macadam (1991) of 752 individuals from a Romano–British site at Poundbury, Dorset, England, 230 had bone changes supporting a diagnosis of anaemia. Infectious disease may have been the main cause. In addition, 173 (75 per cent) had orbital lesions only, 7 (3 per cent) had vault lesions only and 50 (22 per cent) had both. Juveniles had a significantly high prevalence of both orbital and vault lesions, and the lesions were more 'severe'. A similar picture was seen in the analysis of a Medieval Christian population from Upper Nubia derived from two cemeteries (Mittler and Van Gerven, 1994); active lesions of anaemia (unhealed edges to the lesions) were only observed in the young (up to the age of 12 years) and the frequency of lesions decreased after this time. The presence of these active lesions obviously indicates that the individual had not yet adapted to the disease at the time of death. In fact, studies do show that there is an increased mortality in

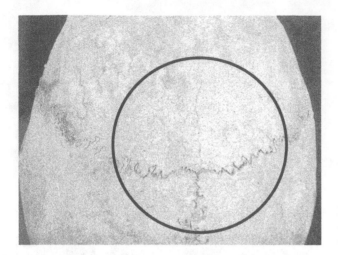

Fig. 8.11. Increased porosity
on frontal and parietal bones
(encircled) (England).

individuals with cribra orbitalia (Huss-Ashmore *et al.*, 1982) compared to those
without. Few studies have explored whether there were differences in anaemia
levels in the past between males and females, although Stuart-Macadam (1998)
provides an overview of data from some past and present population studies. From
this overview she indicates that, before mothers began to rely on wet nurses to feed
their babies, for example, in the Medieval period in Europe, they breastfed their
babies for up to the first four years of life. Consequently, mothers were not
regularly menstruating and there was therefore no excessive blood loss and
subsequent anaemia. The data suggest too that males suffered more anaemia until
the Medieval period and then females had the highest rates (because of repeated
pregnancies, and regular menstruation between them). Cow's milk also has less
iron, and infants can be intolerant to cow's milk, which may lead to gastrointestinal
bleeding (Stuart-Macadam, 1998: 58). With respect to status and the development
of anaemia, some studies have noted a lower frequency in higher-status
individuals, suggesting that perhaps their diet contained more red meat, and/or
that they lived in better conditions and were less susceptible to infection (Larsen,
1997: 39). Novel methods of diagnosing anaemia by measuring the iron content of
the bone and other organic material in skeletons, with and without bone changes of
anaemia, have indicated a correlation between lower iron levels and anaemia
(Fornaciari *et al.*, 1981; Sandford *et al.*, 1983), although some studies have not
(Glen-Haduch *et al.*, 1997). Nevertheless, consideration should always be given to
the possibility of absorption of iron into bone from the grave environment.

Although iron-deficiency anaemia is the most commonly observed anaemia today
(and probably in the past), two **inherited anaemias** characterized by abnormal
haemoglobin should also be discussed. Both are called 'Haemolytic Anaemias' and
are characterized by increased destruction of red blood cells. They produce bone
changes in areas of the skeleton other than the skull but, essentially, the skull
changes are the same for all the anaemias (see Hershkovitz *et al.*, 1997 on
differential diagnostic features of the anaemias). **Thalassaemia** is a genetically

determined disorder caused by a problem of haemoglobin synthesis (Steinbock, 1976). It is named 'alpha' or 'beta' (more common) thalassaemia according to which globin chain of the haemoglobin has the genetic mutation (Aufderheide and Rodríguez-Martín, 1998: 347). Failure or depression of synthesis of the chain leads to pale cells with low haemoglobin content, which are rapidly destroyed once formed. A high frequency of the disorder is seen today around the Mediterranean, in the Middle East and the Far East. There are three types of thalassaemia: minor (symptomless with mild or absent anaemia), intermediate (moderate anaemia) and major (characterized by severe anaemia, and possible bone changes), also termed Cooley's anaemia (Murphy *et al.*, 2002: 428). It is the latter type that may become evident in skeletal remains from archaeological sites, but it has a high infant and childhood mortality (Ortner, 2003: 365). Indeed, Angel (1966b) felt that the porotic hyperostosis he identified in archaeological skeletons from Greek, Cypriot and Turkish contexts, deriving from a marshy environment probably laden with malaria-carrying mosquitoes, was an adaptive response to malaria (along with thalassaemia development). More recent work has explored this theory further by identifying the malaria parasite's (genus *Plasmodium*) ancient DNA (Taylor *et al.*, 1997). While porotic hyperostosis and cribra orbitalia may be an indirect indication of malaria, no bone changes occur in malaria, and therefore ancient DNA analysis is the only method of directly diagnosing malaria in skeletal remains. Malaria is carried from human to human by the bite of the infected female mosquito of the genus *Anopheles* (Dunn, 1993: 855), and *Plasmodium vivax* and *falciparum* today are responsible for most cases and deaths from malaria. It is not appropriate here to discuss the history of the impact of malaria on ancient populations, but a useful review is given in Aufderheide and Rodríguez-Martín (1998). Of course, when trying to differentiate between iron-deficiency anaemia, thalassaemia and sickle-cell anaemia (see below), all of which can lead to cranial changes, postcranial bone changes must also be considered in a diagnosis of thalassaemia and sickle-cell anaemia. Other evidence of thalassaemia comes from Tayles (1996), in Thailand in south-east Asia, who described skeletons with indicative changes dating to 2000–1500 BC. Bone abnormalities in the paranasal sinuses, mastoid processes and facial bones are seen in addition to the vault and orbital lesions already described. The long bones and metacarpals and metatarsals also enlarge with thinning of their cortices (termed dactylitis for the hand and foot changes), generalized osteoporosis of the spine develops, and there is premature closure of epiphyses.

The other type of inherited anaemia is **sickle-cell anaemia**, where abnormal elongation of red blood cells occurs. Here there is a genetic mutation at 'Position 6' on the gene that codes for the haemoglobin beta chain; it results in the substitution of the amino acid valine for glutamate (Aufderheide and Rodríguez-Martín, 1998: 348). Two reactions are precipitated in the skeleton: first, bone changes in the skull (already described), vertebrae, pelvis, hand and foot bones occur due to marrow overactivity and enlargement as the body tries to produce more red blood cells, and, second, necrosis (death) of bone develops due to blockage of the blood vessels by these abnormal cells (Steinbock, 1976). Complications of this condition may include susceptibility to infections, chronic leg ulcers, chronic kidney disease, gallstones and blindness (Murphy *et al.*, 2002: 431). Apart from the macroscopic and radiographic

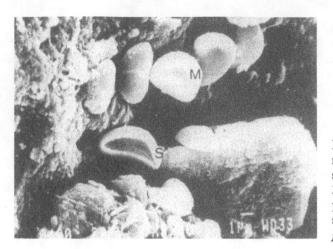

Fig. 8.12. Scanning electron microscopic image of a section from the rib of a 2,000-year-old skeleton with porotic hyperostosis, showing sickled cell (S). *(With permission of George Maat)*

features of sickle-cell anaemia, microscopy has also been used for diagnosis in the past. Maat and Baig (1991) identified fossilized sickle-cells using scanning electron microscopy in bone from a 2,000-year-old skeleton which supported the macroscopic bone lesions of anaemia (Fig. 8.12); without this information, the diagnosis of the type of anaemia would not have been possible. Today, West, Central and East African populations have high rates of sickle-cell anaemia, and it also affects India, the Middle East and Southern Europe (Murphy *et al.*, 2002: 430). Sickle-cell anaemia may be found in up to 4 per cent of Africans, and more than 40 per cent of Africans may carry the sickle-cell trait (Benjamin, 1993).

It has been noted that people with either sickle-cell anaemia or thalassaemia have a resistance to malaria because the infection cannot develop fast enough between the formation and death of the red blood cells during their short life span (Steinbock, 1976: 234). Very few cases of sickle-cell anaemia and thalassaemia have been identified in the archaeological record, perhaps because the cranial changes are so similar for all the anaemias. What is clear, however, is the need to consider the geographic context of skeletal material, which may help with the diagnosis of genetic anaemias in the future. However, the use of ancient DNA analysis has enabled a specific diagnosis of beta-thalassaemia (Filon *et al.*, 1995).

Vitamin C and D deficiencies

Deficiencies of particular vitamins also produce more specific skeletal changes. It might be assumed that in the hunter-gatherer or agriculturalist past, **vitamin C deficiency** was unlikely to occur. This vitamin is found in fresh fruits and uncooked vegetables, natural produce which probably contributed to the staple diet of many past human groups. Nevertheless, even without this fresh produce, scurvy may not develop, for example in Eskimos who eat a lot of uncooked meat (French, 1993: 1000). With the transition to agriculture the availability of vitamin C from fresh foods may have been reduced, together with losses due to cooking of foods and prolonged storage, both common in settled communities. However, scurvy, the clinical manifestation of vitamin C deficiency, is known, albeit rarely, from osteoarchaeological remains. Today scurvy is seen in infants fed boiled milk (cooking destroys the vitamin) and in the elderly who do not eat fresh fruit and vegetables (Elia, 2002: 238).

This vitamin is necessary for the bodily combat of infection and for the absorption of iron, and it is essential for the normal formation of the body tissues (especially collagen). In addition to reducing the resistance to infection, vitamin C deficiency predisposes to bleeding into the skin and beneath the periosteum (membrane surrounding the bones). Apart from faulty formation of the periosteum and the ligaments holding the teeth in the sockets, the cement substance in the blood vessels is defective and predisposes the individual to haemorrhage into the soft tissues, bones (especially the jaws) and joints. The result is the formation of new bone on the skeleton as a response to bleeding. Most commonly the gums swell and bleed, and this leads to the development of periodontal disease (see Chapter 4). Weakness and muscle pain in adults, and irritability, anaemia and pain in children are common signs and symptoms (Elia, 2002: 238).

Until the late 1990s diagnosis of scurvy was often based on generalized new bone formation on long bones. However, Ortner and Ericksen (1997), in their detailed study of the bone changes of scurvy, identified the lesions as occurring in more focused areas of the skull (Figs 8.13 and 8.14), notably bilaterally on the

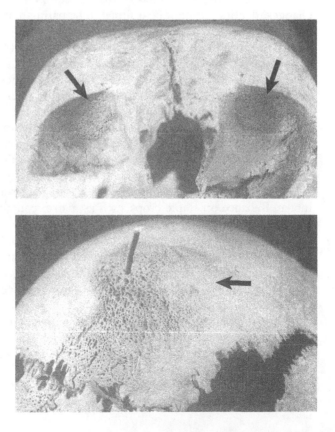

Fig. 8.13. Scorbutic changes in the orbits. *(National Museum of Natural History, Washington DC, United States, 345386, Paimute Eskimo)*

Fig. 8.14. Scorbutic changes on the cranial vault. *(National Museum of Natural History, Washington DC, United States, 345386, Paimute Eskimo)*

greater wing of the sphenoid bone and adjacent bone tissue. This, it is suggested, is the result of haemorrhage from the deep blood vessels associated with the temporalis muscle, which is involved in chewing. In later papers (Ortner *et al.*, 1999), apparent scorbutic skeletal changes were observed in a series of non-adult skulls from Peru, and in North America (Ortner *et al.*, 2001). While Ortner *et al.* (1999: 328) indicate that there has been no supporting clinical evidence for the association of the lesions described with scurvy, they imply that 'chronic bleeding at multiple sites in the skull is the most likely cause of the type and pattern of lesions'. Furthermore, they emphasize that the porous lesions found in the orbital surfaces and usually associated with anaemia may in fact be the result of scurvy or other conditions; evidence of marrow hyperplasia should be a required feature to diagnose anaemia. These skeletal changes are now the focus of many researchers' work, including a recent report from Portugal on a possible case of scurvy from the fourth-century site of Monte da Cegonha (Ferreira, 2002). A more recent view of the subject by Melikian and Waldron (2003: 211) included the study of the skulls of four confirmed cases of scurvy from the Royal College of Surgeons in London. Here they found that 'the changes which we have seen do not conform in any respect to those found in the skulls of clinical cases . . . their relationship to scurvy must be questionable, as must those described by Ortner and his colleagues'. Clearly, there is still much research to be done in this area, although Ortner was careful in his work to emphasize that, although suggestive of scurvy, the skeletal changes identified cannot be claimed to be pathognomonic (yet). Other changes of apparent scurvy have also been described, for example, cracks and staining in the long bones of Dutch seventeenth-century whalers (Maat, 1982, 2004), the latter change being proven to be the result of blood – i.e. haemorrhage (Maat and Uytterschaut, 1984). Recent research has also concentrated on the histological changes of scurvy and the need to consider the microscopic details of sections of pathological bone differentially to diagnose scurvy and anaemia (Schultz, 2001).

Prolonged winters in an inhospitable northern climate in Europe, for example, and the consequent absence of fresh produce for many months would create this scurvy of antiquity. It is proposed that scurvy as a disease would have been more common in settled agricultural communities where gathering of fresh fruit would have been limited and consumption of staple crops would have reduced vitamin C intake. Reliance on staple crops such as maize, containing little vitamin C, would also have predisposed people to scurvy in North America. Certainly, long sea voyages, military operations and the Californian Gold Rush were noted times for the disease and, as is well known, provided observations that were used for the early recognition and treatment of scurvy. James Lind, an English physician in the eighteenth century, is probably the most famous observer and experimenter in the quest to conquer scurvy in sailors. He had three groups of scorbutic people in his experiment, one taking fresh oranges and lemons, one taking cider, and one taking nothing. The first group recovered the quickest, the second less quickly and the third did not improve. His 1753 treatise served as an 'authoritative argument . . . for the use of citrus fruits to prevent scurvy' (French, 1993: 1002), although it was not until the end of the eighteenth century that lime juice was issued to sailors. Other predisposing factors are premature or twin births, infection and feeding with prepared infant foods (Stuart-Macadam, 1989b: 202); this latter cause may not be relevant if one assumes that in most societies in the past children were breast-fed.

For all this, however, scurvy is a palaeopathological rarity, probably due to non-recognition or misdiagnosis in the archaeological record. Evidence in palaeopathology consists of the identification of the bony reaction to haemorrhage; in addition, periodontal disease, ante-mortem tooth loss, haemorrhage into the joints and radio-opaque lines on radiographs of long bones ('scurvy lines') were also highlighted as potential scurvy indicators until the late 1990s and Ortner's work. In the pre-1990s, Ortner (1984) and Roberts (1987) described two of the few convincing cases in the archaeological record. The former was the skull of an 8-year-old child from Alaska with reactive bone change in the orbits and jaws, extending to the anterior portions of the temporal bones, all suggestive of mechanical chewing stress and haemorrhage. Similar changes were observed in a 3–4-year-old child from a cemetery in Britain dated to between 100 BC and AD 43. A final example came from the Netherlands (Maat, 1982, 2004), where historical evidence for scurvy was considered in the examination of fifty whalers' skeletons buried between AD 1642 and the end of the eighteenth century on an island called Zeeusche Uytkyck. Thirty-nine of the fifty skeletons had evidence of scurvy, including bleeding into the joints and gums. Recent work also indicates that scurvy (and rickets) was a problem in children in eighteenth- and nineteenth-century London (Lewis, 2002a). It is suggested that these high social status children would have been weaned onto a diet low in vitamins C and D (Fildes, 1986 in Lewis, 2002a). This high prevalence correlated with reduced stature, thus indicating the effect of disease on growth. The rarity of scurvy in the archaeological record may also be the result of the availability of adequate sources of vitamin C in the past. It is, however, likely that cases are not being recognized or are being misdiagnosed, especially if the orbital lesions are mistaken for the changes of anaemia (as indicated by Ortner et al., 1999). The widespread new bone formation in this deficiency disease may also be a complicating factor, considering the number of disease processes that can initiate this patterning of skeletal abnormalities.

Vitamin D deficiency can also produce chronic abnormalities in the skeleton. This vitamin (more accurately a prohormone) is necessary for the absorption of calcium and phosphorus and the mineralization of osteoid (the organic matrix of bone) and cartilage, and its deficiency leads to a 'softening' of the bones. It is the result of a defect in vitamin D metabolism or availability (Elia, 2002). Inadequate or delayed mineralization of osteoid in cortical and spongy bone is referred to as osteomalacia, while interruption in development and mineralization in the growth plates is rickets (Pitt, 1995: 1885). If this chronic deficiency occurs during the growing period, the disease is called rickets. The weight-bearing bones of the legs become bent and deformed when walking commences (Fig. 8.15); there is no reason not to suspect that the arm bones may also deform when crawling commences. Other bones of the body also deform under the influence of muscular contraction. The ends of the growing long bones expand and, in appearance, resemble the widened end of a trumpet; this reflects excessive unmineralized cartilage causing increase in length and width in the growth plates of the bones. In addition, the costochondral areas of the ribs become nodular prominences (rachitic

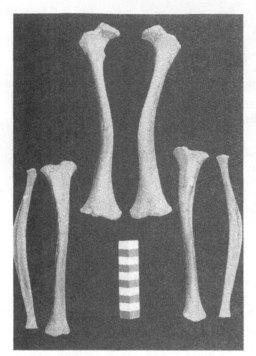

Fig. 8.15. Changes of rickets in the leg bones (FABC B-37, 8-year-old child, First African Baptist Church, AD 1823–1841, Philadelphia, United States). *(With permission of Don Ortner)*

rosary), the pelvis is retarded in growth, dental development and health may be affected and the skull tables may be thinned, usually in the area subject to pressure when the infant is resting (Steinbock, 1976: 266). The squat, bow-legged little figure is not so familiar in England today as he or she was 100 years ago. The woman in labour unable to give birth because of the obstruction of a deformed pelvis was a recognized hazard of past obstetric practice. The child fortunate enough to have survived the precarious neonatal period was pushed further along the rickety road by the inadequacy of the mother's milk. A chronically underfed woman would produce calcium-deficient milk, so imperilling her infant's well-being and reducing her already low health status.

The ingestion of vitamin D from, for example, fish oil and animal fat is not the main source of the vitamin. The human skin is able to effect a chemical change so producing vitamin D from a chemical precursor; 90 per cent of the body's vitamin D requirement is produced in the skin. This change is, however, dependent upon ultraviolet light, and the person must be ingesting adequate levels of calcium and phosphorus (Pitt, 1995: 1897). In 300 BC crooked legs and a hunchback are described in China (Steinbock, 1993: 978), and to Soranus of Ephesus is attributed the first clear description of rickets in the second century AD (Aufderheide and Rodríguez–Martín, 1998: 309). In the past the only source of ultraviolet light was sunshine. Clearly, the children of antiquity, spending their days outside, were unlikely to develop rickets, even during the northern winter months. Urbanization and the later industrial revolution in cities were the sources of such a danger; vitamin D deficiency has been termed a disease of civilization. The crowded, overhanging houses of the city would block out any sunlight that managed to penetrate the barrier of industrial smoke. The poor, often underfed children were compelled to work the daylight hours in the noise, danger and shelter of the factory. In such circumstances rickets was prevalent. In fact, Hess (1929) noted that the prevalence of rickets coincided almost exactly with a deficiency of sunlight. Fildes (1986) indicates that rickets was a common disease in England in the seventeenth and eighteenth centuries ('the English disease'), and Madonna and Child paintings produced in the Netherlands in the fifteenth and sixteenth centuries show characteristic deformities in the form of bowed legs and deformed chests. It was described in seventeenth-century England as a new disease, which does support the lack of evidence before that time in the British archaeological record. Massage and splinting of affected limbs, and the wearing of special boots and long coats to hide deformities were advocated (Fildes, 1986: 128), while the livers of birds and fish, and later (post-1780s) cod liver oil, were dietary recommendations. Of course, cod liver oil is high in vitamin D but it should be remembered that most of this vitamin is formed by the action of sunlight on the skin. It seems that this was not understood until very much later, and the first classic description was in the seventeenth century by Glisson (1650). Today it may be seen in Asian women in western countries where clothing covers most of their skin (and they may not consume enough vitamin D), but anybody who is housebound and not exposing their skin to sunlight is susceptible (Elia, 2002: 584). Furthermore, gastrointestinal, kidney and liver conditions may result in malabsorption of the vitamin, along with renal failure. A further possible factor could be the diet of Asian populations. Chapatti flour is a common dietary component and contains a lot of phytate, which binds to calcium and zinc and results in faecal loss of vitamin D due to decreased absorption (Pitt, 1995: 1897). In other parts of the world with high levels of sunlight, lack of exposure to the sun due to clothing/swaddling of babies/staying indoors appears to be an important factor – for example, in Iran, Africa and Saudi Arabia.

The skeletal evidence of rickets is not plentiful, particularly in the more distant past. Evidence of the disease has been found in Neolithic skeletons from Denmark and Norway (Sigerist, 1951) and more plentiful evidence comes from Hungary during the Roman period (Wells, 1964a). The rarity of this disease in antiquity is attested by Gejvall (1960), who recorded only two cases in his extensive examination of human remains. Møller-Christensen's study (1958) of 800 Medieval skeletons from the Æbelholt Monastery in Denmark revealed only nine cases of rickets. A classic example of rickets has been highlighted in a 7-year-old child from the Medieval cemetery of St Helen-on-the-Walls, York, England (Dawes and Magilton, 1980), and a more recently reported case from Ireland (Power and O'Sullivan, 1992) illustrates well the bending deformities of the lower legs; associated with these deformities were short stature, developmental defects of the teeth and retention of three deciduous teeth. More recent evidence of rickets has been reported in eight individuals (of 687) aged between 3 years and 18 months from the late Medieval site of Wharram Percy in Yorkshire, England (Ortner and Mays, 1998). The classic changes are described. Additionally, Blondiaux et al. (2002) note the association of rickets and child abuse in fourth-century Normandy, France. Prehistoric evidence is, as we might expect, rare, but Pfeiffer and Crowder (2004) report the earliest known case of rickets, deriving from the later Stone Age of Southern Africa and dated to 4820 ± 90 BP, which adds to a probable (inherited) case described by Formicola (1995) from Upper Palaeolithic Italy. Although rickets is, generally speaking, rarely reported in the palaeopathological record, detailed recording of the skeletal changes, possibly alongside radiological and histological techniques of analysis, may identify more evidence (e.g. Schamall, et al., 2003). Perhaps the examination of the later burial grounds of the Industrial Revolution period would even up the balance on the palaeopathology of rickets, but at present this disease of civilization appears to have been a rarity in past populations. It may be that much of the evidence for rickets is lost, since, if deformities were fairly mild in childhood, bone remodelling in adulthood may obscure them from identification (and some adult bones do show abnormal bending deformities to a minor degree). However, recent work on a later (post-Medieval) population of Christ Church, Spitalfields, London, dated to the eighteenth/nineteenth centuries AD (Molleson and Cox, 1993; Lewis, 2002a), showed many children and adults had rickets. Feeding with prepared infant foods, swaddling and keeping infants housebound for the first year of life may all be factors contributing to the prevalence of rickets in this population.

Osteomalacia is the adult counterpart of childhood rickets. Softening of the bones occurs as a result of dietary calcium deficiency, or as a result of abnormal loss of calcium from the body in kidney or intestinal disease. The loss associated with prolonged suckling of infants has already been mentioned, but multiple pregnancies in rapid succession will also deplete calcium stores (Steinbock, 1976: 272). The result of this bone demineralization in adults is not the bending of the bone characteristic of rickets, but rather the collapse and deformity of the vertebrae under weight-bearing stress and the deformity of the pelvis, which is of catastrophic obstetric significance. Bending deformities in the long bones are rare unless it is a severe case, and flaring of the ends of the bones is not present, due to closure of the growth plates. 'Stress fractures' or Looser's zones are also seen perpendicular to the cortices and bilaterally (Pitt, 1995: 1896). The frequency of minor degrees of vertebral collapse in skeletal remains suggests that osteomalacia may have been a common feature of earlier people, but diagnostic precision rests upon the characteristic radiographic or microscopic findings in these early skeletons, as there are many causes of vertebral collapse, such as tuberculosis, osteoporosis and acute trauma.

Harris lines of arrested growth

A less-specific condition (in terms of aetiology) seen in skeletal material is Harris lines of arrested growth. They are seen as dense, opaque transverse lines, particularly on the radiographs of long bones; the tibia, femur and radius tend to be most often affected (Figs 8.16 and 8.17). These lines represent periods of stress when growth in length has been arrested. Nutritional deficiencies or childhood disease, since these lines can only occur when the bones are growing, have been implicated as causes, based on experiments on animals and observations on humans (Harris, 1931). For a line to occur in a bone, the individual has to have recovered from the stress episode, i.e. a person continually malnourished and diseased will not display Harris lines; they are, in effect, 'recovery lines'. These lines mark the ends of the bone when the growth arrest occurred so, in theory, calculation of the age at formation should be possible (Hunt and Hatch, 1981; Hummert and Van Gerven, 1985). However, based on modern growth rates, it has to be assumed that growth occurred at the same rate in the past – not an easy assumption to make. Nevertheless, the study of the age distribution of Harris lines in a population will provide more information on the major stress periods in an individual's life, e.g. weaning or childhood disease (see Goodman and Clarke, 1981 for an example). One of the major problems in interpretation is that, as the individual ages, the lines can become invisible, i.e. remodelled away, because of continual bone turnover.

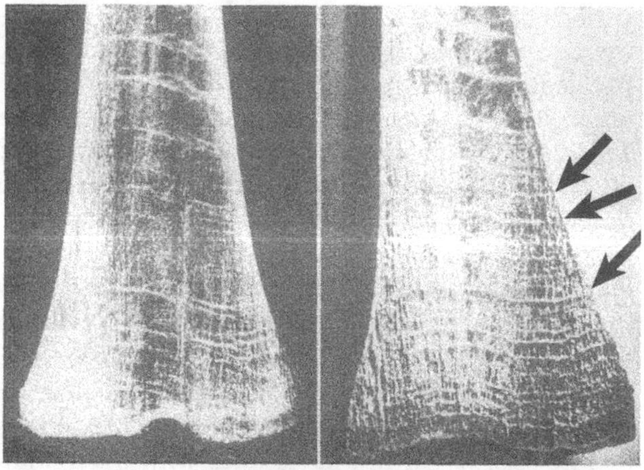

Fig. 8.16. Radiograph of Harris lines of arrested growth in tibiae. *(Calvin Wells Photographic Collection)*

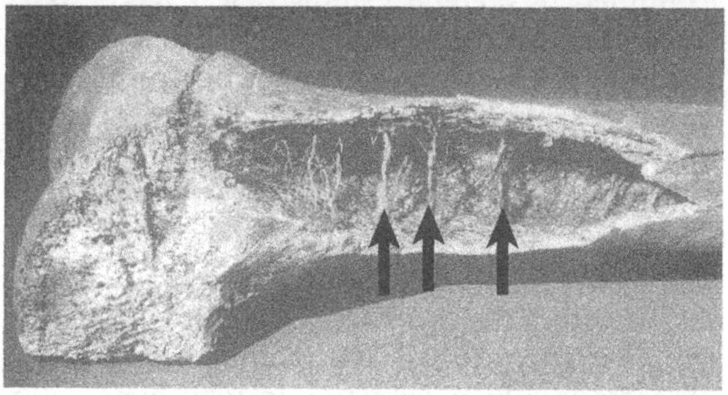

Fig. 8.17. Post-mortem damage to femur, showing Harris lines internally. *(Calvin Wells Photographic Collection)*

The mechanism behind line formation starts with the arrest of cartilage proliferation at the growth plate; the thin layer of cartilage cells below the plate are replaced by osteoblasts which form a thin layer of bone (Steinbock, 1976: 46). When the stress has been overcome, the osteoblasts recover immediately and begin laying down bone, visible on a radiograph as a transverse line. Since Harris lines are formed in the growing years, the study of non-adult individuals would seem to provide the most reliable prevalence rates, but researchers have analysed skeletons over the full age range. However, if the adults are not considered, differences between the sexes cannot be studied (Martin et al., 1985). The recording of Harris lines has its problems too. It appears to be generally accepted that if a line extends 50 per cent or more across the bone shaft it should be recorded. However, if a line was being resorbed at the time of the person's death, it may not extend that far across the bone, so should it be counted? Interobserver error has also been noted as a problem in the recording of Harris lines (Macchiarelli et al., 1994; Grolleau-Raoux et al., 1997). Results of tests showed a substantial interobserver disagreement of Harris line estimates when recording them on radiographs and bone sections. If standardization of recording is not practised, and interobserver error not accounted for between researchers, results cannot be reliably compared. Nevertheless, studies have shown populations subject to regular (or seasonal?)

periods of stress (Caribou Eskimo), because of the even spacing of Harris lines in the bones (e.g. Buikstra, 1976); surprisingly lines have been noted to decrease in frequency in farmers compared to foragers in the past in some populations (when other stress markers such as enamel defects increase) (Cohen and Armelagos, 1984). Clinical studies also indicate that stress episodes in people's lives may not necessarily be reflected in the occurrence of Harris lines, and healthy children may develop them (Larsen, 1997: 43). While a reduction in height may be expected for people who develop Harris lines, Mays (1985) found no reduction in the length of long bones of children from a Romano–British cemetery in England compared to their unaffected peers; this suggests perhaps evidence for catch-up growth. He also found the same result in a study of another site in England but this time from the Medieval period (Mays, 1995). Likewise, Ribot and Roberts (1996) came to the same conclusion in their study of an early Medieval population, also from England.

The association of Harris lines with other indicators of stress has also been examined in skeletal groups (e.g. Clarke, 1982) with inconclusive results, suggesting that the aetiology of these particular 'indicators of stress' is complex, and that the same cause cannot be implicated for all stressors. Although it provides an indication of particularly problematic periods in terms of health during a person's growth, the study of Harris lines has many problems.

Osteoporosis

Osteoporosis is today accepted as the most common of the skeletal metabolic diseases (Resnick and Niwayama, 1995e: 1783); it is also seen in other animals (Sumner et al., 1989). The osteoporoses are 'a heterogeneous set of disorders characterised by a reduction in total bone volume caused by thinning of the cortical walls of the long bones . . . thinning and loss of trabeculae, and increased porosity, principally of cancellous bone' (Burr and Martin, 1989: 197–8). Stini (1995: 397) defines it as 'low bone density associated with increased risk of fractures'. In effect, bone loss is present, and exceeds bone formation. Weaver (1998) adds to this definition by distinguishing between the terms osteoporosis and osteopenia, the former being the most common development of osteopenia. Osteoporosis can be described as a clinical syndrome where there are less than normal amounts of bone of normal quality, which can lead to fracture (or a reduction in bone mass of more than 30 per cent (Ortner, 2003)), while osteopenia is where there are less than normal amounts of bone only. Resnick and Niwayama (1995e: 1783) further discuss the terms and indicate that radiographs of the bones of people with osteoporosis show radiolucency of bone, better termed osteopenia or 'poverty of bone'. However, the presence of osteopenia on a radiograph cannot be taken to be indicative of osteoporosis because it is present with many other conditions – for example, osteomalacia. Osteoporosis is usually diagnosed if decreased bone mass is more than that expected for a given age, sex and ethnicity, and when there is a resulting fracture. Bone mass will obviously depend on peak bone mass attained and the rate of loss during later life (Shipley et al., 2002). Relatively little is known of the frequency of osteoporosis in the past, owing to problems in diagnosis. However, because of increased longevity, a reduction in exercise and an increasing incidence of the disease with age, its prominence is a subject for media attention. Type I osteoporosis is seen mostly in females post-menopausally, while Type II is seen in both sexes and is related to increasing age (senile osteoporosis (Stini, 1995)). Both these types are termed 'primary osteoporosis'. Secondary osteoporosis is usually related to another condition.

Age is the most common correlate of osteoporosis (Woolf and St John Dixon, 1988), but a multitude of disease processes include osteoporosis as one of their many clinical features, e.g. rheumatoid arthritis. Osteoporosis does not seem to select for any particular ethnic group or social class, although studies have shown black groups to have a higher bone mass than white groups (Nelson et al., 1991), and therefore more bone has to be lost before osteoporosis is visible in the former group. Although ageing is the most common underlying factor in osteoporosis, other factors such as lack of calcium or a high protein diet, the female sex, lack of exercise, immobilization, circulating sex hormones, a genetic predisposition, prolonged lactation and a high number of pregnancies, smoking, caffeine and alcohol all have their part to play. Of course, some of these factors may be more significant for some groups both today and in the past, but Stini (1995: 400) states that there is a 'significant environmental influence on the attainment of peak bone density'. During their lives, females always have lower bone mass than males, and the difference increases after the menopause when lower levels of oestrogen circulate around the body. Oestrogen is a hormone which, among other functions, prevents excessive destruction of bone by osteoclasts. The age at menopause today has a mean of 50 years (Woolf and St John Dixon, 1988: 168), and documentary records from classical Greece and Rome (Amundsen and Diers, 1970) suggest that the menopause occurred then around 40 to 50 years of age. This is a factor to bear in mind in the study of past human groups. If, as some researchers suggest, women died in their earlier years, the menopause may not have been a significant factor in the development of osteoporosis. Obviously longevity will vary between groups from different eras and geographic locations.

Diet appears to be another major factor in influencing osteoporosis development. Calcium is the most abundant mineral in the body and it is crucial to the formation of teeth and bones. Disturbances in calcium intake alter the rate of mineralization of new bone matrix formed. A high intake of calcium throughout life is associated with higher bone mass, but the effects of calcium supplementation on osteoporosis development in post-menopausal females varies between studies. Of course, vitamin D is also essential to allow the absorption of calcium (and phosphorus), and a high-protein diet leads to inhibition of calcium absorption and an increase in urinary calcium is seen (Stini, 1990). Calcium depletion may also be caused by factors such as prolonged lactation, frequent pregnancies and reduced access to dairy foods. Furthermore, fluoride may protect against osteoporosis but further studies are needed, and obesity ensures a higher bone mass and prevents osteoporosis (Woolf and St John Dixon, 1988: 46). Finally, higher bone mass is seen in people who exercise regularly. Mechanical demands on the skeleton actively promote increased bone mass; of course, starting exercise post-menopausally after never having exercised before would not prevent osteoporosis. Diet and exercise would be considered (along with age) as relevant factors in osteoporosis development in the past, and quality of diet (Martin et al., 1985, 1987) is an area of study relevant to the consideration of disease in general. Linked with osteoporosis should be an assessment of the frequency of indicators of stress, such as early mortality, reduced stature, enamel defects, Harris lines and the cranial changes of anaemia – a complex aetiological web which may contribute to our understanding of osteoporosis prevalence.

Calcium is available in high quantities in dairy foods (milk and cheese) and vegetables such as broccoli and spinach (in quantity). Thus it may be expected that osteoporosis should be more prevalent in populations practising hunter-gathering rather than agriculture. Some studies show this not to be the case, where cortical thinning, decrease in bone circumference and slowing of growth occurs in a higher frequency in farming groups (Cohen and Armelagos, 1984). However, not all studies show a consistent picture where the protein content of the diet is concerned; it would be expected that earlier hunting groups would have more ready access to protein from hunted animals (the best balanced protein for humans) – could this high protein diet lead to osteoporosis? In this respect, and considering the reduced intake of protein from animals, agricultural communities would be expected to have less osteoporosis. If, as studies show, osteoporosis had a potentially higher frequency in hunter-gatherers because of reduced access to calcium from dairy products but easier access to a high protein diet, perhaps the effect of exercise counteracted its occurrence. Mobile hunter-gatherers would be more likely to undertake regular exercise, thereby strengthening the skeleton throughout their lives, whereas settled farmers may not be so active. However some, but not all, studies comparing hunter-gatherer and agricultural groups show increased rates of osteoarthritis in the latter groups, possibly indicating increased workload. Clearly, osteoporosis can be considered multifactorial in aetiology.

Much osteoporosis is diagnosed today when a person sustains a fracture, especially in the most frequently affected areas of the body in this condition: the wrist (Colles fracture of the radius (Fig. 8.18)), the hip (fractured neck of femur (Fig. 8.19)) and the spine (compression fractures of the thoracic and lumbar vertebral bodies – 'cod fish vertebrae'), leading to kyphotic deformity or 'dowager's hump'. Because trabecular bone has a greater turnover than cortical bone, and is more susceptible to fracture, the areas of the body described above are those most affected. In many respects the skeletal evidence for fractures in the past does highlight a possible underlying osteoporosis. There are a multitude of diagnostic methods available to the modern clinician, but, as Pfeiffer and Lazenby (1994: 36) have pointed out, 'The methods of bone mass quantification applied in the clinical arena may not be easily transferable to dry, long-buried bone tissue.' Methods of

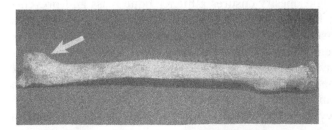

Fig. 8.18. Healed Colles fracture in distal radius (early Medieval Berinsfield 18, Oxfordshire, England); note the posterior displacement of the distal fragment ('dinner fork deformity').

diagnosis in the clinical arena include radiography (bone density and thickness), single and dual photon absorptiometry (SPA and DPA), dual-energy X-ray analysis (DEXA, for bone mineral content and density), computed tomography, calculating the metacarpal index from radiographs, and blood, urine and faecal analysis (bone mineral turnover). While all these methods are non-invasive (good for archaeological studies of bone), not all of them can be used by palaeopathologists. Further-more, diagenetic change leading to bone loss and alteration may not be identified using many of these methods.

Radiography is probably the most common non-invasive diagnostic tool used in palaeopathology, but it suffers from a number of limitations; the most common of these are the effects of burial in the ground on the body and on loss of bone, i.e. post-mortem effects. What a person sees on a radiograph as bone loss may purely be the result of post-mortem damage. Invasive methods, such as examining the microscopic structure of bone (histomorphometry) or assessing

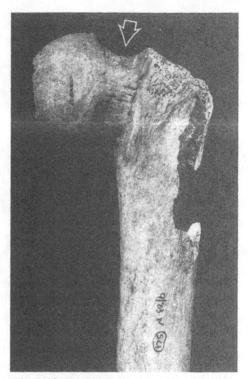

Fig. 8.19. Healed fracture to the neck of the femur (Romano-British, fourth century AD, Gambier-Parry Lodge 521, Gloucester, Gloucestershire, England).

bone mass (cortical thickness, cortical area and bone mineral content), have been applied to archaeological populations to assess bone loss (Martin *et al.*, 1985). The use of these methods is very much determined by the preservation of the skeletal material being studied (as for radiography). Work has also shown the value of scanning electron microscopy (SEM) in assessing osteoporotic changes in bones from archaeological populations (Roberts and Wakely, 1992). SEM records the topographic features of bone, and excessive bone resorption, with reduced formation, may be identified in sections of bone (Fig. 8.20). The presence of healing microfractures in the trabeculae of vertebrae also suggests that these increase with age and osteoporosis (Vernon-Roberts and Pirie, 1973; Mosekilde, 1990). These can be interpreted as a repair mechanism to preserve the bone integrity. It is suggested that these features could be used to diagnose osteoporosis before any more significant changes in the skeleton occur, such as reduction in mineral density or structural collapse of bone. Low-angle X-ray scattering analysis (LAXS) of bone mineral density has also been used in archaeological contexts (Farquharson and Brickley, 1997; Farquharson *et al.*, 1997), and stereophotogrammetry to assess trabecular bone structure (Brickley and Howell, 1999). Weaver (1998) recommends the use of microradiography to assess density, and histological analysis to consider bone turnover and metabolism.

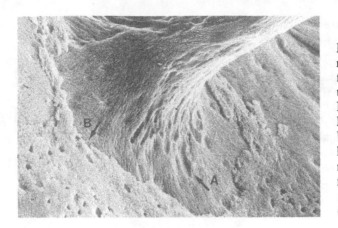

Fig. 8.20. Scanning electron micrograph of rib section from 79-year-old female from the Terry Collection, National Museum of Natural History, Washington DC, United States. A: Howship's lacunae (osteoclast resorption); B: new bone formation (osteoblasts). *(With permission of Don Ortner)*

Reports of osteoporosis in archaeologically derived skeletal remains are rare, however, and, apart from the methodologically driven studies already described, consist of descriptions of individuals with osteoporosis-related fractures (e.g. Foldes *et al.*, 1995). Here a middle-aged female dated to the sixth century AD from the Negev Desert in Israel had compression fractures to the spine but was also subject to radiological, photon densitometrical and histomorphometric analyses to confirm the diagnosis. DEXA was used to assess bone mineral density in prehistoric pre-Hispanic individuals from Gran Canaria, with the result that a high proportion of osteopenia was found, and it increased with age (González-Reimers *et al.*, 2002). Furthermore, Macchiarelli and Bondioli (1994) used densitometry of radiographs to assess femoral bone loss in 66 males and females from the Terry Collection (modern early twentieth century and curated in the Natural History Museum, Smithsonian Institution), with a view to using the technique for age-at-death estimation in archaeological and forensic contexts. However, their research suggested that bone loss with age as visualized on radiographs appears to be too variable to provide accurate individual age at death assessments. This suggests that the use of radiography to assess osteopenia and osteoporosis in archaeological populations is fraught with problems, even after the effects of diagenesis have been considered. Of some note is the work of Mays and colleagues, who have considered the non-invasive technique of measuring the metacarpal index using radiographs of the second metacarpal. Mays initially (1996b) considered the Medieval site of Wharram Percy in North Yorkshire, England, and radiographed the metacarpals of 83 males and 71 females. He found significant bone loss in females but not males, and the magnitude of bone loss for the older females was similar to age-matched living individuals. The results of this research were supported by later work by Mays *et al.* (1998), where DEXA was used on the proximal femora. It was suggested that this was a surprising result considering the assumed more active lifestyle of people in the past. However, it may be that different aetiological factors were at play in inducing bone loss in the archaeological group compared to the modern group, the under-activity of today not being the key predisposing factor. More recent research on the known-age males and females from the post-Medieval site of Christ Church, Spitalfields, London, had similar results. Using metacarpal index data again, although the female peak cortical thickness was less than for modern counterparts, loss of bone occurred at a similar rate, thus supporting the results of the Medieval study (Mays, 2000; Mays, 2001). Recent research has indicated that metacarpal radiography is a robust technique to assess cortical bone loss when diagnosing osteoporosis, although film type differences and measurement position may introduce problems (Ives and Brickley, 2004). A more novel approach to studying osteopenia was described by White and Armelagos (1997), where stable carbon and nitrogen isotopes were analysed in both normal and ostepenic male and female individuals from the X-Group Sudanese Nubian population. They found that females with osteopenia had elevated nitrogen levels, which may signify physiological differences contributing to the development of bone loss. Certainly this approach contributes to the methods available for identifying osteopenia and osteoporosis in archaeologically derived human skeletal remains. The study of osteoporosis in archaeological populations has great potential, considering its incidence today, as seen in Agarwal and Stout (2003).

ENDOCRINE DISEASE

The endocrine diseases are rarely seen in palaeopathological contexts and are therefore not discussed in detail here; the interested reader is referred to Ortner (2003) for archaeological data and Resnick (1995a) for clinical descriptions and detailed bone changes. However, they warrant brief consideration in this chapter.

The endocrine system consists of a series of ductless glands whose cells secrete hormones into the blood. Hormones are chemical substances, formed in a body organ or gland, which are carried by the blood to influence growth, function and nutrition elsewhere in the body. Over- and undersecretion of hormones leads to endocrine disease. Although there are several endocrine glands (pituitary, thyroid, parathyroids, adrenals, ovaries, testes and pancreas), the pituitary and thyroid glands are the ones most relevant to palaeopathology, because they control skeletal growth (pituitary) and maturation (thyroid). The pituitary gland lies inside the skull and the thyroid gland is situated in the neck.

Hyperpituitarism is characterized by excessive production of growth hormone by the pituitary gland. Gigantism or acromegaly may occur, producing taller than normal individuals. Hyperpituitarism occurring during growth produces gigantism, and in adulthood acromegaly. In acromegaly bone deposition occurs and leads to enlargement of bones, an increase in thickness of the skull vault, enlarged frontal sinuses, spinal osteophytes, prominent tendinous and ligamentous insertions and extreme height. Few convincing cases have been described in palaeopathology. **Hypopituitarism**, or a deficiency in growth hormone during growth, leads to dwarfism. Tumours, infection or injury to the pituitary gland and genetic factors may be implicated for the abnormality. It is a cause of a large percentage of people with short stature today. Stunted growth, delayed development of the dentition and fusion of the secondary ossification centres, and a short, gracile, proportional skeleton results. Disproportionate dwarfism, e.g. achondroplasia, can be differentiated relatively easily from this condition (see Chapter 3). There are many causes of short, proportional stature, such as chronic infection, but the distribution

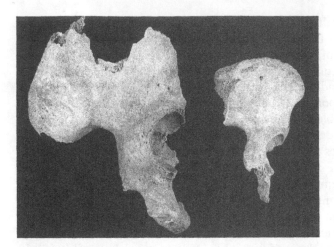

Fig. 8.21. Innominate bone of pituitary dwarf compared to normal size (Romano-British, fourth century AD, Gambier-Parry Lodge 557, Gloucester, Gloucestershire, England).

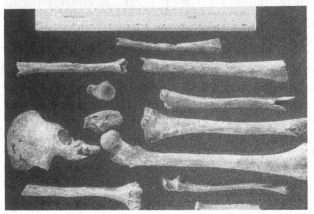

Fig. 8.22. Long bones of same individual in Fig. 8.21 with scale.

and character of bony abnormalities seen in pituitary dwarfism should differentiate these conditions in skeletal remains (if not always in artistic representation). Two probable cases have been described by Ortner and Putschar (1981: 302–3) and Roberts (1988b). In the latter case a proportionately short female adult skeleton, excavated from a fourth-century AD cemetery in Gloucester, England, was diagnosed as having pituitary dwarfism (Figs 8.21 and 8.22). This was based on delayed fusion of the secondary ossification centres, a gracile skeleton, abnormalities of the dentition and a reduced stature (131.2cm compared to the mean for females in that cemetery of 153cm). Interestingly, the only possible cause of this disorder identified on the skeleton was in the form of long-standing plaques of new bone on the endocranial surface of the skull, suggesting possible infection.

Hyperthyroidism, or thyrotoxicosis, is characterized by excessive amounts of thyroxine produced by the thyroid gland. Iodine is necessary for the formation of thyroxine, and there appear to be several areas of the world where iodine deficiency exists in groundwater, e.g. Switzerland, parts of the United States and England (Bloom, 1975: 202). Today about 30 per cent of the world population is at risk from iodine deficiency (Dobson, 1998), and 10 per cent of the world population is affected (Cotran *et al.*, 1989: 1227). Enlargement of the gland (goitre) may result from excessive iodine in the diet, which stimulates overproduction of thyroxine (toxic goitre). However, a lack of iodine can also lead to swelling of the gland, yet no hyperactivity (non-toxic goitre), even though there may be an increase in thyroid-stimulating hormone (TSH) by the pituitary gland. Increased bone resorption and osteoporosis, with cartilage calcification, characterize the disorder, with fatigue, nervousness, weight loss and palpitations as some of the signs and symptoms. Although there have been many representations of goitre in art, no cases of thyrotoxicosis have been reported palaeopathologically, except in an eighteenth-century Sicilian mummy where an enlarged thyroid gland was found (Ciranni *et al.*, 1999). **Hypothyroidism** (cretinism in the young and myxoedema in adults) involves a thyroxine deficiency. This may be the result of wasting, atrophy or destruction of either the thyroid or pituitary gland, or a deficiency in iodine in local water. Bone changes may consist of delayed maturation of the skeleton, irregular fragmentary ossification centres, prominent cranial sutures and wormian bones, accompanied by generalized osteoporosis (Ortner, 2003). The individual (if affected in the growing years) is short but proportionately so. The clinical features of the disease are very much opposite to those of thyrotoxicosis – mental retardation, constipation, lethargy, slow heart rate, decreased sweating and weight gain. Although there are some differences in the skeletal changes compared to pituitary dwarfism, in archaeological populations diagnosis of one of the two conditions may prove difficult. In fact, no cases of hypothyroidism have been reported to date.

Related to the pituitary gland disorders is hyperostosis of the endocranial surface of the frontal bone of the skull (**hyperostosis frontalis interna**). Prominent thickening, and formation of nodules of new bone on the frontal bone occurs, most frequently, in post-menopausal females (Fig. 8.23). These changes are probably the result of altered pituitary gland secretion of hormones (Ortner and Putschar, 1981: 294) but males can also have the condition; it is most commonly found in people over 60 years of age (Hershkovitz *et al.*, 1999). In archaeological populations it has been rarely reported (but see Armelagos and Chrisman, 1988; Anderson, 1994b). More recent research has described the condition in fossil hominids dated to 1.5 million years ago (Antón, 1997). The lack of evidence has been suggested to be because radiographic diagnosis is not commonly used (Barber *et al.*, 1997).

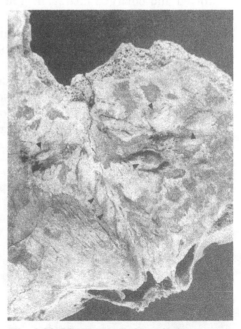

Fig. 8.23. Hyperostosis frontalis interna (early Medieval, eighth–tenth centuries AD, Raunds, Northamptonshire, England).

PAGET'S DISEASE

A final condition to consider in this chapter is Paget's disease, osteitis deformans or 'matrix metabolic madness' (Cotran *et al.*, 1989: 1328). It was first described by James Paget in 1877, and, although of unknown cause, a slow viral infection is implicated (Aufderheide and Rodríguez-Martín, 1998: 413; Resnick and Niwayama, 1995f: 1925). Another rarely reported condition in the palaeo-pathological literature, it does deserve discussion because of its frequency in modern populations; Caucasians in Europe, North America, Australia and New Zealand are most commonly affected, and frequencies of 10 per cent in males and 15 per cent in females are apparent by the ninth decade of life (Cotran *et al.*, 1989: 1329). People with Paget's disease tend to be lethargic and withdrawn, and they have an increased heart rate and blood flow, leading to a very warm skin. Today, it tends to affect mainly males over 50 years of age. Its prevalence in the past was likely to have been of the same order, but numerically it was probably not as common as today if a reduced longevity is assumed.

The disease is slow and progressive, and is characterized by pain in the affected part and by increasing deformity of the bone due to 'softening'. A localized increased bone turnover rate characterizes the disease, resulting in a 'mosaic' patterning of the bone, both radiologically and histologically; this is the result of irregular and excessive woven and lamellar bone formation. The normally demarcated cortex (compact bone) and medullary cavity of bone are less precise. The cortex becomes thickened and spongy and the whole bone assumes a distorted and enlarged character. The sacrum, spine, femora and skull are the most commonly affected bones. Head enlargement due to skull thickening is a startling feature, and prominent meningeal vessel grooves on the endocranial skull surface, representing increased blood flow, are obvious (Fig. 8.24). There may be spinal deformity (kyphosis) and long bone bowing. The whole picture of bone deformity is complicated by frequent spontaneous bone fracture, and by the occasional development of an osteosarcoma, osteoarthritis and neurological symptoms due to pressure on the body systems from enlargement of bone. However, many of these sequelae are rare findings in skeletal remains. The usual

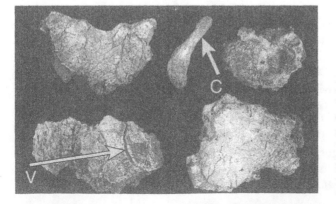

Fig. 8.24. Skull fragments with vessel impressions (V) on the endocranial surface, and part of the clavicle (C) with an unhealed fracture; Paget's Disease (post-Medieval, St Albans, Hertfordshire, England).

presentation is a fairly localized bone swelling and deformity, neither of which were of significance to their possessor. However, neuromuscular complications are quite common e.g. muscle weakness, paralysis and incontinence (Resnick and Niwayama, 1995f: 1924), as well as heart failure.

Reports of the disease in palaeopathological contexts do occur, but at present the earliest example is a femur of French Neolithic date from Lozère (Pales, 1929); much younger examples from France (fourth and eleventh centuries AD) have also recently been reported (Roches *et al.*, 2002). One of the most complete and convincing examples was discovered in the early Medieval monastic cemetery at Jarrow, England, and dated to AD 950; in this case the disease affected almost all the bones in this male body. An abnormally large skull was supported on a deformed spine. The long bones of the legs and arms were twisted, thickened and deformed. The left femur was fractured as a consequence of the underlying disorganized bone weakness of the disease (Wells and Woodhouse, 1975). Other cases have been reported from a Medieval site in Norwich, England (Stirland, 1991b) and a sixteenth-century grave at Wells Cathedral in the south-west of England (Aaron *et al.*, 1992). Of note in England today, Paget's disease is seen most frequently in the north-west (8.3 per cent rate compared to between 3.5 and 4.5 per cent in high prevalence parts of the world (Altman, 1993: 911)). Few cases have been reported there from the archaeological record, although a recent report identified six affected individuals from a Medieval cemetery at Norton Priory (Boylston, 2003). Diagnosis of Paget's disease requires radiographic and histological analytical confirmation, as in most of the cases described here.

Paget's disease is a condition that does not, on the basis of skeletal evidence, appear to have been as frequent in the past as today, but some of the preceding disease processes discussed in the metabolic disease classification were very common. This perhaps reflects the multifactorial nature of these 'indicators of stress' and the more precise (but as yet unknown) aetiology of Paget's disease. The metabolic diseases provide a fascinating and exciting insight into past human adaptation and the factors responsible for their occurrence in human populations of earlier periods. Their potential in future palaeopathological studies is acknowledged.

CHAPTER 9

Neoplastic Disease

Environmental carcinogens undoubtedly have a long history but both the number and the concentration of these agents have changed in recent human history, often to the disadvantage of human groups. (Ortner, 2003: 504)

INTRODUCTION

In the developed countries of the world today, everyone is familiar with the problem of cancer. For example, in 1997 the World Health Organization listed cancer as the second biggest killer (6.3 million deaths annually) after heart disease at 7.2 million; more than 10 million people in the world are diagnosed with cancer every year. In England and Wales it is also the main cause of death (Swerdlow *et al.*, 1997: 30). Between 1950 and 1999 lung, prostate and colon (males) and breast, colon and lung (females) made up 50 per cent of the 220,000 new cases and 135,000 deaths from cancer annually (Quinn and Babb, 1999); many cases were identified in the lower social classes. Furthermore, since 1971 cancer incidence has risen by 20 per cent in men and 30 per cent in women. Of course, screening for breast cancer in women, for example, and developments in radiotherapy and chemotherapy have improved survival rates.

Although, today, the word tumour is, to most people, synonymous with the term new growth, this has not always been so. In strict terms of derivation, the word should be applied to all swellings and, until the early nineteenth century, inflammatory swellings, cysts and new growths (both benign and malignant) were all considered as tumours. Neoplasms or new growths are in essence the uncontrolled growth of tissue cells (bone, cartilage, fibrous tissue or blood/marrow (Ortner, 2003: 503) and also fat and nerve cells). By definition, a neoplasm is an abnormal mass of tissue (Fig. 9.1), the growth of which exceeds and is uncoordinated with that of the normal tissues and persists in the same excessive manner after cessation of the stimulus which evoked the change (Cotran *et al.*, 1989). They may arise in any tissue of the body, in any organ of the body and in any individual without consideration of age, sex, ethnicity, health status or social group. However, the incidence of specific neoplasms may vary within these groups for reasons ill-understood in many cases.

Individual neoplasms may consist of differentiated cells characteristic of the original tissue, or alternatively the growth may consist of totally undifferentiated cells not resembling any specific organ of the body. Neoplasms are considered as either benign or malignant. Benign neoplasms are those that remain solely at their site of origin and tend to spread only locally without a generalized bodily effect.

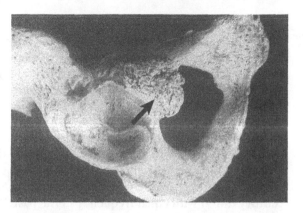

Fig. 9.1. Bone tumour in pelvic bone. *(National Museum of Natural History, Washington DC, United States, 256474)*

The cells comprising benign neoplasms are generally well differentiated. They are clinically insignificant when compared to malignant neoplasms. Any symptoms from a benign neoplasm are due to the local effect of the growth on the surrounding body structures and to the sheer size of the growth itself. The malignant neoplasms are characterized by the uncontrolled local spread of the primary growth into and onto other organs of the body, and by the more sinister generalized spread of cells to distant organs of the body. This spread is achieved through the bloodstream and the lymphatic channels, and by the direct implantation of cells in such zones as the pleural and peritoneal cavities from the original growth. This autonomy of the malignant neoplasm results in the dissemination of these secondary deposits, the so-called metastases, in almost any organ of the body, with the complete disturbance and breakdown of that organ function. Without the control of the *milieu intérieur*, the relentless unchecked growth of the primary malignant neoplasm and its metastases results ultimately in the death of the individual. There is clearly a resemblance of effect between the biological suicide of bacterial parasites and malignant neoplasms.

Diagnosis of neoplastic disease in skeletal remains can prove difficult and relies on identification of macroscopic lesions affecting specific bones in particular age and sex groups. For example, the benign tumour called osteoid osteoma affects males twice as much as females and more than 50 per cent of cases are in the 11–20-year-old age group; a quarter of cases affect the femur and a quarter affect the tibia. Ideally, radiographic analysis should be undertaken to ensure that internal lesions are identified, but this is rarely achieved. However, Rothschild and Rothschild (1995), in their study of cancer in skeletons from the Hamann Todd Skeletal Collection in Cleveland, Ohio, United States, found more evidence of cancer in skeletons subject to radiography than if visual inspection was used.

The following overview considers benign and malignant neoplasms of bone, cartilage, fibrous tissue and blood/marrow. The latter group includes only malignant tumours (myeloma, leukaemia and Ewing's sarcoma). Those affecting cartilage include the osteochondroma (benign) and chondrosarcoma (malignant), and, in the bone, the ivory osteoma, osteoclastoma and osteoid osteoma (benign) and osteosarcoma (malignant); the benign tumour of fibrous tissue is that of the fibrous cortical defect.

BENIGN NEOPLASMS

The multitude of soft tissue benign neoplasms, the 'warts and everything' of Oliver Cromwell, generally leave no evidence in skeletal remains. With few exceptions, only the benign neoplasms of bone itself will be manifest in skeletal remains. These lesions, which remain discrete, albeit of varying size, can be seen in skeletal remains of antiquity. As has been noted earlier, cartilage is an essential component of developing bone and neoplasms are found originating from it. For the present discussion only the more common or the more spectacular true benign neoplasms will be considered. Indeed, the full range of benign growths known today is not recognized in palaeopathological material as yet. Of course, it is quite likely that the benign neoplasms which affect humans in the twenty-first century did so with equal frequency in the past.

One of the first descriptions of a bony excrescence was in the femur of a *Homo erectus* of Middle Pleistocene date (Brothwell, 1967b). This bony tumour is, in fact, a post-traumatic ossification ('myositis ossificans') similar to that from the pelvis of seventeenth-century date illustrated in Fig. 5.2. This is due to trauma to the muscle and is not a neoplasm of bone and confusion has occurred in diagnosis. An excrescence of similar outward appearance has been noted at the lower end of a femur from an Egyptian individual of the V Dynasty (Brothwell, 1967b). This lesion, an **osteochondroma** (Fig. 9.2), is one of the most common benign bone tumours diagnosed in modern clinical practice. Although traditionally considered neoplastic, osteochondromas are, strictly, developmental aberrations caused by faulty ossification of the growth plate rather than true neoplasms. Radiographic analysis shows continuity of the cancellous tissue into the lesion. The onset of the lesion is during the growing period of childhood development and the tumour arises from the growing cartilaginous plate towards the end of the bone. By and large the only sign is the inconvenience of a localized swelling on a limb. The palaeopathological literature includes a number of notable cases (Bennike, 1985; Roberts, 1985; Gregg and Gregg, 1987; Chamberlain *et al.*, 1992; Gladykowska-Rzeczycka, 1997). Growth of the tumour ceases on completion of childhood growth. Although the osteochondroma is a single tumour, more rarely multiple and apparently similar bony swellings may be found (Ortner, 1981; Katzenberg *et al.*, 1982). These lesions,

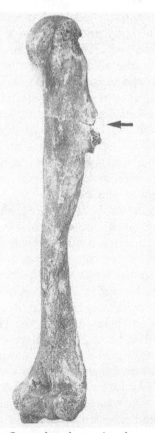

Fig. 9.2. Osteochondroma in a humerus (Roman, Derby Racecourse cemetery, Derby, Derbyshire, England).

widespread throughout the skeleton, are part of an hereditary abnormality of development called diaphyseal aclasia or exostosis multiplex (Figs 9.3 and 9.4). A particularly dramatic and fatal example of this latter condition has been reported from a Danish Medieval cemetery (Sjøvold *et al.*, 1974). The subject was a young pregnant woman. Her multiple bony excrescences were sufficiently large and ill-placed within her pelvis to prevent childbirth. The fetus contained within this poor woman's body was at full term, but both mother and unborn child perished because of the condition (seen in both individuals).

A particularly common finding in terms of neoplasm in skeletal remains is a small, round, smooth projection of dense lamellar bone known descriptively as an **ivory osteoma**. These lesions are sometimes no larger than a pinhead but sometimes reach almost tennis-ball diameter, and are found most frequently on the outer surface of the frontal and parietal bones of the skull (Fig. 9.5), although they have been found in other places – for example, the facial sinuses and the mandible (Anderson, 1997). No doubt they were entirely symptomless and are today, just as in antiquity, of no consequence, and occur in 1 per cent of autopsies (Ortner, 2003: 506), but 38 per cent of modern and 41 per cent of archaeological black, white, male and female populations are reported as being affected

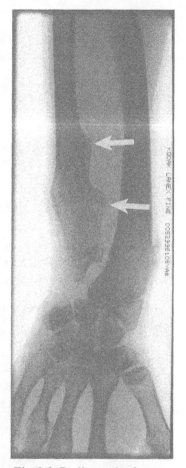

Fig. 9.3. Radiograph of diaphyseal aclasia seen here in the forearm bones.

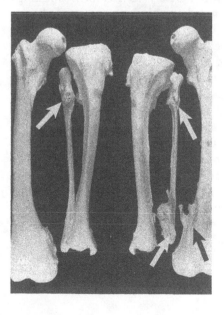

Fig. 9.4. Diaphyseal aclasia in the lower leg bones. *(Terry Collection 1270, National Museum of Natural History, Washington DC, United States)*

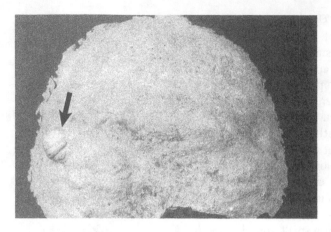

Fig. 9.5. Ivory osteoma on the occipital bone (late Medieval, twelfth–sixteenth centuries AD, St Helen-on-the-Walls, York)

(Eshed *et al.*, 2002). While the lesion is usually solitary, some skeletal remains have multiple osteomas. For example, at the late Medieval site of Fishergate, York (Stroud and Kemp, 1993), of the seventeen individuals with osteomas, six had between two and six each, and one had twenty. A less common, but equally benign, bone-forming neoplasm of bone, termed **osteoid osteoma**, has also been identified in skeletal remains (Gladykowska-Rzeczycka and Myśliwski, 1985). These lesions, commonly of the young, develop in the cortex and are of woven bone, usually towards the ends of the tibia or femur and appear palaeopathologically as fusiform swellings which, on radiography, present a radiolucent interior (Fig. 9.6). Symptomatically, they are noted for producing considerable pain in the bone and it is easy to imagine the distressed child of antiquity with unremitting, constant and boring pain in the leg, unassuaged by the benefits of modern analgesia.

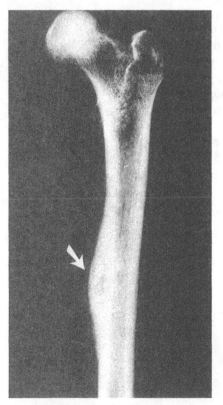

Fig. 9.6. Radiograph of an osteoid osteoma on the femur, showing radiolucent interior. *(Calvin Wells Photographic Collection)*

The **osteoclastoma**, a benign tumour of bone, is one of the most common primary bone tumours (Ortner, 2003: 512), and is seen in adolescents and young adults. It is seen in the ends of the bones at the knee joint, proximal humerus and distal radius. The tumour tends to destroy the ends of the bone and a new periosteal shell is formed. The fibrous cortical defect is a common lesion seen in the skeleton and affects males twice as much as females (Jaffe, 1958, in

Ortner, 2003); 1950s data suggest it occurs in one-third of all children. It develops in the periosteum, adjacent to the growth plate, and a dense layer of bone separates it from the medullary cavity. The femur is most often affected at its distal end, and lesions are often multiple and symmetrical.

Very rarely appearing in palaeopathological specimens, a tumour of soft tissue may produce a bony reaction which itself resembles a neoplasm. This accounts for about 15–20 per cent of all intra-cranial tumours (Waldron, 1998: 213). Such is the case with a growth of the membranous covering of the brain. This neoplasm, called a **meningioma**, may induce, albeit rarely, a most alarming growth of the skull overlying the lesion accompanied by destructive changes of the inner table (Rogers, 1949; Anderson, 1991; Jónsdóttir *et al.*, 2003). A specimen of the XX Dynasty has such an extensive skull reaction that it is suggested that the meningioma was itself malignant. Clearly this could be confused, as will be seen, with a primary malignant neoplasm of bone. A single case of a reactive bony excrescence in a skull secondary to a neoplasm of the wall of a blood vessel has also been noted, of prehistoric date (Manchester, 1980b).

MALIGNANT NEOPLASMS

The malignant neoplasms of bone are of the greatest palaeopathological interest, having the most terrifying clinical symptomatology and the most revealing epidemiological significance. And yet, in spite of their interest and their possible significance for modern cancer research, the malignant neoplasms of bone, both primary and secondary, are uncommon findings in palaeopathology (Ortner and Putschar, 1981; Micozzi, 1991; Strouhal, 1994). They are either sarcomas (bone and muscle) or carcinomas (epithelial tissue); both can spread to other places in the body, and are termed metastases (Ortner, 2003: 503).

It is a quirk of nature that the most malign and deadly tumours of humans are the malignant neoplasms affecting the young. One of the most common primary malignant neoplasms of bone, **osteosarcoma**, is no exception. This cancer, sometimes known as osteogenic sarcoma, arises *de novo* from the cells constituting bone tissue; it occurs principally during the growing period of life, and after the age of 30 years is comparatively rare. There is, however, a second peak of tumour development accounting for some 6–10 per cent of osteosarcomas (Cotran *et al.*, 1989). This second peak, occurring in the elderly, may be associated with Paget's disease in such people. Males more than females are affected and the distal femur, proximal tibia and humerus are mostly involved. The metaphyseal areas of the growth plate are the sites where the tumour develops, extending through the cortex into the soft tissues (Ortner, 2003: 524). The bone is woven in nature, and bone formed may appear 'sunburst'. An osteosarcoma is so highly malignant that in the absence of treatment early death results. No doubt such was the case in antiquity before the advent of effective and radical surgery and radiotherapy, and before the introduction of cancer chemotherapy. A constant, severe, boring pain, deep in the affected bone, is the presenting symptom. This may be followed by spontaneous bone fracture at the site of the neoplasm, so-called pathological fracture. The early spread of neoplastic cells to other parts of the body seals the miserable fate of the victim of this most pernicious disease.

Although there are other primary sarcomas of bone known to modern practice, hitherto only the osteosarcoma is certainly recognized in palaeopathology. Perhaps the earliest example is found in a humerus of Iron Age date from Munsingen, Switzerland. The craggy disorganized growth, with spicules of bone developing at right angles to the original bone axis, is characteristic. A burst of frenzied and uncontrolled bone growth is captured in this single humerus, which doubtless from its secondary spread was responsible for death. A possible osteosarcoma has been described from the pelvis of a mature man from Westerhus (Gejvall, 1960), but there is clearly doubt concerning this diagnosis. More certain and more dramatic is the diagnosis of an early Medieval individual from Standlake, Oxfordshire, England. An enormous osteosarcoma measuring about 25cm × 27cm was found at the right knee (Brothwell, 1967b). A pathological fracture had occurred and the individual was probably bedridden and in excruciating pain, but may have been cared for during the terminal illness. Surely this is testimony to the fortitude of our ancestors, who were denied the benefit of powerful modern pain relief. The diagnosed cases of osteosarcoma in the archaeological record are few (Suzuki, 1987). As stated, this is a tumour of the young and it is perhaps surprising, and maybe aetiologically significant, that the prevalence in antiquity was not greater, although the survival of young individuals in the archaeological record is not always good enough for observing diseases affecting this age group.

The **chondrosarcoma** is the second most common malignant tumour and occurs in the metaphyses of long bone extremities (Ortner, 2003: 526). The ends of the femur, proximal humerus and pelvis are the most common sites affected in the skeleton, and the malignant cartilage is nodular in appearance with destruction of the cancellous bone. If the tumour calcifies or ossifies, then it may be recognizable in the skeleton.

A primary bone neoplasm of similar type but differing in the cells and site of origin is **Ewing's sarcoma**, the third most common malignant tumour of bone. Whereas the osteosarcoma develops from the bone cortex, Ewing's sarcoma develops in cells in the interior of the bone. The result is a swelling, with the expanding tumour eventually breaking through the cortex. It is seen more commonly in young individuals in long bone extremities or the pelvis (Ortner, 2003: 526). The tumour destroys the marrow spaces and may attack the cortex, spreading into the periosteum, producing new bone formation, either of 'sunburst' appearance or as multiple layers of bone ('onion skin'). Although no definite diagnosis of this tumour in antiquity has been made, it seems possible that an example exists in the pelvis of an Egyptian of the Roman period (Ruffer and Willmore, 1914). The diagnosis has yet to be substantiated.

If the young are unfortunate in their susceptibility to the osteosarcoma, the elderly are rather more unfortunate in their primary malignant bone neoplasm. The neoplasm known as **myeloma** is, strictly speaking, not a new growth of bone cells but a new growth originating in the plasma cells in the blood-forming tissues of the bone marrow. Myelomatosis, or multiple myeloma, so called because the neoplastic lesions are widespread and multifocal in origin in many marrow cavities throughout the skeleton, is the most common of the primary malignant tumours of the skeleton. The tumour is rarely found in people below the age of 40 years, and 90 per cent of cases are found in individuals between the ages of 50 and 60 years. Males more than females are affected. Although solitary lesions do occur, the condition usually appears as multiple lesions, which probably arise as independent developments in a systematized neoplastic bone marrow disease, rather than as secondary deposits from a single primary source. The result is a rarefaction of the bone, perforation of the cortex and possible pathological fracture. Most commonly involved sites are the vertebrae, skull, ribs and pelvis. Since the skull bones are relatively thin, perforation of the skull is perhaps an early feature (Figs 9.7 and 9.8). At least in skeletal remains, it is the feature upon which the diagnosis is usually based. The multiple and clearly destructive nature of these skull perforations distinguishes them from the perforations of chronic infections such as venereal syphilis and from the perforations of trauma. What is more difficult in palaeopathological diagnosis is the separation of these myelomatous lesions in the skull from the skull perforations of secondary cancer (Cattaneo *et al.*, 1994), but see Rothschild *et al.* (1998) for a discussion. In some individuals doubt as to their specific diagnosis remains (Strouhal, 1976).

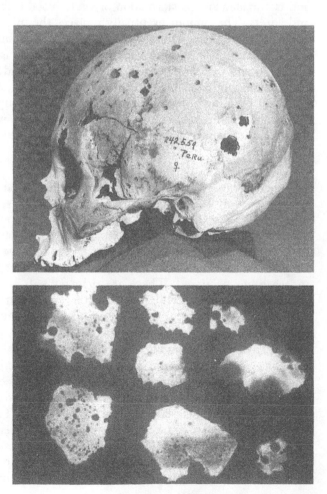

Fig. 9.7. Multiple myeloma of the skull vault, shown by multiple perforations (National Museum of Natural History, Washington DC, United States, 242559, adult female, prehistoric AD 500–1530, Caudiville, Peru, South America). *(With permission of Don Ortner)*

Fig. 9.8. Radiograph of lesions, probably the result of multiple myeloma (early Medieval Addingham, West Yorkshire, England).

At present there are several cases of multiple myeloma in the palaeopathological record. In view of the expectation of longevity in antiquity discussed in an earlier chapter, it might (or might not) be thought that the neoplasm was a rarity in the past, but in prehistoric native American Indian populations it was not rare at all (Morse *et al.*, 1974). In palaeopathological research the first recognition of the disease in early skeletal material was in a pre-Columbian Indian (Ritchie and Warren, 1932). The bone-destructive lesions, which were demonstrated by radiography, were widespread, being found in the skull, vertebrae, ribs, sternum, femur, pelvis and scapula. Since that time the geographic and time spread of the disease have been extended (e.g. a fourteenth- to sixteenth-century female from Abingdon, Oxfordshire, England (Wakely *et al.*, 1998)). The earliest case so far recorded is of the fourth century BC from Kentucky (Steinbock, 1976) and the condition extends through the Old and the New World (Alt and Adler, 1992). The modern practitioner familiar with the myelomatous patient who, without treatment, is likely to die within two years from infection and kidney failure must understand the suffering of the elderly in the past. **Leukaemia**, a malignant tumour, also affects the bone marrow, and is a malignant transformation of white blood cells, occurring in both children and adults. The tumour eventually replaces the marrow spaces of the body. The skeletal changes may include loss of bone mass and small destructive lesions in the cortex (Ortner, 2003: 376). A narrow radiolucent line is seen at the metaphyseal side of the growth plate in children, accompanied by widening of the foramina of the blood vessels and grooving and porosity of the cortex. A recent study by Rothschild *et al.* (1997) documented these and other changes in skeletons from the Hamann–Todd Collection of two people diagnosed with leukaemia. However, no individuals from antiquity have yet been diagnosed with this condition.

SECONDARY CANCER

The prevalence of cancer suggested by the palaeopathological record does demonstrate an overall increase in malignant disease from the distant past until today. If, as seems likely, environmental changes in pollution and atmosphere, and changes in diet, have brought about an increase in cancer, this increase is unlikely to be of the primary bone neoplasms arising *de novo* in bone cells. It is surely in the cancers of lung, stomach, bowel, skin and breast, among others, that the increase has occurred. These are primary soft-tissue neoplasms. Their only manifestation in bone is by virtue of their secondary spread (Galasko, 1986), or more rarely their local bone invasion. Consequently the primary growths themselves are rarely in evidence in skeletal remains.

Neither must it be forgotten that death may occur before spread of the cancer to the bones. Death may ensue from intercurrent infection in the early stages of the malignant disease. In modern practice the infections occurring in the early stages of malignant disease are treated, and it is noted that today 20 per cent of fatal cancer cases possess bone metastatic deposits (Willis, 1973). Therefore, because in antiquity the individual may have succumbed earlier in his or her cancerous illness, this figure of 20 per cent may be too high for past societies. It must also be remembered that not all cancers have the same tendency to spread to bone. Cancers of the breast, lung, stomach, thyroid gland, prostate and kidney are most likely to produce bone metastases. These metastases do not tend to be uniformly distributed throughout the whole skeleton. As was first recorded by Von Recklinghausen in 1891, the vertebrae, sternum, ribs, skull, pelvis and upper ends of femur and humerus are perhaps the most commonly affected, although the sites do vary from neoplasm to neoplasm.

A further problem in palaeopathological recognition is the fact that the secondary growths commence in the marrow cavities deep inside the bones and only later destroy and perforate the cortex to the bone exterior. Mere inspection of bones may fail to reveal these deep growths, which may only be demonstrated by radiography of the bone. Ideally, therefore, in order to assess the true pattern of malignant disease in antiquity, radiography of all skeletons from archaeological excavations should be carried out, but funding does not allow this to happen. At present palaeopathological diagnosis rests upon finding the irregularly eroded and perforated bone surface, the skull being most commonly involved and observed (Waldron, 1987b). The lesions are usually multiple, and, because of the similarity, confusion with multiple myeloma may occur. With the exception of cancer of the prostate, most secondary deposits cause loss of bone substance with consequent weakening. The bone at the site of the deposit is liable to fracture. Cancer of the prostate usually causes bone secondaries which themselves produce bone, albeit of a widespread, disorganized and functionless nature (Tkocz and Bierring, 1984; Anderson *et al.*, 1992; Wakely *et al.*, 1995; Mays *et al.*, 1996; Waldron, 1997b). Prostate cancer was first described in the nineteenth century, and the condition does not appear to have been common in the past; it occurs in older males today. It also affects people most in north-west Europe and North America, and is rarer in the Far East (Waldron, 1997b: 244). It seems to be associated more with some religious groups and with higher social classes.

Metastatic cancer of bone as a result of primary cancer in another part of the body is the most common cause of tumours affecting the skeleton, with most being destructive of bone (Ortner, 2003: 533). Bone destruction is usually the result of cancer of the lung, breast, gastrointestinal tract, thyroid gland and kidney, while bone-forming lesions are caused by prostate cancer in males and cancer of the breast, uterus and ovary in females (Ortner, 2003: 533). The axial skeleton, plus the proximal humeri and femora, are most affected (Fig. 9.9). The tumour cells destroy the marrow, followed by destruction of bone, and sometimes formation.

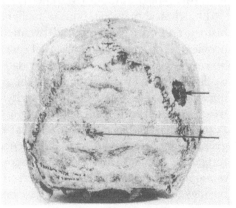

Fig. 9.9. Skull showing perforations of secondary cancer (arrowed) (early Medieval, sixth–eighth centuries AD, Eccles, Kent, England)

Occasionally in skeletal material evidence of both primary and secondary growths is found. An Egyptian skull of III–V Dynasty date exhibits invasive destruction of a primary cancer of the nasopharynx. In addition, the skull vault is perforated by a number of secondary deposits from this primary nasopharyngeal cancer (Wells, 1963). Scarcely can we imagine the suffering of this individual with a foul, fungating cancer relentlessly advancing through the roof of the mouth to protrude into the mouth itself. Death must surely have been a welcome release from this bleeding, ulcerated obstruction to swallowing, talking and decent life.

Perhaps the first analytical and clinical study of metastatic cancer in a skeleton of archaeological context was that by Møller and Møller-Christensen (1952). Secondary deposits were noted in the skull of a woman from the Medieval cemetery at Aebelholt, Denmark. By analogy with modern studies it was suggested that the individual may have died as a result of a primary cancer of the breast and its metastases. Other Medieval examples of skull metastases have been described (Gejvall, 1960; Wells, 1964d), and indeed the span of examples, both in time and distribution, is increasing (Brothwell, 1967b; Steinbock, 1976; Allison *et al.*, 1980; Ortner and Putschar, 1981; Manchester, 1983a; Gregg and Gregg, 1987; Grupe, 1988; Ortner *et al.*, 1991). The earliest example known at present is from the European Bronze Age. A female skull, dated to 1900–1600 BC from Mokrin, in the former Yugoslavia, shows perforating lesions characteristic of cancer metastases, which it is suggested originated from a primary cancer of the breast (Soulié, 1980). Notwithstanding the increasing number of reports, the cases of malignancy recognized in the skeletal remains of the past are few (Micozzi, 1991), although examples are being reported in increasing frequency and have been reported to increase through time (e.g. in Slovakia, Šefčáková *et al.*, 2001). Malignant disease has, of course, been recognized in mummified remains too. An example of a malignant disease called malignant melanoma, rare today and in the past, has been noted in pre-Columbian Inca mummies from Peru (Urteaga and Pack, 1966). This pigmented growth resulted in small, dark masses within the mummy skin and in multiple pigmented lesions in the skull bones. Furthermore, in an Italian mummy dated to 1431–94 (the King of Naples), a pelvic tumour of the appearance of an adenocarcinoma was identified through histological analysis; further biomolecular analysis identified a mutation in the K-*ras* gene, compatible with this type of tumour (Marchetti *et al.*, 1996, in Aufderheide, 2003).

The clinical manifestations of malignancy have probably not changed throughout history, and only from the mid-twentieth-century did therapy begin to alleviate the problem. The surgical treatment of cancer is not exclusively a modern phenomenon, however. A skull of twelfth-century date from Caen exhibits an enormous fungating malignant tumour projecting from the right side of the facial skeleton and extending into the eye-socket and the nasal cavity. An attempt, albeit unsuccessful, at surgical treatment had been made by cutting a hole in the adjacent bone (Dastugue, 1965). Perhaps the Medieval patient felt that the attempted cure of the disease was more grievous than its endurance. The general ill-health, weight loss and anaemia, the fungating, offensive and bleeding tumour, the pain and the eventual death were just as much features of the Medieval person as they might be of the twenty-first-century business executive. Malignant disease has no respect for creed or class.

That cancer is a disease of advancing years is well recognized today. It has been noted in an earlier chapter that the expectation of life in antiquity may not have been as great as today. Maybe the number of individuals in the past surviving to the age of 'cancer prevalence' was not as great. However, cancer is also a problem of younger age groups today, and therefore the presumed reduced life expectancy in antiquity cannot be the sole reason for the rarity of palaeopathological evidence. If, as seems likely, there has been an increase in malignant disease in recent times, the reasons may be related to the changing environment throughout history. Physical (ultraviolet light), chemical (chemicals that are carcinogens) and viral agents (e.g. hepatitis B virus can cause liver cancer) as well as diet (e.g. fatty foods) all have their part to play today in the development of cancers. Lack of fibre in the diet and excess fat and protein are believed today also to lead to colon cancer. However, the woodsmoke-filled cave environment, naturally occurring gases such as radon and uranium, specific dietary components and toxic fumes induced by metalworking in the past may all have contributed to the development of neoplastic disease. That certain substances may induce cancer of the scrotum was first noted by Percival Pott in 1775 in respect of soot. Since then many agents have been found to stimulate malignant change. Most of these agents are the products of modern industrial development and would not have been encountered in the village or town life of pre-industrial societies. An entirely recent hazard, too, is the effect of radiation. The peaceful and military use of radioactive materials, which are potentially cancer inducing, is an aspect of life, welcome or otherwise, totally unknown to earlier peoples. The incidence of lung cancer in western society rose steeply after the Second World War. The relationship between lung cancer and cigarette smoking is well attested, with a likely association also with the pollution of modern cities. But what of the cancers of the breast, prostate, stomach and so on, for which no definite environmental association or cancer-inducing agent is known? It is recognized that nasopharyngeal cancer has a higher incidence in North Africa than in other parts of the world, and similar tumour associations occur with various ethnic groups. Blood-group association with cancer has already been mentioned and is a well-recognized, but hitherto ill-explained, phenomenon. However, this does not explain the apparent increase in this dreaded disease from the sparse palaeopathological evidence of distant antiquity to the feared high incidence of today. With increasing excavation and research, perhaps the recognition of cancer in antiquity and its correlation to the socio-economic context of the time may help to elucidate the cause of malignant disease in the past. Indeed, Waldron (1996) did go some way to explaining the frequency of malignant tumours of the skeleton. From the model he proposed, using data from the 1901–5 Annual Reports of the Registrar General for England, the number of tumours expected for a past population was, as expected, low. However, he cautions that this may be a function of low sample size and small expected numbers.

CHAPTER 10

Conclusions: The Next Ten Years

The intricate relationship between a people's way of life and the diseases they endure is the chief reason for the study of palaeopathology. (Wells, 1964a: 18)

INTRODUCTION

The year 1983 saw the first edition of this book (Manchester, 1983b), 1995 saw the second edition (Roberts and Manchester, 1995), and ten or so years later comes the third edition. There have been many developments in the study of palaeopathology since the nineteenth century and a concentration on case studies, even since the 1980s. Since 1995 population-based studies of health have increased and there is more consideration for placing health data in cultural context. The 'biocultural', or more recently termed 'bioarchaeological', approach to reconstructing past human health is much more productive and more relevant to archaeology as a whole. Furthermore, analysing skeletal remains for disease from the perspective of testing hypotheses and answering questions has been recognized as essential.

In the 1983 edition Sandison's (1968) recommendations for the development of palaeopathology were returned to; here, again, we review these recommendations and then consider future prospects. The **establishment of a central registry for palaeopathological examples** has not advanced much at all. Some researchers have websites, and some palaeopathological data, including images, are published on websites, but there is no single website or other medium of publication that is central. However, the increasing use of electronic media over the last ten years has provided many more people with the opportunity to access data. Skeletal data on disease, of course, are published to a certain extent in cemetery site reports but may also appear in microfiche, on microfilm, on a compact disk or on a website. For example, data from the 'Western Hemisphere Health' project (studying the health of 12,520 individuals from 5000 BC to the late nineteenth century in the Americas) have recently been made available to all on a website (Website 2), following its publication (Steckel and Rose, 2002). Data from a current project focusing on the 'History of Health in Europe', also coordinated by Richard Steckel, will similarly be made available to scholars in the future when it has been published. With regard to a **bibliography**, the Paleopathology Association in 1997 published a hard copy of a bibliography of palaeopathology and provides regular updates on disk (Tyson, 1997). The **publication and recording of classic pathological cases** in skeletal remains are a continuous process with significant contributions through journals such as the *American Association of Physical Anthropology*, but also in texts such as those by Ortner (2003) and Aufderheide and Rodríguez Martín (1998). It is perhaps a worrying development that pathology museums holding classic documented cases of dry bone pathologies may be under threat of survival; they are not always considered as important for educational purposes as they used to be, and, again, electronic media are taking over in storing images and text for access to all.

THE PAST (SINCE 1995)

The biocultural/bioarchaeological population approach to palaeopathology

It is fair to say that since 1995 more population studies of disease patterning have been published than before that time. Additionally, no person working in palaeopathology can fail to ignore the importance of the integration of biological data on disease with cultural context. For example, being aware of the type of living environment a population experienced will help us to interpret and explain the disease patterns we see. A person living in an overcrowded environment might be expected to contract population-density-dependent diseases such as tuberculosis. Diagnosis of disease has also advanced but still remains a challenge.

Diagnosis and interpretation of disease

Diagnosis of disease in skeletal remains, for it is skeletal remains with which the palaeopathologist mostly deals, can still prove difficult. The use of clinical data to diagnose disease in a skeleton is the base from which all palaeopathologists work, but these data may not always be appropriate for the task in hand, something that should be remembered. For example, very subtle changes in disease-affected bones from archaeological sites may not be described in clinical literature as part of the diagnostic criteria for a disease even though they may be important. This is the case for new bone formation on ribs that is probably the result of lung infection; because the change does not show radiographically, it is not detected by clinicians and therefore it is not documented. The skeletal collections with known causes of death and medical histories in North America (the Hamann-Todd Collection in Cleveland, Ohio, and the Terry Collection in the Smithsonian Institution, Washington DC), and Portugal (Coimbra Identified Skeletal Collection, Coimbra, and that in Lisbon), particularly, can help us significantly in our understanding of the skeletal changes of disease. Nevertheless, our increasing use of electronic media to communicate information and images about pathological cases in order to achieve a more accurate diagnosis has meant more people get a chance to comment on problematic cases.

The main point expressed in both the 1983 and 1995 editions of this book was that developments in palaeopathology would lie in the application of the scientific techniques of microscopy, radiology and biochemical analysis to diagnose disease in skeletal remains. However, even now researchers in the discipline should not think that the application of methods of analysis beyond visual/macroscopic description and diagnosis of pathological conditions will answer all our palaeopathological problems. Nevertheless, biomolecular analysis (i.e. mainly that of extracting and amplifying ancient DNA of micro-organisms) has of course been used over the last ten years increasingly to answer specific questions about health, but also to diagnose disease *per se* (e.g. plague, malaria, Spanish influenza, tuberculosis, leprosy, treponemal disease and other infections). This has allowed disease to be diagnosed when bone changes do not occur (e.g. malaria (Taylor *et al.*, 1997) and plague (Drancourt *et al.*, 1998)), and also to diagnose disease in people who died before bone changes occurred (e.g. see Faerman *et al.*, 1999). More sophisticated approaches have also involved trying to identify the strain of an organism, for example whether a person had tuberculosis of the human or bovine form (Mays *et al.*, 2001). However, there is still a lot of basic groundwork to do in the recording of palaeopathology in skeletal populations. In financial terms visual recording of pathological lesions is a lot less expensive than biomolecular analysis, for example, but grant-giving bodies have generally seemed interested in funding only 'high-tech' media-attracting research, certainly in Britain, in recent years. Elsewhere in the world there appears to be more sympathy with the need to fund basic palaeopathological recording on large skeletal samples.

The practitioners

At the time of the second edition in 1995 it was noted that people working in palaeopathology came from a variety of backgrounds, and many were medically trained. An increasing trend of graduates in archaeology and anthropology was being seen in the mid-1990s, and this has continued to rise into the new millennium. In Britain, for example, the number of graduates taking Master's level courses in 'physical anthropology' and related subjects, including palaeopathology, increased through the late 1990s, with more universities providing relevant courses (in Britain: Bradford, Bournemouth, Durham, Sheffield and Southampton). Additionally, related M.Sc. courses such as that between the University of Sheffield and the University of Manchester (M.Sc. in Biomolecular Archaeology) have generated graduates who are knowledgeable about the diagnosis of disease using biomolecular techniques. Nevertheless, each person with his or her own particular background can contribute expertise to enhance our knowledge of the evolution and palaeoepidemiology of disease. As an extension to the burgeoning number of Master's courses, and Ph.D. graduates in the discipline, the UK particularly has also seen more academic posts being created over the last ten years, mainly in archaeology departments in universities. We believe that this is because the value of research on human remains to the archaeological and anthropological community is being more widely recognized.

Ambitious projects on disease

Probably the most ambitious project so far in the history of palaeopathological study has been the 'Western Hemisphere Health Project', originally conceived in 1990 by Richard Steckel and Jerome Rose (2002). Funded variously by the Ohio State University, the Wenner Gren Foundation and the National Science Foundation, the project brought together health data on 12,520 skeletons in 18 studies from 218 sites in North, Central and South America. This project had in its sights the publication by Mark Cohen and George Armelagos on health at the transition to agriculture in various parts of the world (1984). However, as Steckel and Rose pointed out, the papers in that 1984 study were not comparable in terms of the data that were presented. In the 2002 study a common data-reporting format was used that made comparison between populations possible. In addition, many more skeletons were used, the time span was greater, and interdisciplinary perspectives were used to interpret and explain the data. In addition, the concept of a 'Health Index' was used for the first time. A multi-attribute system was used to assess aspects of the quality of life (Steckel *et al.*, 2002: 68). A number of health variables were considered (stature, enamel hypoplasia, anaemia, infection (periostitis), degenerative joint disease and trauma), and all were weighted equally in the index. While details of this Index should be accessed in Steckel *et al.* (2002), it should be noted that health levels varied greatly by region and time period, but Native Americans were both the healthiest and the least healthy (Steckel *et al.*, 2002: 74). This is an interesting change to the usual methods of presenting health data, although it may be criticized in some respects. For example, condensing down a number of health indicators with differing aetiologies to one number can be seen to simplify the way in which disease affects a person, and, as we have already noted, a person or population's experience of the same disease will vary. Nevertheless, the next project on 'Health in Europe' will prove to be even more sophisticated and incorporate larger data samples.

Standardization of palaeopathological data recording

There have been considerable advances in the recording of skeletal changes in disease, an area that needs to be maintained and enhanced if comparisons of populations are to be made with any degree of accuracy (and any reinterpretations of data made). These advances were initiated with the publication of Buikstra and Ubelaker (1994), which documented the standards needed for recording skeletal remains to aid the identification of sex and age at death, and to record metrical and non-metrical data, and pathological conditions. Don Ortner has also for many years emphasized in his writings (e.g. 1991), and also through the Paleopathology Workshops at the Annual Meetings of the Paleopathology Association in North America, the need to describe abnormal changes accurately in the skeleton before an attempt at a differential diagnosis is made. Ultimately, however, Buikstra and Ubelaker (1994) was produced because of the threat of repatriation and reburial of native American skeletal populations that had not been recorded, or not very well (see Rose *et al.*, 1996 on the Native American Graves Protection and Repatriation Act of 1990). In Britain in 2001 at the Annual

Meeting of the British Association of Biological Anthropology and Osteoarchaeology at the University of Durham, Roberts and Cox (2003) also underlined the problem of non-comparable data on pathology in Britain from archaeological sites. Following that meeting in November 2001, a working party met to discuss the problem and in 2004 a document was published on line by the Institute of Field Archaeologists outlining recommendations for recording skeletal remains in Britain (Brickley and McKinley, 2004). The 'History of Health in Europe' project will, likewise, be using a standard recording system so that skeletal data will be recorded in a comparable manner. These advances are significant and it is recommended that future work in palaeopathology adheres to these recommendations to benefit the discipline of palaeopathology overall. A related area of concern is the format and content of skeletal reports. Recent steps have been taken to address this concern in Britain with the publication of guidelines for producing reports (English Heritage 2002; Brickley and McKinley, 2004).

Research on specific diseases or themes

Since 1994 we have seen conferences particularly focused on one disease. This allows a much more detailed appraisal of diagnostic criteria, and the extant evidence, than is normal at most conferences. For example, venereal syphilis in Europe (Dutour et al., 1994), tuberculosis (Pálfi et al., 1999), leprosy (Roberts et al., 2002) and the plague in Marseilles, France, in 2001 have been considered. Publications have also appeared that cover themes such as violence in the past (Martin and Frayer, 1998), health at transitions (Swedlund and Armelagos, 1990), health at European contact in the Americas (Larsen and Milner, 1994), and differences in health between males and females (Grauer and Stuart-Macadam, 1998) and in children (e.g. Lewis, 2002a); some of these themes were noted for attention in 1995. Themed works in palaeopathology allow researchers to explore the evidence from a number of perspectives, as do multidisciplinary perspectives on mortality and morbidity. For example, two notable publications considered both skeletal and historical data of recent populations, mostly from North America (Grauer, 1995; Saunders and Herring, 1995).

Of course, papers have also appeared that consider specific diseases, especially those that are less common such as neoplastic and congenital disease. In the 1995 edition these conditions were noted to be rare, if publications are to be believed. Since that time the data have not changed this belief, with case study approaches being the common method for disseminating information, although some collective data from Britain have been commented upon regarding aetiology (Roberts and Cox, 2003). There have, however, been few comments about the possible factors leading to either congenital or neoplastic disease in specific populations. Physical, chemical and viral agents have been labelled as responsible for neoplastic disease today. However, although we are aware of increasing social complexity through time (including the presence of factors such as toxic fumes from metalworking, and woodsmoke in houses that could be potentially carcinogenic), there has been little attempt to link occurrence with causative factors. The same can be said of congenital disease. While there are few cases reported archaeologically of congenital disease, there were potential aetiological factors in people's environments. Both neoplastic and congenital disease have seen few population studies, most literature concentrating on individual skeletons. Considering the multifactorial aetiology of both conditions, some large population studies would be informative. However, as Rothschild and Rothschild's (1995) study showed, detecting actual frequency rates for neoplastic disease, for example, requires at the very least radiographic analysis, a methodology that is rarely available or cheap enough to be applied to every skeleton from an archaeological site. The other rare find from archaeological sites noted in 1995 was calcified tissue such as bladder, kidney and gall stones; there has been no advance in the study and interpretation of these tissues since then.

However, there have been advances in the diagnosis of specific pathological conditions since the mid-1990s. Particular attention has been paid to the joint diseases by Juliet Rogers and Tony Waldron (Rogers and Waldron, 1995), but there has been a distressing burgeoning of studies of 'occupationally related' osteoarthritis in the archaeological record, despite the multifactorial aetiology of this joint disease (see Jurmain, 1999 for a detailed analysis of the data, both clinical and archaeological). In fact, the use of musculo-skeletal markers of stress (MSMs), such as enthesopathies and osteoarthritis, has been a frequent research tool in physical anthropology to explore (usually uncritically) the presence and nature of activity in past human populations. Perhaps the most promising avenue of research in this area is biomechanical analysis (Ruff, 2000). Another research focus has developed the diagnosic criteria for the metabolic diseases of scurvy and rickets. Don Ortner of the Smithsonian Institution, Washington DC, has been instrumental in this respect (Ortner and Ericksen, 1997; Ortner and Mays, 1998). Developing the diagnostic criteria for osteoporosis has also seen attention, particularly from Megan Brickley (2000), and this was an area of study recommended for future work in the 1995 edition. There have also been increasing interest in the diagnosis and interpretation of non-specific infective changes in focal areas of the body – for example, maxillary sinusitis (Roberts *et al.*, 1998; Merrett and Pfeiffer, 2000), endocranial new bone formation (Lewis, 2004), and new bone formation on ribs (Roberts, 1999; Lambert, 2002).

Methodological advances

In terms of methodological advances, some biomolecular analyses have already been discussed, although assessing palaeodietary status using stable isotope analysis of carbon and nitrogen has increased markedly over the last ten years (e.g. Katzenberg, 2000; Lillie and Richards, 2000). While a direct link between dietary status and health is not usually the focus of such studies, the relevance is clear: 'you are what you eat.' The analysis of stable isotopes of oxygen, strontium and lead to track mobility has also shown great potential (Sealy *et al.*, 1995; Price *et al.*, 2001; Budd *et al.*, 2004; Hodell *et al.*, 2004), and has relevance for future studies of palaeopathology. Palaeohistological analyses have also made advances in helping to secure more precise diagnoses (e.g. see Pfeiffer, 2000; Schultz, 2001), although all these methods of analysis involve destruction of bone or teeth, something to bear in mind for the future integrity of skeletal collections. A noted methodological advance, although rare, has been the reconstruction of faces (Wilkinson and Neave, 2003) and heads affected by abnormal change (Kustár, 1999). It has proved of use to see the person's face as they were living, which should provide a useful insight to possible associated stigma and ostracism in the past. Of course, much facial reconstruction in archaeology is for museum purposes to bring back to life the person whose skull has been reconstructed. However, the media attention on the study of human remains from archaeological sites has also been considerable over the last ten years, and facial reconstructions have been popular with the public (e.g. *Meet the Ancestors* on BBC2 in Britain). So what of the future? What lies in store for those who wish to continue to contribute to our understanding of the history of disease?

THE PRESENT AND FUTURE

Standardization of recording and reporting, and access to palaeopathological data

There are a number of very important areas that need discussion with respect to future developments in palaeopathology. We believe that, paramount to our understanding of the experience of disease by our ancestors, is the continued effort aimed at standardization of recording of pathological changes, with detailed descriptions of lesions being made before differential diagnoses are made. This allows re-evaluation of data and possible re-diagnosis by future researchers and makes the data more transparent. The archiving of these detailed data in a form that is accessible to those who require it is also essential, unless the full details are to be published. It is anticipated that increasing use will be made of the World Wide Web as more people have access to this form of communication globally. The 'History of Health in Europe' project will be another major advance in achieving these recommendations.

It is hoped too that less data on the health of past populations will remain in the 'grey literature'. For example, a recent collation and interpretation of data on health in Britain through time found that, of the data from 311 cemetery sites used for the project, nearly 40 per cent of sites were unpublished, with many reports having been written up to twenty years previously (Roberts and Cox, 2003). We would suggest that this appears to reflect the structure and workings of archaeology as a discipline in Britain, and we are also aware that it is not only human skeletal reports that suffer from not being published; other 'specialisms' in archaeology have similar problems (including the non-standardization of reporting).

Access to good quality and large amounts of comparative data allows researchers to move the discipline forward in terms of taking overviews of data from a regional, temporal or even specific disease perspective. Additional to this, a central database, perhaps within each country of the world, where these data can be stored and accessed, would be useful (but it would need to be continually updated). Related to this would be details for each cemetery site recorded: the location of the site (map reference, whether it is coastal, inland, on an island, rural, urban, highland, lowland, etc.), the year excavated, the period of time, the site type (e.g. poor or monastic cemetery), the number of skeletal remains analysed (males, females, unsexed adults and juveniles), preservation state of the remains, phasing of the site, details of whether the data have been published, relevant information such as the pH of the site, hydrology, etc., whether the skeletal remains are still above ground and whether they are accessible and where (and contact details), and finally a bibliography of the publications.

The practitioners, organizations and conferences, and the media

It is anticipated that the people working in palaeopathology in the future will increasingly be those graduating with archaeology and anthropology degrees, and those who also go on to take a Master's and/or Ph.D. degree in a subject concerned with the study of human remains from archaeological sites. We believe that they may be the most appropriate people to promote the study of human remains from a biocultural perspective, having a good archaeological/ anthropological background. This is not to say that medically trained researchers in palaeopathology cannot contribute. They contribute enormously in our understanding of the epidemiology of disease and help us to understand the impact of disease on individuals and populations; they also provide caution in diagnosis and interpretation of the impact of disease in the past.

Additionally, we believe that the discipline of medical anthropology has a large part to play in our understanding of past population health. 'Medical anthropology studies human health in a variety of environmental and cultural contexts, ranging from isolated tribal peoples to modern urban communities. A subfield called medical ecology views health and disease as reflections of relationships within a population, between neighbouring populations, and among life forms and physical components of a habitat' (McElroy and Townsend, 1996: 2). Some researchers in palaeopathology have conducted medical anthropological research themselves and used the data to contribute to the understanding of palaeopathological data on the same condition observed (e.g. Goodman *et al.*, 1987; Goodman and Rose, 1990), but this is quite rare to date. While we use clinical data as a base from which to work, we are often using data collected from living populations following a westernized lifestyle. Much medical anthropological research is based on groups of people living a rather more traditional life, which may reflect the situation for our past populations (e.g. Huijbers *et al.*, 1996). We think that certain areas of palaeopathology would benefit considerably from using a medical anthropological perspective – for example, the study of activity-related changes in the skeleton.

There are a number of organizations that promote the study of palaeopathology, and these will continue to have a significant impact on its development. The most important is the Paleopathology Association founded in 1973; its quarterly Newsletter and its annual, and biennial European, meetings enable dissemination of knowledge, exchange of ideas and the meeting of people working in palaeopathology. The Dental Anthropology Association, the American Association of Physical Anthropologists, the European Anthropological Association and the British Association of Biological Anthropology and Osteoarchaeology are also organized groups who promote the study of physical anthropology generally, including palaeopathology. Finally, one could also say that the media in recent years, as already noted, have acquired a fascination for portraying our discipline in television and radio programmes. If these programmes are made in a scientific and sound way, with respect to the human remains being portrayed, without outrageous interpretation being based on data that cannot support it, the media could continue to provide publicity to our important research.

Palaeopathological studies

As reiterated time and again, we consider that the main thrust of palaeopathological research advancement should lie in the study of *population* health, and not solely in case studies of interesting pathological conditions (see Mays, 1997 on a comparison of palaeopathological studies in the UK, Japan, Germany and the USA). While these individual cases are interesting in their own right, because they are usually rare, their real value emerges when the data are collated and interpreted in cultural context. The large collective studies of the 'Western Hemisphere Health' project and the 'History of Health in Europe' project allow a much broader perspective on health at the population level to be considered through long periods of time. The bioarchaeology/biocultural approach to palaeopathology of course is paramount to our understanding of our data; without considering our biological data on health within the cultural context from which they derive, our discipline will be much poorer. We also believe that the consideration of palaeopathological data within themes will allow us to exploit those cultural contextual data to their full potential.

More studies should be undertaken that consider broad themes: for example, the effect of social status on health (e.g. see Cohen, 1998; Robb et al., 2001), the effects of biological sex and gender on health (e.g. see Grauer and Stuart-Macadam, 1998), including considerations of how males and females perceive their health and whether they access health care (e.g. see medical anthropological studies such as Kettel, 1996; Gijsbers van Wijk et al., 1999; Pollard and Hyatt, 1999; Courtenay, 2000), and the effect of climate (e.g. see Lukacs and Walimbe, 1998; Martens, 1998), diet (e.g. Larsen, 1995), environment (e.g. see Roberts et al., 1998), work (e.g. for a balanced view of potential see Jurmain, 1999) and migration on health (Kaplan, 1988; Armelagos, 1990; Dobyns, 1993). We also consider highly important the development of the study of the palaeopathology of other animals so that we can better understand the relationship of humans to their wild and domesticated animals with respect to zoonoses (an area of study emphasized continually by Don Brothwell – e.g. Brothwell, 1991 – but also described by others – e.g. O'Connor, 2000). We also hope that, stimulated by the excellent review by Aufderheide (2003), more data on the palaeopathology of mummified bodies may be forthcoming in the future.

Our resource, and analytical developments

There are many extant skeletal collections, large and small, curated in museums and institutions; they derive from different periods and geographical regions of the world, and from a variety of archaeological contexts. They provide practitioners with a large and valuable resource for research and teaching. In terms of teaching, it allows us to teach students at all levels about the evolution, presence and change in disease through very long periods of time; it provides a temporal and geographical perspective that is essential in allowing us to understand disease today. Having skeletons available that derive from a variety of populations also enables us to show how differently disease may affect a person. In addition to variation in skeletal involvement in disease, we can observe the great variation in the skeleton's appearance from one person to another and from one population to another. Retaining and curating these skeletal samples with respect and care are vital to generating knowledge about our past, which continually evolves as ideas change and analytical methodology develops (e.g. see Buikstra and Gordon, 1981).

In some parts of the world skeletal remains have been repatriated to the care of native populations, and many have been reburied. Australian aboriginal populations, native Americans and the Maori have, in many people's eyes, rightly claimed their ancestors' remains from curating institutions. In some cases repatriation has led to retention of skeletal remains in holding places that are accessible to *bona fide* researchers, but in other cases the skeletons have been reburied. This latter situation of course makes skeletal material inaccessible for further study, and it emphasizes the need to make sure data are recorded properly and accurately. As indicated above, Buikstra and Ubelaker (1994) was produced with this in mind. In Britain there have also been recent moves by the British government's Department of Culture, Media and Sport to look at issues surrounding the storage of human remains in museums (DCMS, 2004), and also by the Cathedrals and Church Buildings Division of the Church of England and English Heritage Human Remains Working Group (Church of England and English Heritage, 2005). This latter group has looked at ethical, legal and scientific issues to agree guidelines that would cover excavation and treatment of Christian burials in archaeological projects, and reburial. With all this in mind, there is an urgent need to acquire reliable palaeopathological data that are comparable between sites, but there is also a need to curate skeletal material with respect and care in order that it is not compromised (see Caffell *et al.*, 2001; Janaway *et al.*, 2001; Bowron, 2003).

Our resource is very precious, and with the development of new (often destructive) methods of analysis, we must be ever careful of maintaining the integrity of that resource. If samples are to be taken for biomolecular and/or histological analyses, then the research projects must have clearly defined hypotheses and objectives. It is without doubt, we believe, that biomolecular analyses will continue to be at the forefront of developments in diagnosis in palaeopathology, and will contribute in the future to our understanding not only of genetic disease and relatedness in archaeological samples (see Weiss, 1993 for a clinical perspective), but also of changes in the structure of micro-organisms. Relatedness between individuals in a cemetery has already been studied using ancient DNA analysis (e.g. Cappellini *et al.*, 2004) and also dental non-metric traits (e.g. Alt *et al.*, 1997; Corruccini *et al.*, 2002), but this needs now to be applied to exploring whether related people had the same diseases. It is likely that researchers will also start to consider the use of stable isotopes for analysing the origin of disease and the effect of migration on disease transmission, but studies of palaeodiet will also continue (perhaps linking dietary status and disease). Likewise, histological analyses will continue to contribute in the future to diagnosis. Perhaps one major point to be made is that we should perhaps develop further our understanding of the taphonomic factors affecting the survival of microscopic structures and biomolecules in bone and teeth (for example, with more studies such as Haynes *et al.*, 2002; Banerjee and Brown, 2004; Jans *et al.*, 2004); if we could predict their survival (as has been done in India (Kumar *et al.*, 2000)), this may prevent unnecessary destruction of valuable bones and teeth.

Palaeopathology has an excellent future, backed up by a solid base of research that is increasing by the day. While it does have many limitations, as described earlier in this book, it is not alone in this respect; as long as we are aware of these limitations when we come to record, analyse and interpret our data, then we can contribute considerably to everybody's understanding of the impact of disease on populations through very long periods of our history and in different parts of the world. The study of palaeopathology can also highlight what we might expect to see in the future if we change our diet, work patterns, climate or living conditions. It is a science that is multidisciplinary in nature and must work from the premiss of understanding the biological data on disease with respect to cultural context. Wells's (1964a: 17) words ring true even today:

> The pattern of disease or injury that affects any group of people is never a matter of chance. It is invariably the expression of stresses and strains to which they were exposed, to everything in their environment and behaviour. It reflects their genetic inheritance (which is their internal environment), the climate in which they lived, the soil that gave them sustenance and the animals and plants that shared their homeland. It is influenced by their daily occupations, their habits of diet, their choice of dwellings and clothes, their social structure, even their folklore and mythology.

References

Aaron, J.E., Rogers, J. and Kanis, J.A. 1992. Paleohistology of Paget's disease in 2 medieval skeletons. *Am. J. Phys. Anthrop.* 89: 325–31.

Ackerknecht, E.H. 1967. Primitive surgery. In D. Brothwell and A.T. Sandison (eds), *Diseases in antiquity*. Springfield, Ill., Charles Thomas, pp. 635–50.

Aegerter, E. and Kirkpatrick, J.A. 1975. *Orthopaedic diseases: physiology, pathology, radiology*. Philadelphia, W.B. Saunders.

Agarwal, S.C. and Stout, S.D. 2003. *Bone loss and osteoporosis: an anthropological perspective*. New York, Kluwer Academic/Plenum Publishers.

Ainsworth, G.C. 1993. Fungus infections (mycoses). In K. Kiple (ed.), *The Cambridge world history of human disease*. Cambridge, Cambridge University Press, pp. 730–6.

Aird, I. and Bentall, H.H. 1953. A relationship between cancer of the stomach and the ABO blood groups. *Br. Med. J.* 1: 799–801.

Allen, T. 2003. Perception is everything. *New Scientist* 1 March: 25.

Allison, M.J., Gerszten, E., Shadomy, J.H., Munizaga, J. and Gonzalez, M. 1979. Paracoccidiomycosis in a northern Chilean mummy. *Bull. New York Acad. Med.* 56: 670–83.

Allison, M.J., Gerszten, E., Munizaga, J. and Santoro, C. 1980. Metastatic tumor of bone in a Tiahuanaco female. *Bull. New York Acad. Med.* 56: 581–7.

Allison, M.J., Gerszten, E., Munizaga, J., Santoro, C. and Mendoza, D. 1981. Tuberculosis in pre-Columbian Andean populations. In J.E. Buikstra (ed.), *Prehistoric tuberculosis in the Americas*. Evanston, Ill., Northwestern University, pp. 49–61.

Alt, K.W. and Adler, C.P. 1992. Multiple myeloma in an early medieval skeleton. *Int. J. Osteoarchaeology* 2: 205–9.

Alt, K.W., Pichler, S., Vach, W., Klíma, B., Vlček, E. and Sedlmeier, J. 1997. Twenty-five thousand year old triple burial from Dolní Věstonice: an Ice-Age family? *Am. J. Phys. Anthrop.* 102: 123–31.

Alter, G.C. and Carmichael, A.G. 1999. Classifying the dead: toward a history of registration of causes of death. *J. Social History of Medicine* 54: 114–32.

Altman, R.D. 1993. Paget's disease of bone. In K. Kiple (ed.), *The Cambridge world history of human disease*. Cambridge, Cambridge University Press, pp. 911–13.

Alvrus, A. 1996. Fracture patterns among the Nubians of Semna South, Sudan. MA Thesis, Arizona State University.

Alvrus, A. 1999. Fracture patterns among the Nubians of Semna South, Sudanese Nubia. *Int. J. Osteoarchaeology* 9: 417–29.

American Association of Physical Anthropologists 1996. AAPA statement on biological aspects of race. *Am. J. Phys. Anthrop.* 101: 569–70.

Amundsen, D.A. and Diers, C.J. 1970. The age of menopause in Classical Greece and Rome. *Hum. Biol.* 42: 79–86.

Anasthaswamy, A. 2003. Death in the sun. *New Scientist* 26 July: 12–13.

Andahl, R.O. 1978. The examination of saw marks. *J. For. Sci. Soc.* 18: 31–46.

Andersen, J.G. 1969. *Studies in the medieval diagnosis of leprosy in Denmark*. Copenhagen, Costers Bogtrykkeri.

Andersen, J.G. and Manchester, K. 1987. Grooving of the proximal phalanx in leprosy: a palaeopathological and radiological study. *J. Archaeological Science* 14: 77–82.

Andersen, J.G. and Manchester, K. 1988. Dorsal tarsal exostoses in leprosy: a palaeopathological and radiological study. *J. Archaeological Science* 15: 51–6.

Andersen, J.G. and Manchester, K. 1992. The rhinomaxillary syndrome in leprosy: a clinical, radiological and palaeopathological study. *Int. J. Osteoarchaeology* 2: 121–9.

Andersen, J.G., Manchester, K. and Ali, R.S. 1992. Diaphyseal remodelling in leprosy: a radiological and palaeopathological study. *Int. J. Osteoarchaeology* 2(3): 211–21.

Andersen, J.G., Manchester, K. and Roberts, C. 1994. Septic bone changes in leprosy: a clinical, radiological and palaeopathological study. *Int. J. Osteoarchaeology* 4: 21–30.

Anderson, T. 1991. A medieval example of meningiomatous hyperostosis. *Br. J. Neurosurg.* 5: 499–504.

Anderson, T. 1994a. Medieval example of cleft lip and palate from St Gregory's Priory, Canterbury. *Cleft Palate-Craniofacial J.* 31(6): 466–72.

Anderson, T. 1994b. An Anglo-Saxon case of hyperostosis frontalis interna from Sarre, Kent. *J. Paleopathology* 6(1): 29–34.

Anderson, T. 1997. A probable osteoma of the mandible from Northamptonshire, Great Britain. *J. Paleopathology* 9(2): 69–72.

Anderson, T. 2000. Congenital conditions and neoplastic disease in palaeopathology. In M. Cox and S. Mays (eds), *Human osteology in archaeology and forensic science*. London, Greenwich Medical Media, pp. 199–225.

Anderson, T. and Carter, A.R. 1995. The first archaeological case of Madelung's deformity? *Int. J. Osteoarchaeology* 5: 168–73.

Anderson, T. and Thomas, T.G. 1997. A possible case of arthrogryposis multiplex from medieval Canterbury. *Int. J. Osteoarchaeology* 7: 171–85.

Anderson, T., Arcini, C., Anda, S., Tangerud, A. and Robertsen, G. 1986. Suspected endemic syphilis (Treponarid) in sixteenth century Norway. *Med. Hist.* 30: 341–50.

Anderson, T., Wakely, J. and Carter, A. 1992. Medieval example of metastatic carcinoma: a dry bone, radiological and SEM study. *Am. J. Phys. Anthrop.* 89: 309–23.

Angel, J.L. 1966a. Early skeletons from Tranquillity, California. *Smithsonian Contributions to Anthropology* Washington, Smithsonian Institution Press 2(1): 1–19.

Angel, J.L. 1966b. Porotic hyperostosis, anaemias, malarias, and marshes in the prehistoric eastern Mediterranean. *Science* 153: 760–3.

Angel, J.L. 1974. Patterns of fractures from Neolithic to modern times. *Anthrop. Kozl.* 18: 9–18.

Anon. 1999. Congenital anomaly statistics: notifications 1998 England and Wales. *Health Statistics Quarterly* 4: 46–50.

Anon. 2000. Congenital anomaly statistics: notifications 1999 England and Wales. *Health Statistics Quarterly* 8: 87–90.

Anon. 2001. Population review of 1999: England and Wales. *Health Statistics Quarterly* 9: 2.

Antón, S. 1997. Endocranial hyperostosis in Sangiran 2, Gibraltar 1, and Shanidar 5. *Am. J. Phys. Anthrop.* 102: 111–22.

Arce, A.L. 2003. Furniture and spinal joint disease: a new etiological factor that contributed to the deterioration of the spine in the past. Poster presented at the Annual British Association of Biological Anthropology and Osteoarchaeology Conference, University of Southampton.

Arcini, C. 1990. Evidence of leprosy in 10th century Lund: the earliest known cases of leprosy in the Nordic Countries. Paper presented at the 8th Paleopathology Association European Meeting, Cambridge.

Armelagos, G.J. 1990. Health and disease in prehistoric populations in transition. In A.C. Swedlund and G.J. Armelagos (eds), *Disease in populations in transition: anthropological and epidemiological perspectives.* New York, Bergin and Garvey, pp. 127–46.

Armelagos, G.J. and Chrisman, O.D. 1988. Hyperostosis frontalis interna: a Nubian case. *Am. J. Phys. Anthrop.* 76: 25–8.

Armentano, N., Malgosa, A. and Campillo, D. 1999. A case of frontal sinusitis from the Bronze Age site of Can Filuà (Barcelona). *Int. J. Osteoarchaeology* 9: 438–42.

Arnott, R., Finger, S. and Smith, C.U.M. 2003. *Trepanation: history, discovery, theory.* Lisse, Swets and Zeitlinger.

Arriaza, B.T. 1997. Spondylolysis in prehistoric human remains from Guam and its possible etiology. *Am. J. Phys. Anthrop.* 104: 393–7.

Arrizabalaga, J., Henderson, J. and French, R. 1997. *The great pox: the French Disease in Renaissance Europe.* London, Yale University Press.

Aufderheide, A.C. 2003. *The scientific study of mummies.* Cambridge, Cambridge University Press.

Aufderheide, A.C. and Rodríguez-Martín, C. 1998. *The Cambridge encyclopaedia of human palaeopathology.* Cambridge, Cambridge University Press.

Awofeso, N. 1995. Effect of socio-cultural beliefs on patients' perception of leprosy. *Tropical and Geographical Medicine* 47(4): 175–8.

Aykroyd, R.G., Lucy, D., Pollard, A.M. and Roberts, C.A. 1999. Nasty, brutish, but not necessarily short: a reconsideration of the statistical methods used to calculate age at death from adult human skeletal and dental age indicators. *American Antiquity* 64(1): 55–70.

Backay, L. 1985. *An early history of craniotomy: from antiquity to the Napoleonic era.* Springfield, Ill., Charles Thomas.

Bahn, P. 1989. Early teething troubles. *Nature* 337: 693.

Baker, B. 1999. Early manifestations of tuberculosis in the skeleton. In G. Pálfi, O. Dutour, J. Deák and I. Hutás (eds), *Tuberculosis: past and present.* Budapest/Szeged, Golden Book Publishers and Tuberculosis Foundation, pp. 301–7.

Baker, B. and Armelagos, G.J. 1988. Origin and antiquity of syphilis: a paleopathological diagnosis and interpretation. *Curr. Anthrop.* 29(5): 703–37.

Balasegaram, S., Majeed, A. and Fitz-Clarence, H. 2000. Trends in hospital admissions for fractures in England 1989/90 to 1997/8. *Health Statistics Quarterly* 7: 10–17.

Banerjee, M. and Brown, T.A. 2004. Non-random DNA damage resulting from heat treatment: implications for sequence analysis of ancient DNA. *J. Archaeological Science* 31: 59–63.

Barber, G., Watt, I. and Rogers, J. 1997. A comparison of radiological and palaeopathological diagnostic criteria for hyperostosis frontalis interna. *Int. J. Osteoarchaeology* 7: 157–64.

Barnes, E. 1994. *Developmental defects of the axial skeleton in palaeopathology.* Boulder, Colo., University Press of Colorado.

Barrett, R., Kuzawa, C.W., McDade, T. and Armelagos, G.J. 1998. Emerging and re-emerging infectious diseases: the third epidemiologic transition. *Ann. Rev. Anthrop.* 27: 247–71.

Bass, W.M. 1987. *Human osteology: a field guide and manual.* Missouri, Archaeological Society.

Bates, J.H. and Stead, W.W. 1993. The history of tuberculosis as a global epidemic. *Medical Clinics of North America* 77(6): 1205–17.

Bathurst, R. and Barta, J.L. 2004. Molecular evidence of tuberculosis induced hypertrophic osteopathy in a 16th century Iroquoian dog. *J. Archaeological Science* 31(7): 917–25.

Bayliss, A., Shepherd Popescu, E.S., Beavan-Athfield, N., Bronk Ramsay, C., Cook, G.T. and Locker, A. 2004. The potential significance of dietary offsets for the interpretation of radiocarbon dates: an archaeologically significant example from Medieval Norwich. *J. Archaeological Science* 31: 563–75.

Beattie, O. and Geiger, J. 1987. *Frozen in time.* London, Bloomsbury Publishing Ltd.

Becker, M.J. 1994. Etruscan dental appliances: origins and functions as indicated by an example from Orvieto, Italy in the Danish National Museum. *Dent. Anthrop. Newsletter* 8(3): 2–8.

Bedford, M.E., Russell, K.F., Lovejoy, C.O., Meindl, R.S., Simpson, S.W. and Stuart-Macadam, P. 1993. Test of the multifactorial aging method using skeletons with known ages-at-death from the Grant Collection. *Am. J. Phys. Anthrop.* 91: 287–97.

Bell, L. 1990. Palaeopathology and diagenesis: an SEM evaluation of structural changes using backscattered electron imaging. *J. Archaeological Science* 17: 85–102.

Bell, L. and Piper, L. 2000. An introduction to palaeohistology. In M. Cox and S. Mays (eds), *Human osteology in archaeology and forensic science*. London, Greenwich Medical Media, pp. 255–74.

Benítez, J.T. 1988. Otopathology of Egyptian mummy PUM II: final report. *J. Laryngology and Otology* 102: 485–90.

Benjamin, G.C. 1993. Sickle-cell anaemia. In K. Kiple (ed.), *Cambridge world history of human disease*. Cambridge, Cambridge University Press, pp. 1006–8.

Benjamin, N., Rawlins, M. and Vale, J.A. 2002. Drug therapy and poisoning. In P. Kumar and M. Clark (eds), *Clinical medicine*. 5th edn, Edinburgh, W.B. Saunders, pp. 957–90.

Bennike, P. 1985. *Palaeopathology of Danish skeletons: a comparative study of demography, disease and injury*. Copenhagen, Akademisk Forlag.

Bennike, P. 2002. Vilhelm Møller-Christensen: his work and legacy. In C.A. Roberts, M.E. Lewis and K. Manchester (eds), *The past and present of leprosy: archaeological, historical, palaeopathological and clinical approaches*. British Archaeological Reports International Series 1054. Oxford, Archaeopress, pp. 135–44.

Bennike, P. and Fredebo, L. 1986. Dental treatment in the Stone Age. *Bull. Hist. Dent.* 34(2): 81–7.

Beñus, R., Masnicová, S. and Lietava, J. 1999. Intentional cranial vault deformation in a Slavonic population from the Medieval cemetery in Devín (Slovakia). *Int. J. Osteoarchaeology* 9: 267–70.

Berger, T.D. and Trinkaus, E. 1995. Patterns of trauma among Neandertals. *J. Archaeological Science* 22: 841–52.

Bernard, M-C. 2003. Tuberculosis in 20th century Britain: a demographic and social study of admissions to a children's sanatorium in Stannington, Northumberland. Ph.D. Thesis, University of Durham.

Berry, A.C. and Berry, R.J. 1967. Epigenetic variation in the human cranium. *J. Anat.* 101(2): 361–79.

Berryman, H.E. and Haun, S.J. 1996. Applying forensic techniques to interpret cranial fracture patterns in an archaeological specimen. *Int. J. Osteoarchaeology* 6: 2–9.

Bintliff, J.L. and Sbonias, K. (eds) 1999. *Reconstructing past population trends in Mediterranean Europe (3000 BC–AD 1800)*. Oxford, Oxbow Books.

Björnstig, U., Eriksson, A. and Örnehult, L. 1991. Injuries caused by animals. *Injury* 22(4): 295–8.

Black, F.L. 1975. Infectious diseases in primitive societies. *Science* 187: 515–18.

Black, J. 1982. A stitch in time 1: the history of sutures. *Nursing Times* 78: 619–23.

Blau, S., Kennedy, B.J. and Kim, J.Y. 2002. An investigation of possible fluorosis in human dentition using synchrotron radiation. *J. Archaeological Science* 29: 811–17.

Blondiaux, G., Blondiaux, J., Secousse, F., Cotton, A., Danze, P-M. and Flipo, R-M. 2002. Rickets and child abuse: the case of a two year old girl from the 4th century in Lisieux (Normandy). *Int. J. Osteoarchaeology* 12: 209–15.

Blondiaux, J. 1989. *Le cimetière Mérovingien de Neuville-sur-Escaut*. Musée Municipal de Demain.

Blondiaux, J., Dürr, J., Khouchaf, L. and Eisenberg, L. 2002. Microscopic study and X-ray analysis of two 5th century cases of leprosy: palaeoepidemiological inferences. In C.A. Roberts, M.E. Lewis and K. Manchester (eds), *The past and present of leprosy: archaeological, historical, palaeopathological and clinical approaches*. British Archaeological Reports International Series 1054. Oxford, Archaeopress, pp. 105–10.

Blondiaux, J., Duvette, J-F., Vatteon, S. and Eisenberg, L. 1994. Microradiographs of leprosy from osteoarchaeological contexts. *Int. J. Osteoarchaeology* 4: 13–20.

Bloom, A. (ed.) 1975. *Toohey's medicine for nurses.* 11th edn, Edinburgh, Churchill Livingstone.

Bloom, A.I., Bloom, R.A., Kahila, G., Eisenberg, E. and Smith, P. 1995. Amputation of the hand in the 3600-year-old skeletal remains of an adult male: the first case reported from Israel. *Int. J. Osteoarchaeology* 5: 188–91.

Bogin, B. 1988. *Patterns of human growth.* Cambridge, Cambridge University Press.

Bogin, B. 2000. The tall and the short of it. In A.H. Goodman, D.L. Dufour and G.H. Pelto (eds), *Nutritional anthropology: biocultural perspectives on food and nutrition.* Mountain View, California, Mayfield Publishing Company, pp. 192–5.

Bonn, D. 2000. Maggot therapy: an alternative for wound infection. *Lancet* 356: 1174.

Bonser, W. 1963. *Medical background to Anglo-Saxon England.* London, Wellcome Institute.

Boocock, P., Roberts, C.A. and Manchester, K. 1995. Maxillary sinusitis in Medieval Chichester, England. *Am. J. Phys. Anthrop.* 98(4): 483–95.

Botting, B. and Abrahams, C. 2000. Linking congenital anomaly and birth records. *Health Statistics Quarterly* 8: 36–40.

Botting, B., Skjaerven, R., Alberman, E. and Abrahams, C. 1999. Multiple congenital anomalies in England and Wales 1992–7. *Health Statistics Quarterly* 3: 24–9.

Boulestin, B. and Gomez de Soto, J. 1995. *Le cannibalisme au Néolithique: réalité et sens, 'La Mort': Passé, Présent, Conditionel.* La Roche-sur-Yon, Groupe Vendéen d'Etudes Préhistoriques, pp. 59–68.

Bouman, A. and Brown, T.A. 2005. The limits of biomolecular palaeopathology: ancient DNA cannot be used to study venereal syphilis. *J. Archaeological Science* 32: 703–13.

Bowron, E.L. 2003. A new approach to the storage of human skeletal remains. *The Conservator* 27: 95–106.

Boylston, A. 2000. Evidence for weapon-related trauma in British archaeological samples. In M. Cox and S. Mays (eds), *Human osteology in archaeology and forensic science.* London, Greenwich Medical Media, pp. 357–80.

Boylston, A. 2001. Physical anthropology. In V. Fiorato, A. Boylston and C. Knüsel (eds), *Blood red roses: the archaeology of a mass grave from the Battle of Towton AD 1461.* Oxford, Oxbow Books, pp. 45–59.

Boylston, A. 2003. Paget's Disease ancient and modern: discussion of six cases from Norton Priory. Paper presented at the Annual Conference of the British Association of Biological Anthropology and Osteoarchaeology, University of Southampton, September 2003.

Boylston, A., Knüsel, C.J. and Roberts, C.A. 2000. Investigation of a Romano-British rural ritual in Bedford, England. *J. Archaeological Science* 27: 241–54.

Brickley, M. 2000. The diagnosis of metabolic disease in archaeological bone. In M. Cox and S. Mays (eds), *Human osteology in archaeology and forensic science.* London, Greenwich Medical Media, pp. 183–98.

Brickley, M. and Howell, P.G.T. 1999. Measurement of changes in trabecular bone structure with age in an archaeological population. *J. Archaeological Science* 26: 151–7.

Brickley, M. and McKinley, J. 2004 (eds). *Guidelines to the standards for recording human remains.* Reading, Institute of Field Archaeologists Paper Number 7.

Bridges, P.S. 1989. Changes in activities with the shift to agriculture in the southeastern U.S. *Curr. Anthrop.* 30(3): 385–94.

Bridges, P.S. 1991. Degenerative joint disease in hunter-gatherers and agriculturists from the southeastern U.S. *Am. J. Phys. Anthrop.* 85: 379–91.

Bridges, P.S. 1994. Vertebral arthritis and physical activities in the prehistoric United States. *Am. J. Phys. Anthrop.* 93: 83–93.

Bridges, P.S., Blitz, J.H. and Solano, M.C. 2000. Changes in long bone diaphyseal strength with horticulture intensification in West-Central Illinois. *Am. J. Phys. Anthrop.* 112: 217–38.

Brimblecombe, P. 1976. Attitudes and responses towards air pollution in medieval England. *J. Air Pollution Control Assoc.* 26(10): 941–5.

Brimblecombe, P. 1982. Early urban climate and atmosphere. In A.R. Hall and H.K. Kenward (eds), *Environmental archaeology in the urban context*. Council for British Archaeology Research Report 43. London, Council for British Archaeology, pp. 10–25.

Brooks, S.T. and Hohenthal, W.D. 1963. Archeological defective palate crania from California. *Am. J. Phys. Anthrop.* 21(1): 25–32.

Brosch, R., Gordon, S.V., Marmiesse, M., Brodin, P., Buchrieseer, C. and ten other authors. 2002. A new evolutionary sequence for the *Mycobacterium tuberculosis* complex. *Proc. Nat. Acad. Sci.* 99(6): 3684–9.

Brothwell, D. 1960. A possible case of mongolism in a Saxon population. *Ann. Human Genet.* 24: 141–50.

Brothwell, D. 1967a. Major congenital anomalies of the skeleton: evidence from earlier populations. In D. Brothwell and A.T. Sandison (eds), *Diseases in antiquity*. Springfield, Ill., Charles Thomas, pp. 423–44.

Brothwell, D. 1967b. The evidence for neoplasms. In D.R. Brothwell and A.T. Sandison (eds), *Diseases in antiquity*. Springfield, Ill., Charles Thomas, pp. 320–45.

Brothwell, D. 1970. The real history of syphilis. *Science* 6(9): 27–33.

Brothwell, D. 1981. *Digging up bones*. London, British Museum (Natural History).

Brothwell, D. 1986. *The bog man and the archaeology of people*. London, British Museum (Natural History).

Brothwell, D. 1989. The relationship of tooth wear to aging. In M.Y. Iscan (ed.), *Age markers in the human skeleton*. Springfield, Ill., Charles Thomas, pp. 306–16.

Brothwell, D. 1991. On the zoonoses and their relevance to paleopathology. In D. Ortner and A. Aufderheide (eds), *Human paleopathology: current syntheses and future options*. Washington, Smithsonian Institution Press, pp. 18–22.

Brothwell, D. and Brothwell, P. 1969. *Food in antiquity: a survey of the diet of early peoples*. Expanded edition. Baltimore, Md, Johns Hopkins University Press.

Brothwell, D. and Browne, S. 1994. Pathology. In J.M. Lilley, G. Stroud, D.R. Brothwell and M.H. Williamson (eds), *The Jewish burial ground at Jewbury: the archaeology of York*. The Medieval cemeteries 12/3. York, Council for British Archaeology for York Archaeological Trust, pp. 457–94.

Brothwell, D. and Browne, S. 2002. Skeletal atrophy and the problem of the differential diagnosis of conditions causing paralysis. *Antropologia Portuguesa* 19: 5–17.

Brothwell, D. and Møller-Christensen, V. 1963. Medico-historical aspects of an early case of mutilation. *Danish Med. Bull.* 10: 21–7.

Brothwell, D. and Powers, R. 1968. Congenital malformations of the skeleton in earlier man. In D.R. Brothwell (ed.), *Skeletal biology of earlier human populations*. Symposia of the Society for the study of Human Biology Volume 8. London, Pergamon Press, pp. 173–203.

Brothwell, D. and Sandison, A.T. 1967 (eds). *Diseases in antiquity*. Springfield, Ill., Charles Thomas.

Brown, K. 2000. Ancient DNA applications in human osteoarchaeology. In M. Cox and S. Mays (eds), *Human osteology in archaeology and forensic science*. London, Greenwich Medical Media, pp. 455–73.

Brown, K. 2001. Identifying the sex of human remains by ancient DNA analysis. *Ancient Biomolecules* 3: 215–25.

Brown, P. 2002. Test tube drama. *New Scientist* 16 March: 17.

Brown, P.J. 1998. *Understanding and applying medical anthropology*. London, Mayfield Publishing Company.

Brown, P.J., Inhorn, M.C. and Smith, D.J. 1996. Disease, ecology and human behavior. In C.F. Sargent and T.F. Johnson (eds), *Medical anthropology: contemporary theory and method*. London, Praeger, pp. 183–218.

Bruintjes, T. 1990. The auditory ossicles in human skeletal remains from a leper cemetery in Chichester, England. *J. Archaeological Science* 17: 627–33.

Bryceson, A. and Pfaltzgraaf, R.E. 1990. *Leprosy.* Edinburgh, Churchill Livingstone.

Buchanan, W.W. and Laurent, R.M. 1990. Rheumatoid arthritis: an example of ecological succession. *Can. Bull. Med. Hist.* 7: 77–91.

Buckley, R. 1994. *World population: the biggest problem of all?* London, European Schoolbooks Publishing Limited.

Buckley, H. 2000. A possible fatal wounding in the prehistoric Pacific islands. *Int. J. Osteoarchaeology* 10: 135–41.

Buckley, H.R. and Dias, G.J. 2002. The distribution of skeletal lesions in treponemal disease: is the lymphatic system responsible? *Int. J. Osteoarchaeology* 12: 178–88.

Buckley, H.R. and Tayles, N.G. 2003. The functional cost of tertiary yaws (*Treponema pertenue*) in a prehistoric Pacific Island skeletal sample. *J. Archaeological Science* 30: 1301–14.

Budd, P., Montgomery, J., Evans, J. and Trickett, M. 2003. Human lead exposure in England from approximately 5500 BP to the 16th century AD. *Science of the Total Environment* 318: 45–58.

Budd, P., Millard, A., Chenery, C., Lucy, S. and Roberts, C. 2004. Investigating population movement by stable isotope analysis: a report from Britain. *Antiquity* 78: 127–41.

Bueschgen, W.D. and Case, D.T. 1996. Evidence of prehistoric scalping at Vosberg, Central Arizona. *Int. J. Osteoarchaeology* 6: 230–48.

Buhr, A.J. and Cooke, A.M. 1959. Fracture patterns. *Lancet* 1: 531–6.

Buikstra, J.E. 1976. The Caribou Eskimo: general and specific disease. *Am. J. Phys. Anthrop.* 45: 351–68.

Buikstra, J.E. (ed.) 1981. *Prehistoric tuberculosis in the Americas.* Chicago, Ill., Northwestern University Archeological Program.

Buikstra, J.E. and Cook, D.C. 1980. Paleopathology: an American account. *Ann. Rev. Anthrop.* 9: 433–70.

Buikstra, J.E. and Gordon, C.C. 1981. The study and restudy of human skeletal series: the importance of long term curation. *Ann. New York Acad. Sci.* 376: 449–65.

Buikstra, J. and Konigsberg, L. 1985. Paleodemography: critiques and controversies. *American Anthropologist* 87: 316–33.

Buikstra, J. and Mielke, J.H. 1985. Demography, diet and health. In R.I. Gilbert and J.H. Mielke (eds), *Analysis of prehistoric diets.* London, Academic Press, pp. 359–422.

Buikstra, J.E. and Milner, G.R. 1991. Isotopic and archaeological interpretations of diet in the central Mississippi valley. *J. Archaeological Science* 18: 319–29.

Buikstra, J.E. and Ubelaker, D. 1994. *Standards for data collection from human skeletal remains.* Arkansas Archeological Survey Research Series, No. 44.

Burkitt, D.P., Walker, A.R.P. and Palmer, N.S. 1972. Effect of dietary fibre on stools and transit times, and its role in the causation of disease. *Lancet* 2: 1408–12.

Burr, D.B. and Martin, B. 1989. Errors in bone remodeling: toward a unified theory of metabolic bone disease. *Am. J. Anat.* 186: 186–216.

Bush, H. 1991. Concepts of health and stress. In H. Bush and M. Zvelebil (eds), *Health in past societies: biocultural interpretations of human skeletal remains in archaeological contexts.* British Archaeological Reports International Series 567. Oxford, Tempus Reparatum, pp. 11–21.

Byers, S.N. and Roberts, C.A. 2003. Bayes' Theorem in palaeopathological diagnosis. *Amer. J. Phys. Anthrop.* 121(1): 1–9.

Caffell, A.C., Roberts, C.A. Janaway, R.C. and Wilson, A.S. 2001. Pressures on osteological collections – the importance of damage limitation. In E. Williams (ed.), *Human remains: conservation, retrieval and analysis.* Proceedings of a conference held in Williamsburg, VA, 7–11 November 1999. British Archaeological Reports International Series 934. Oxford, Archaeopress, pp. 187–97.

Camuffo, D., Daffara, C. and Sghedoni, M. 2000. Archaeometry of air pollution: urban emission in Italy during the 17th century. *J. Archaeological Science* 27: 685–90.

Canci, A., Minozzi, S. and Borgognini Tarli, S.M. 1994. Osteomyelitis: elements for differential diagnosis on skeletal material. In O. Dutour, G. Pálfi, J. Bérato and J.-P. Brun (eds), *L'origine de la syphilis en Europe: avant ou après 1493?* Toulon, Centre Archéologique du Var, Éditions Errance, pp. 88–90.

Canci, A., Minozzi, S. and Borgognini Tarli, S. 1996. New evidence of tuberculous spondylitis from Neolithic Liguria. *Int. J. Osteoarchaeology* 6: 497–501.

Capasso, L. 1998. Lice buried under the ashes of Herculaneum. *Lancet* 351 (9107): 992.

Capasso, L. 1999. Brucellosis at Herculaneum (79 AD). *Int. J. Osteoarchaeology* 9: 277–88.

Capasso, L., Kennedy, K.A.R. and Wilczak, C. 1999. *Atlas of occupational markers on human remains.* Teramo, Italy, Edigrafital S.p.A.

Cappellini, E., Chiarelli, B., Sineo, L., Casoli, A., Di Gioia, A., Vernesi, C., Biella, M.C. and Caramelli, D. 2004. Biomolecular study of the human remains from tomb 5859 in the Etruscan necropolis of Monterozzi, Tarquinia (Veiterbo, Italy). *J. Archaeological Science* 31: 603–12.

Cardy, A. 1997. The environmental material. The human bones. In P. Hill (ed.), *Whithorn and St Ninian: the excavation of a monastic town 1984–91.* Stroud, Sutton Publishing, pp. 519–62.

Carlson, D.S., Armelagos, G.J. and Van Gerven, D.P. 1974. Factors influencing the etiology of cribra orbitalia in prehistoric Nubia. *J. Hum. Evol.* 4: 405–10.

Carroll, G.A. 1972. Traditional medical cures along the Yukon. *Alaska Medicine* 14: 50–3.

Cattaneo, C. 1991. Direct genetic and immunological information in the reconstruction of health and biocultural conditions of past populations: a new prospect for archaeology. In H. Bush and M. Zvelebil (eds), *Health in past societies: biocultural interpretations of human skeletal remains in archaeological contents.* British Archaeological Reports International Series 567. Oxford, Tempus Reparatum, pp. 39–53.

Cattaneo, C., Gelsthorpe, K., Phillips, P., Waldron, T., Booth, J.R. and Sokol, R.J. 1994. Immunological diagnosis of multiple myeloma in a medieval bone. *Int. J. Osteoarchaeology* 4: 1–2.

Centurion-Lara, A., Castro, C., Castillo, R. Shaffer, J., Van Voorhis, W. and Lukehart, S. 1998. The flanking region sequences of the 15-kDa lipoprotein gene differentiate pathogenic treponemes. *J. Infectious Diseases* 177: 1036–40.

Chadwick Hawkes, S.C. and Wells, C. 1975. An Anglo-Saxon obstetric calamity from Kingsworthy, Hampshire. *Med. Biol. Ill.* 25: 47–51.

Chakrabarty, A. and Dastidar, S. 1989. Correlation between occurrence of leprosy and fossil fuels: role of fossil fuel bacteria in the origin and global epidemiology of leprosy. *Indian J. Exper. Biol.* 27: 483–96.

Chamberlain, A. 2000. Problems and prospects in palaeodemography. In M. Cox and S. Mays (eds), *Human osteology in archaeology and forensic science.* London, Greenwich Medical Media, pp. 101–15.

Chamberlain, A. 2001. Palaeodemography. In D. Brothwell and A.M. Pollard (eds), *Handbook of archaeological science.* Chichester, John Wiley and Sons Ltd, pp. 259–68.

Chamberlain, A.T., Rogers, S. and Romanowski, C.A. 1992. Osteochondroma in a British Neolithic skeleton. *Br. J. Hosp. Med.* 47(1): 51–3.

Chaussinand, R. 1953. Tuberculosis and leprosy: mutually antagonistic diseases. *Leprosy Review* 24: 90–4.

Cherniack, M. 1992. Diseases of unusual occupations: an historical perspective. *Occupational Med.* 7(3): 369–84.

Church of England and English Heritage 2005. *Guidance on best practice for treatment of human remains excavated from Christian burial grounds in England.* Swindon, English Heritage and Church of England.

Ciaraldi, M. 2000. Drug preparation in evidence? An unusual plant and bone assemblage from the Pompeian countryside, Italy. *Veget. Hist. Archaeobot.* 9: 91–8.

Ciranni, R., Castagna, M. and Fornaciari, G. 1999. Goiter in an 18th century Sicilian mummy. *Am. J. Phys. Anthrop.* 108: 427–32.

Clairet, D. and Dagorn, J. 1994. Skeletal disorders acquired in syphilis: radiographic study and differential diagnosis. In O. Dutour, G. Pálfi, J. Bérato and J.-P. Brun (eds), *L'origine de la syphilis en Europe: avant ou après 1493?* Toulon, Centre Archéologique du Var, Éditions Errance, pp. 32–5.

Clark, W.A. 1937. History of fracture treatment up to the 16th century. *J. Bone Joint Surgery* 19(1): 47–63.

Clark, G.A., Kelley, M.A., Grange, J.M. and Hill, M.C. 1987. The evolution of mycobacterial disease in human populations. *Curr. Anthrop.* 28(1): 45–62.

Clarke, N.G. and Hirsch, R.S. 1991. Physiological, pulpal and periodontal factors influencing alveolar bone. In M. Kelley and C.S. Larsen (eds), *Advances in dental anthropology.* New York, Alan Liss, pp. 241–66.

Clarke, S.K. 1982. The association of early childhood enamel hypoplasias and radiopaque transverse lines in a culturally diverse prehistoric skeletal sample. *Hum. Biol.* 54(1): 77–84.

Clarkson, L. 1975. *Death, disease and famine in preindustrial England.* Dublin, Gill and Macmillan.

Coale, A.J. 1974. The history of the human population. In D. Flanagan (ed.), *The human population.* San Francisco, W.H. Freeman.

Cockburn, A. 1961. The origin of the treponematoses. *Bull. WHO* 24: 221–8.

Cockburn, A., Barraco, R.A., Reyman, T.A. and Peck, W.H. 1975. Autopsy of an Egyptian mummy. *Science* 187(4182): 1155–60.

Cogbill, T.H., Steenlage, E.S., Landercasper, J. and Strutt, P.J. 1991. Death and disability from agricultural injuries in Wisconsin: a 12 year experience with 739 patients. *J. Trauma* 31(12): 1632–7.

Coghlan, A. 2002. GM row delays food aid. *New Scientist* 3 August: 4–5.

Cohen, M.M., Gorlin, A.J., Berkman, M.D. and Feingold, M. 1971. Facial variability in Apert type acrocephalosyndactyly. In D. Bergsma (ed.), *Third conference on the clinical delineation of birth defects. Part II.* New York, National Foundation for the March of Dimes, pp. 143–6.

Cohen, M.N. 1989. *Health and the rise of civilisation.* London, Yale University Press.

Cohen, M.N. 1998. The emergence of health and social inequalities in the archaeological record. In S.S. Strickland and P.S. Shetty (eds), *Human biology and socal inequality.* Cambridge, Cambridge University Press, pp. 249–71.

Cohen, M.N. and Armelagos, G.J. 1984 (eds). *Paleopathology at the origins of agriculture.* London, Academic Press.

Cohen, P. 2002. Key gene in cleft lip traced. *New Scientist* 7 September: 16.

Cohen, P. 2003. Recipes for bioterror. *New Scientist* 18 January: 10–11.

Congdon, R.T. 1931. Spondylolisthesis and vertebral anomalies in skeletons of American Aborigines: with clinical notes on spondylolisthesis. *J. Bone Joint Surgery* 14B: 511–24.

Constandse-Westermann, T.S. and Newell, R.R. 1989. Limb lateralization and social stratification in western European Mesolithic societies. In I. Hershkovitz (ed.), *People and culture change.* Proceedings of the 2nd Symposium on Upper Palaeolithic, Mesolithic and Neolithic populations of Europe and the Mediterranean Basin. British Archaeological Reports International Series 508(i). Oxford, BAR, pp. 405–33.

Cook, D.C. 1994. Dental evidence for congenital syphilis (and its absence) before and after the conquest of the New World. In O. Dutour, G. Pálfi, J. Bérato and J.-P. Brun (eds), *L'origine de la syphilis en Europe: avant ou après 1493?* Toulon, Centre Archéologique du Var, Éditions Errance, pp. 169–75.

Cook, D.C. 2002. Rhinomaxillary syndrome in the absence of leprosy: an exercise in differential diagnosis. In C.A. Roberts, M.E. Lewis and K. Manchester (eds), *The past and present of leprosy: archaeological, historical, palaeopathological and clinical approaches.* British Archaeological Reports International Series 1054. Oxford, Archaeopress, pp. 81–8.

Cook, J. 1986. Marked human bones from Gough's cave, Somerset. *Proceedings of the University of Bristol Speleological Society* 17(3): 275–85.

Copeman, W.S. 1970. Historical aspects of gout. *Clinical Orthopaedics and Related Research* 74: 14–22.

Coren, S. and Porac, C. 1977. Fifty centuries of right handedness: the historical record. *Science* 198: 632–3.

Corruccini, R.S., Handler, J.S. and Jacobs, K.P. 1985. Chronological distribution of enamel hypoplasias and weaning in a Caribbean slave population. *Hum. Biol.* 57(4): 699–711.

Corruccini, R.S., Shimada, I. and Shinoda, K-I. 2002. Dental and ntDNA relatedness among thousand-year-old remains from Huaca Loro, Peru. *Dent. Anthrop.* 16(1): 9–14.

Cosivi, O. Meslin, F-X., Daborn, C.J. and Grange, J.M. 1995. Epidemiology of *M. bovis* infection in animals and humans with particular reference to Africa. *Rev. Sci. Tech. Off. Int. Epiz.* 14(3): 733–46.

Cotran, R.S., Kumar, V. and Robbins, S.L. 1989. *Robbins pathologic basis of disease.* 4th edn, London, W.B. Saunders.

Coughlan, J. and Holst, M. 2001. Health status. In V. Fiorato, A. Boylston and C. Knüsel (eds), *Blood red roses: the archaeology of a mass grave from the Battle of Towton AD 1461.* Oxford, Oxbow Books, pp. 60–76.

Courtenay, W.H. 2000. Constructions of masculinity and their influence on men's well-being: a theory of gender and health. *Soc. Sci. Med.* 50: 1385–401.

Courville, C.B. 1965. War wounds of the cranium in the Middle Ages: 1. As disclosed in the skeletal material from the Battle of Wisby (1361 AD). *Bull. Los Angeles Neurolog. Soc.* 30: 27–33.

Cox, G., Sealy, J., Schrire, C. and Morris, A. 2001. Stable carbon and nitrogen isotopic analyses of the underclass at the colonial Cape of Good Hope in the 18th and 19th centuries. *World Archaeology* 33(1): 73–97.

Cox, M. 2000a. Assessment of parturition. In M. Cox and S. Mays (eds), *Human osteology in archaeology and forensic science.* London, Greenwich Medical Media, pp. 131–42.

Cox, M. 2000b. Ageing adults from the skeleton. In M. Cox and S. Mays (eds), *Human osteology in archaeology and forensic science.* London, Greenwich Medical Media, pp. 61–81.

Crane-Kramer, G.M.M. 2002. Was there a Medieval diagnostic confusion between leprosy and syphilis? An examination of the skeletal evidence. In C.A. Roberts, M.E. Lewis and K. Manchester (eds), *The past and present of leprosy: archaeological, historical, palaeopathological and clinical approaches.* British Archaeological Reports International Series 1054. Oxford, Archaeopress, pp. 111–19.

Crawford-Adams, J. 1983. *Outline of fractures.* 8th edn, Edinburgh, Churchill Livingstone.

Crawfurd, R. 1911. *The King's Evil.* Oxford, Oxford University Press.

Cronk, C.E. 1993. Down's syndrome. In K. Kiple (ed.), *The Cambridge world history of human disease.* Cambridge, Cambridge University Press, pp. 683–6.

Crosby, A.W. 1993. Smallpox. In K. Kiple (ed.), *The Cambridge world history of human disease.* Cambridge, Cambridge University Press, pp. 1008–13.

Crubézy, E. and Trinkhaus, E. 1992. Shanidar 1: a case of hyperostotic disease (DISH) in the Middle Paleolithic. *Am. J. Phys. Anthrop.* 89: 411–20.

Cucina, A. and Tiesler, V. 2003. Dental caries and ante-mortem tooth loss in the Northern Peten area, Mexico: a biocultural perspective on social status differences among the Classic Maya. *Am. J. Phys. Anthrop.* 122: 1–10.

Cunha, E., Fily, M-L., Clisson, I., Santos, A.L., Silva, A.M., Umbelino, C., César, P., Corte-Real, A., Crubézy, E. and Ludes, B. 2000. Children at the convent: comparing historical data, morphology and DNA extracted from ancient tissues for sex diagnosis at Santa Clara-a-Velha (Coumbra, Portugal). *J. Archaeological Science* 27: 949–52.

Curry, J.D. 1970. The mechanical properties of bone. *Clinical Orthopaedics* 73: 210–31.

Czarnetski, A. 1980. *A possible trisomy 21 from the Late Hallstatt Period.* Proceedings of the 3rd European Paleopathology Association Meeting, Caen, France, 1980.

Dalby, G. 1994. Middle ear disease in antiquity. Unpublished Ph.D. thesis, University of Bradford.

Dalby, G., Manchester, K. and Roberts, C.A. 1993. Otosclerosis and stapedial footplate fixation in archaeological material. *Int. J. Osteoarchaeology* 3: 207–12.

Daly, M. and Wilson, M. 1984. A sociobiological analysis of human infanticide. In G. Hausfater and S. Blaffer (eds), *Infanticide: comparative and evolutionary perspective.* New York, Aldine Publishing Company, pp. 487–500.

Daniel, H.J., Schmidt, R.T., Fulghum, R.S. and Ruckriegal, L. 1988. Otitis media: a problem for the physical anthropologist. *Yearbook of Phys. Anthrop.* 31: 143–67.

Danielsen, K. 1970. Odontodysplasia in Danish medieval skeletons. *Saertryk af Tandlaegebladet* 74: 603–25.

Danielson, D.R. and Reinhard, K.J. 1998. Human dental microwear caused by calcium oxalate phytoliths in prehistoric diet of the Lower Pecos region, Texas. *Am. J. Phys. Anthrop.* 107: 297–304.

Dasen, V. 1988. Dwarfism in Egypt and Classical antiquity: iconography and medical history. *Med. Hist.* 32: 253–76.

Dastugue, J. 1965. Tumeur maxillaire sur un crâne du moyen-âge. *Bull. du Cancer* 52(1): 69–72.

Davidson, P.M. 1993. *M. avium* complex, *M. kanasii, M. fortuitum,* and other mycobacteria causing human disease. In L.B. Reichman and E.S. Hershfield (eds), *Tuberculosis: a comprehensive international approach, Vol. 66: lung biology in health and disease.* New York, Marcel Dekker, pp. 505–30.

Davies, D.M., Picton, D.C.A. and Alexander, A.G. 1969. An objective method of assessing the periodontal condition in human skulls. *J. Periodontal Res.* 4: 74–7.

Dawes, J.D. and Magilton, J.R. 1980. *The cemetery of St Helen-on-the-Walls, Aldwark.* The archaeology of York. The Medieval Cemeteries 12/1. London, Council for British Archaeology for York Archaeological Trust.

Day, M.H. 1977. *Guide to fossil man.* London, Cassell.

De Garine, I. 1993. Culture, seasons and stress in two traditional African cultures (Massa and Mussey). In S.J. Ulijaszek and S.S. Strickland (eds), *Seasonality and human ecology.* Cambridge, Cambridge University Press, pp. 184–201.

Dean, V.L. 1995. Sinus and meningeal vessel pattern changes induced by artificial cranial deformation: a pilot study. *Int. J. Osteoarchaeology* 5: 1–14.

Dean, V.L. 1996. Comparative endocranial vascular changes due to craniosynostosis and artificial cranial deformation. *Am. J. Phys. Anthrop.* 110: 369–85.

Dean, V.L. 2004. Effects of different kinds of cranial deformation on the incidence of wormian bones. *Am. J. Phys. Anthrop.* 123: 146–55.

DeGusta, D. 1999. Fijian cannibalism: osteological evidence from Navatu. *Am. J. Phys. Anthrop.* 110: 215–41.

DeGusta, D. 2000. Fijian cannibalism and mortuary ritual: bioarchaeological evidence from Vunda. *Int. J. Osteoarchaeology* 10: 76–92.

DeGusta, D. 2002. Comparative skeletal pathology and the case for conspecific care in Middle Pleistocene hominids. *J. Archaeological Science* 29: 1435–8.

DeGusta, D. 2003. Aubesier 11 is not evidence of Neanderthal conspecific care. *J. Hum. Evol.* 43(1): 821–30.

Denny, N. and Filmer-Sankey, J. 1966. *The Bayeux Tapestry: the story of the Norman Conquest: 1066.* London, Collins.

Department of Media, Culture and Sport 2004. *Care of historic human remains: a consultation on the Report of the Working Group on Human Remains.* London, DCMS.

Dequecker, J. 1977. Arthritis in Flemish paintings (1400–1700). *Br. Med. J.* 1: 1203.

Derry, D.E. 1913. A case of hydrocephalus in an Egyptian of the Roman Period. *J. Anat. (London)* 48: 436–58.

Derums, V.J. 1979. Extensive trepanation of the skull in ancient Latvia. *Bull. Hist. Med.* 53: 459–64.

Dettwyler, K. 1991. Can paleopathology provide evidence for 'compassion'? *Am. J. Phys. Anthrop.* 84: 375–84.

Dharmendra. 1947. Leprosy in ancient Indian medicine. *Int. J. Leprosy* 15: 424–30.

Dias, G. and Tayles, N. 1997. 'Abscess cavity' – a misnomer. *Int. J. Osteoarchaeology* 7: 548–54.

Dickel, D.N. and Doran, G.H. 1989. Severe neural tube defect syndrome from early archaic Florida. *Am. J. Phys. Anthrop.* 80: 325–34.

Dietz, A., Sennewald, E. and Maier, H. 1995. Indoor air pollution by emissions of fossil fuel single stoves: possibly a hitherto underrated risk factor in the development of carcinomas in the head and neck. *Otolaryngology – head and neck surgery* 112(2): 308–15.

Dobney, K. and Brothwell, D. 1987. A method for evaluating the amount of dental calculus on teeth from archaeological sites. *J. Archaeological Science* 14: 343–51.

Dobney, K. and Brothwell, D. 1988. A scanning electron microscope study of archaeological dental calculus. In S.L. Olsen (ed.), *Scanning electron microscopy in archaeology.* British Archaeological Reports International Series 452. Oxford, BAR, pp. 372–85.

Dobney, K. and Goodman, A.H. 1991. Epidemiological studies of dental enamel hypoplasias in Mexico and Bradford: their relevance to archaeological skeletal material. In H. Bush and M. Zvelebil (eds), *Health in past societies: biocultural interpretations of human skeletal remains in archaeological contexts.* British Archaeological Reports International Series 567. Oxford, Tempus Reparatum, pp. 81–100.

Dobson, J.E. 1998. The iodine factor in health and evolution. *The Geographical Review* 88(1): 1–28.

Dobson, M. 1994. Malaria in England: a geographical and historical perspective. *Parassitologia* 36: 35–60.

Dobyns, H.F. 1993. Disease transfer at contact. *Ann. Rev. Anthrop.* 22: 273–91.

Dols, M.W. 1979. Leprosy in medieval Arabic medicine. *J. Hist. Med.* 34(3): 314–33.

Donaldson, L.J., Cook, A. and Thomson, R. 1990. Incidence of fractures in a geographically defined population. *J. Epidemiology and Community Health* 44: 241–5.

Dooley, J.R. and Binford, C.H. 1976. Treponematoses. In C.H. Binford and D.H. Connor (eds), *Pathology of tropical and extraordinary diseases.* Washington, Armed Forces Institute of Pathology, pp. 110–17.

Dorland's Pocket Medical Dictionary. 1995. London, W.B. Saunders.

Drancourt, M., Aboudhaaram, G., Signoli, M, Dutour, O. and Raolut, D. 1998. Detection of 400-year-old *Yersinia pestis* DNA in human dental pulp: an approach to the diagnosis of ancient septicemia. *Proc. Nat. Acad. Sci. USA* 95: 12637–40.

Drinkall, G. and Foreman, M. 1998. *The Anglo-Saxon cemetery at Castledyke South, Barton-on-Humber.* Sheffield, Academic Press.

Drury, P.L. and Howlett, T.A. 2002. Endocrine disease. In P. Kumar and M. Clark (eds), *Clinical medicine.* 5th edn, Edinburgh, W.B. Saunders, pp. 999–1068.

Duncan, H. and Leisen, J.C.C. 1993. Arthritis (rheumatoid). In K. Kiple (ed.), *The Cambridge world history of human disease.* Cambridge, Cambridge University Press, pp. 599–602.

Duncan, K. 1994. Climate and the decline of leprosy in Britain. *Proc. Royal Coll. Physicians, Edinburgh* 24:114–20.

Dunn, F.L. 1993. Malaria. In K. Kiple (ed.), *The Cambridge world history of human disease.* Cambridge, Cambridge University Press, pp. 855–62.

Dupras, T.L., Schwarcz, H.P. and Fairgrieve, S.I. 2001. Infant feeding and weaning practices in Roman Egypt. *Am. J. Phys. Anthrop.* 115: 204–12.

Duray, S. 1990. Deciduous enamel defects and caries susceptibility in a prehistoric Ohio population. *Am. J. Phys. Anthrop.* 81: 27–34.

Duray, S. 1996. Dental indicators of stress and reduced age at death in prehistoric native Indians. *Am. J. Phys. Anthrop.* 99: 275–86.

Dutour, O., Pálfi, G., Bérato, J. and Brun, J.-P. 1994 (eds). *L'origine de la syphilis en Europe: avant ou après 1493?* Toulon, Centre Archéologique du Var, Éditions Errance.

Dyer, C. 1989. *Standards of living in the Middle Ages: social change in England c. 1200–1520.* Cambridge, Cambridge University Press.

Dzierzykray-Rogalski, T. 1980. Palaeopathology of the Ptolemaic inhabitants of Dakhleh Oasis (Egypt). *J. Hum. Evol.* 9: 71–4.

Edwards, R. 2002. The road from Rio. *New Scientist* 17 August: 30–43.

Effros, B. 2000. Skeletal sex and gender in Merovingian mortuary archaeology. *Antiquity* 74: 632–9.

Eisenstein, S. 1978. Spondylolysis. *J. Bone Joint Surgery* 64B(4): 488–94.

Elia, M. 2002. Nutrition. In P. Kumar and M. Clark (eds), *Clinical medicine.* 5th edn, Edinburgh, W.B. Saunders, pp. 221–51.

Elliot-Smith, G. 1908. The most ancient splints. *Br. Med. J.* 1: 732–73.

Elliot-Smith, G. and Dawson, W.R. 1924. *Egyptian mummies.* New York, Dial Press.

Elliot-Smith, G. and Wood Jones, F. 1910. *The archaeological survey of Nubia 1907–8*, Vol. 2. *Report on the human remains.* Cairo, National Printing Department.

Elmahi, A.T. 2000. Prehistoric population controls in the Sudanese Nile Valley: a consideration of infanticide. *Beiträge zur Sudanforschug* 7: 103–18.

El-Najjar, M.Y. 1979. Human treponematosis and tuberculosis: evidence from the New World. *Am. J. Phys. Anthrop.* 51: 599–618.

El-Najjar, M.Y. and Mulinski, T.M.J. 1980. Mummies and mummification practices in the Southwestern and Southern United States. In A. Cockburn and E. Cockburn (eds), *Mummies, disease and ancient cultures.* Cambridge, Cambridge University Press, pp. 103–17.

Enderle, A., Meyerhofer, D. and Unverfehrt, G. 1994. *Small people – great art: restricted growth from an artistic and medical viewpoint.* Germany, Artcolor Verlag.

English Heritage. 2002. *Centre for Archaeology Guidelines. Human bones from archaeological sites. Guidelines for producing assessment documents and analytical reports.* Swindon, English Heritage.

Epstein, S. 1937. Art, history and the crutch. *Ann. Med. Hist.* 9: 304–13.

Ermene, B. and Dolene, A. 1999. Possibilities of comparing clinical and post-mortem diagnoses. *For. Sci. Int.* 103: S7–S12.

Eshed, V., Latimer, B., Greenwald, C.M., Jellema, L.M., Rothschild, B.M., Wish-Baratz, S. and Hershkovitz, I. 2002. Button osteoma: its etiology and pathophysiology. *Am. J. Phys. Anthrop.* 118: 217–30.

Eshed, V., Gopher, A., Galili, E. and Hershkovitz, I. 2004. Musculoskeletal stress markers in Natufian hunter-gatherers and Neolithic farmers in the Levant: the upper limb. *Am. J. Phys. Anthrop.* 123: 303–15.

Etxeberria, F. 1994. Vertebral epiphysitis: early signs of brucellar disease. *J. Paleopathology* 6(1): 41–9.

Evans, C.C. 1998. Historical background. In P.D.O. Davies (ed.), *Tuberculosis.* 2nd edn, London, Chapman and Hall Medical, pp. 1–19.

Evans, F.G. 1973. *Mechanical properties of bone.* Springfield, Ill., Charles C. Thomas.

Eversley, D.E.C., Laslett, P. and Wrigley, E.A. 1966. *An introduction to English historical demography.* London, Weidenfeld and Nicolson.

Ezzati, M. and Kammen, D. 2001. Indoor air pollution from biomass combustion and acute respiratory infections in Kenya: an exposure-response study. *Lancet* 358(9282): 619–20.

Faerman, M., Kahila, G., Smith, P., Greenblatt, C., Stager, L., Filon, D. and Oppenheim, A. 1997. DNA analysis reveals the sex of infanticide victims. *Nature* 385: 212–13.

Faerman, M., Jankauskas, R., Gorski, A., Becovier, H. and Greenblatt, Ch.L. 1999. Detecting *Mycobacterium tuberculosis* in Medieval skeletal remains from Lithuania. In G. Pálfi, O. Dutour, J. Deák and I. Hutás (eds), *Tuberculosis: past and present.* Budapest/Szeged, Golden Book Publishers and Tuberculosis Foundation, pp. 371–6.

Farmer, P. 1996. Social inequalities and emerging infectious diseases. *Emerging Infectious Diseases* 2(4): 259–69.

Farquharson, M.J. and Brickley, M. 1997. Determination of mineral composition of archaeological bone using energy-dispersive low-angle X-ray scattering. *Int. J. Osteoarchaeology* 7: 95–9.

Farquharson, M.J., Speller, R.D. and Brickley, M. 1997. Measuring bone mineral density in archaeological bone using energy-dispersive low-angle X-ray scattering techniques. *J. Archaeological Science* 24: 765–72.

Farwell, D.E. and Molleson, T. 1993. *Poundbury Volume 2: the cemeteries.* Dorset Natural History and Archaeological Society Monograph Series 11. Dorchester, Dorset Natural History and Archaeological Society.

Faulkner, R.A., Howson, C.S., Bailey, D.A., Drinkwater, D.T., McKay, H.A. and Wilkinson, A.A. 1993. Comparison of bone mineral content and bone mineral density between dominant and nondominant limbs in children 8–16 years of age. *Am. J. Hum. Biol.* 5: 491–9.

Fein, O. 1995. The influence of social class on health status: American and British research on health inequalities. *J. Gen. Intern. Med.* 10: 577–86.

Fernando-Jalvo, Y., Carlos Díez, J., Cáceres, I. and Rosell, J. 1999. Human cannibalism in the early Pleistocene of Europe (Gran Dolina, Sierra de Atapuerca, Burgos, Spain). *J. Hum. Evol.* 37: 591–622.

Ferreira, M.T. 2002. A scurvy case in an infant from Monte da Cegonha (Vidigueira – Portugal). *Antropologia Portuguesa* 19: 57–63.

Fife, D. and Barancik, J.I. 1985. Northeastern Ohio trauma study III: incidence of fractures. *Ann. Emerg. Med.* 14(3): 244–8.

Fife, D., Barancik, J.I. and Chatterjee, B.F. 1984. Northeastern Ohio trauma study II: injury rates by age, sex and cause. *Am. J. Pub. Health* 74(5): 473–8.

Fildes, V.A. 1986. 'The English Disease': infantile rickets and scurvy in pre-Industrial England. In J. Cule and T. Turner (eds), *Child care through the centuries.* London, British Society for the History of Medicine, pp. 121–34.

Filon, D., Faerman, M., Smith, P. and Oppenheim, A. 1995. Sequence analysis reveals a ß-thalassaemia mutation in the DNA of skeletal remains from the archaeological site of Akhziv, Israel. *Nature Genetics* 9: 365–8.

Fine, P.E.M. 1984. Leprosy and tuberculosis – an epidemiological comparison. *Tubercle* 65: 137–53.

Fine, P.E.M. 1995. Variation in protection by BCG: implications of and for heterologous immunity. *Lancet* 346: 1339–45.

Finnegan, M. 1978. Non-metrical variation of the intracranial skeleton. *J. Anatomy* 125(1): 23–37.

Fiorato, V., Boylston, A. and Knüsel, C. 2001. *Blood red roses: the archaeology of a mass grave from the Battle of Towton AD 1461.* Oxford, Oxbow Books.

Fitzpatrick, J., Griffiths, C. and Kelleher, M. 2000. Geographic inequalities in mortality in the United Kingdom during the 1990s. *Health Statistics Quarterly* 7: 19–31.

Foldes, A.J., Moscovici, A., Popovtzer, M.M., Mogle, P., Urman, D. and Zias, J. 1995. Extreme osteoporosis in a sixth-century skeleton from the Negev Desert. *Int. J. Osteoarchaeology* 5: 157–62.

Forestier, J. and Rotès-Querol, J. 1950. Senile ankylosing hyperostosis of the spine. *Ann. Rheumat. Dis.* 9: 321–30.

Formicola, V. 1995. X-linked hypophosphotemic rickets: a probable case from Upper Paleolithic. *Am. J. Phys. Anthrop.* 98(4): 403–9.

Formicola, V.Q., Milanesi, C. and Scarsini, C. 1987. Evidence of spinal tuberculosis at the beginning of the fourth millennium BC from Arena Candide Cave (Liguria, Italy). *Am. J. Phys. Anthrop.* 72: 1–7.

Fornaciari, G. and Marchetti, A. 1986. Italian smallpox of the 16th century. *Lancet* 2: 1469–70.

Fornaciari, G., Mallegni, F., Bertini, D. and Nuti, V. 1981. Cribra orbitalia and elemental bone in the Punics of Carthage. *Ossa* 8: 63–77.

Fortuine, R. 1984. Traditional surgery among the Alaska natives. *Alaska Med.* 26(1): 22–5.

Fox, C.L., Juan, J. and Albert, R.M. 1996. Phytolith analysis on dental calculus, enamel surface, and burial soil: information about diet and paleoenvironment. *Am. J. Phys. Anthrop.* 101: 101–13.

Frayer, D.W., Horton, W.A., Macchiarelli, R. and Mussi, M. 1987. Dwarfism in an adolescent from the Italian late Upper Palaeolithic. *Nature* 330: 60–1.

French, R. 1993. Scurvy. In K. Kiple (ed.), *The Cambridge world history of human disease*. Cambridge, Cambridge University Press, pp. 1000–5.

Fricker, E.J., Spigelman, M. and Fricker, C.R. 1997. The detection of *Escheria coli* DNA in the ancient remains of Lindow Man using the polymerase chain reaction. *Letters in Applied Microbiology* 24: 351–4.

Froment, A. 1994. Epidemiology of African endemic treponematoses in tropical forest and savanna. In O. Dutour, G. Pálfi, J. Bérato and J.-P. Brun (eds), *L'origine de la syphilis en Europe: avant ou après 1493?* Toulon, Centre Archéologique du Var, Éditions Errance, pp. 41–7.

Froment, A. 2001. Evolutionary biology and health of hunter-gatherer populations. In C. Panter-Brick, R.H. Layton and P. Rowley-Conwy (eds), *Hunter-gatherers: an inter-disciplinary perspective*. Cambridge, Cambridge University Press, pp. 239–66.

Fuller, B.T., Richards, M.P. and Mays, S.A. 2003. Stable carbon and nitrogen isotope variations in tooth dentine and serial sections from Wharram Percy. *J. Archaeological Science* 30: 1673–84.

Galasko, C.S.B. 1986. *Skeletal metastases*. London, Butterworth.

Gejvall, N.-G. 1960. *Westerhus, Medieval population and church in light of their skeletal remains*. Lund, Hakak Ohlssons Boktryckeri.

Gelis, J. 1991. *History of childbirth*. Cambridge, Polity Press.

Gernaey, A. and Minnikin, D. 2000. Chemical methods in palaeopathology. In M. Cox and S. Mays (eds), *Human osteology in archaeology and forensic science*. London, Greenwich Medical Media, pp. 239–53.

Gernaey, A.M., Minnikin, D.E., Copley, M.S., Dixon, R.A., Middleton, J.C. and Roberts, C.A. 2001. Mycolic acids and ancient DNA confirm an osteological diagnosis of tuberculosis. *Tuberculosis* 81(4): 259–65.

Gerszten, P.C. and Gerszten, E. 1995. Intentional cranial deformation: a disappearing form of self-mutilation. *Neurosurgery* 37(3): 374–82.

Gijsbers van Wijk, C.M.T., Huisman, H. and Kolk, A.M. 1999. Gender differences in physical symptoms and illness behavior: a health diary study. *Soc. Sci. Med.* 49: 1061–74.

Gilbert, R.I. and Mielke, J.H. 1985 (eds). *Analysis of prehistoric diets*. London, Academic Press.

Gjestland, T. 1955. The Oslo study of untreated syphilis: an epidemiological investigation of the natural course of the syphilitic infection based upon a re-study of the Boeck-Bruusgaard material. *Acat Dermato-Venerologica*. Volume 35. Supplementum 34.

Gladykowska-Rzeczycka, J. 1980. Remains of achondroplastic dwarf from Legnica of XI–XIIth century. *Ossa* 7: 71–4.

Gladykowska-Rzeczycka, J. 1994. Syphilis in ancient and medieval Poland. In O. Dutour, G. Pálfi, J. Bérato and J.-P. Brun (eds), *L'origine de la syphilis en Europe: avant ou après 1493?* Toulon, Centre Archéologique du Var, Éditions Errance, pp. 116–18.

Gladykowska-Rzeczycka, J. 1997. Osteosarcoma and ostechondroma from Polish Medieval cemeteries. *J. Paleopathology* 9(1): 47–53.

Gladykowska-Rzeczycka, J. and Myśliwski, A. 1985. Osteoid-osteoma from Middle Ages cemetery in Poland. *Ossa* 12: 33–9.

Glencross, B. and Stuart-Macadam, P. 2000. Childhood trauma in the archaeological record. *Int. J. Osteoarchaeology* 10: 198–209.

Glen-Haduch, E., Szostek, K. and Glab, H. 1997. Cribra orbitalia and trace element content in human teeth from Neolithic and early Bronze Age graves in southern Poland. *Am. J. Phys. Anthrop.* 103: 201–7.

Glisson, F. 1650. *De rachitide sive morbo puerili qui vulgo The Rickets Dicitur Tractatus. Adscitis in operas societatem Georgio Bate et Ahasuero Regemortero*. London, G. Du-Gardi.

Glob, P.V. 1973. *The bog people*. London, Book Club Associates.

Goldman, A.B. 1995. Heritable diseases of connective tissue, epiphysial dysplasias, and related conditions. In D. Resnick (ed.), *Diagnosis of bone and joint disorders.* 3rd edn, London, W.B. Saunders, pp. 4095–162.

Goldmeier, D. and Gualler, C. 2003. Syphilis: an update. *Clin. Med.* 3(3): 209–11.

Goldstein, M.S. 1957. Skeletal pathology of early Indians in Texas. *Am. J. Phys. Anthrop.* 15: 299–311.

González-Reimers, E., Velasco-Vázquez, J., Arnay-de-la-Rosa, M., Santolaria-Fernández, F., Gómez-Rodríguez, M.A. and Machado-Calvo, M. 2002. Double-energy X-ray absorptiometry in the diagnosis of osteopenia in ancient skeletal remains. *Am. J. Phys. Anthrop.* 118: 134–45.

Goodman, A.H. 1991. Stress, adaptation and enamel developmental defects. In D. Ortner and A. Aufderheide (eds), *Human paleopathology: current syntheses and future options.* Washington, Smithsonian Institution Press, pp. 280–7.

Goodman, A.H. and Capasso, L. 1992 (eds). *Recent contributions to the study of enamel developmental defects.* Journal of Paleopathology Monographic Publications 2, Teramo, Italy, Edigrafital.

Goodman, A.H. and Clarke, G.A. 1981. Harris lines as indicators of stress in prehistoric Illinois populations. In D.L. Martin and P. Bumsted (eds), *Biocultural adaptation: comprehensive approaches to skeletal analysis.* Amherst, University of Massachusetts Research Reports 20, pp. 35–46.

Goodman, A.H. and Martin, D.L. 2002. Reconstructing health profiles from skeletal remains. In R. Steckel and J. Rose (eds), *The backbone of history: health and nutrition in the Western Hemisphere.* Cambridge, Cambridge University Press, pp. 11–60.

Goodman, A.H. and Rose, J. 1990. Assessment of systemic physiological perturbations from dental enamel hypoplasias and associated histological structures. *Am. J. Phys. Anthrop.* 33: 59–110.

Goodman, A.H. and Rose, J.C. 1991. Dental enamel hypoplasias as indicators of nutritional status. In M.A. Kelley and C.S. Larsen (eds), *Advances in dental anthropology.* New York, Wiley-Liss, pp. 279–93.

Goodman, A.H., Lallo, J., Armelagos, G.J. and Rose, J.C. 1984. Health changes at Dickson Mounds, Illinois (AD 950–1300). In M.N. Cohen and G.J. Armelagos (eds), *Paleopathology at the origins of agriculture.* London, Academic Press, pp. 271–306.

Goodman, A.H., Allen, L.H., Hernandez, G.P., Amador, A., Arriola, L.V., Chavez, A. and Pelto, G.H. 1987. Prevalence and age at development of enamel hypoplasias in Mexican schoolchildren. *Am. J. Phys. Anthrop.* 72: 7–19.

Goodman, A.H., Brooke Thomas, R. Swedlund, A.C. and Armelagos, G.J. 1988. Biocultural perspectives on stress in prehistorical, historical and contemporary population research. *Yearbook of Phys. Anthrop.* 31: 169–202.

Gordon, I., Shapiro, H. and Berson, S. 1988. *Forensic medicine: a guide to principles.* Edinburgh, Churchill Livingstone.

Gould, M.I. and Moon, G. 2000. Problems of providing health care in British island communities. *Soc. Sci. Med.* 50: 1081–90.

Gowland, R.L. and Chamberlain, A.T. 2002. A Bayesian approach to ageing perinatal skeletal material from archaeological sites: implications for the evidence for infanticide in Roman Britain. *J. Archaeological Science* 29: 677–85.

Gowland, R.L. and Chamberlain, A.T. 2005. Detecting plague: palaeodemographic characterisation of a catastrophic death assemblage. *Antiquity* 79: 146–57.

Grange, J.M. 1995. Human aspects of *Mycobacterium bovis* infection. In C.O. Thoen and J.H. Steele (eds), *Mycobacterium bovis infection in animals and humans.* Ames, Iowa State University Press, pp. 29–46.

Grange, J.M. 1999. The global burden of tuberculosis. In J.G.H. Porter and J.M. Grange (eds), *Tuberculosis: an interdisciplinary perspective.* London, Imperial College Press, pp. 3–11.

Grauer, A.L. 1991. Patterns of life and death: the palaeodemography of medieval York. In H. Bush and M. Zvelebil (eds), *Health in past societies: biocultural interpretations of human skeletal remains in archaeological contexts.* British Archaeological Reports International Series 567. Oxford, Tempus Reparatum, pp. 67–80.

Grauer, A. 1993. Patterns of anemia and infection from Medieval York. *Am. J. Phys. Anthrop.* 91: 203–13.

Grauer, A. 1995 (ed.). *Bodies of evidence: reconstructing history through skeletal analysis.* New York, Wiley-Liss.

Grauer, A. and Roberts, C.A. 1996. Paleoepidemiology, healing and possible treatment of trauma in the Medieval cemetery population of St Helen-on-the-Walls, York, England. *Am. J. Phys. Anthrop.* 100: 531–44.

Grauer, A. and Stuart-Macadam, P. 1998 (eds). *Sex and gender in paleopathological perspective.* Cambridge, Cambridge University Press.

Gray, P.H. 1969. A case of osteogenesis imperfecta associated with dentinogenesis imperfecta, dating from antiquity. *Clin. Radiol.* 21: 106–8.

Green, V.H.H. 1971. *Medieval civilisation in Western Europe.* London, Edward Arnold.

Gregg, J.B. and Gregg, P.S. 1987. *Dry bones: Dakota Territory reflected.* Sioux Falls, SD, Sioux Printing.

Grmek, M. 1983. *Les maladies à l'aube de la civilisation occidentale.* Paris, Payot.

Grmek, M. 1989. *Histoire du SIDA.* Paris, France Loisirs.

Grmek, M. 1992. La lèpre a-t-elle été représentée dans l'iconographie antique? *Pact* 34: 147–56.

Grmek, M.D. 1994. Discussion. In O. Dutour, G. Pálfi, J. Bérato and J.-P. Brun (eds), *L'origine de la syphilis en Europe: avant ou après 1493?* Toulon, Centre Archéologique du Var, Éditions Errance, p. 283.

Grolleau-Raoux, J.-L., Crubézy, E., Rouge, D., Brugne, J.-F. and Saunders, S.R. 1997. Harris lines: a study of age-associated bias in counting and interpretation. *Am. J. Phys. Anthrop.* 103: 209–17.

Gron, K. 1973. Leprosy in literature and art. *Int. J. Leprosy* 41(2): 249–83.

Groves, S.E., Roberts, C.A., Johnstone, C., Hall, R. and Dobney, K. 2003. A high status burial from Ripon Cathedral, North Yorkshire: differential diagnosis of a chest deformity. *Int. J. Osteoarchaeology* 13: 358–68.

Grupe, G. 1988. Metastasizing carcinoma in a medieval skeleton: differential diagnosis and etiology. *Am. J. Phys. Anthrop.* 75: 369–74.

Gunnell, D., Rogers, J. and Dieppe, P. 2001. Height and health: predicting longevity from bone length in archaeological remains. *J. Epidemiology and Community Health* 55: 505–7.

Gurdjian, E.S. 1973. Prevention and mitigation of head injury from antiquity to the present. *J. Trauma* 13(11): 931–45.

Gurdjian, E.S., Webster, J.E. and Lissner, H.R. 1950. The mechanism of skull fracture. *J. Neurosurg.* 7: 106–14.

Guy, H., Masset, C. and Baud, C-A. 1997. Infant taphonomy. *Int. J. Osteoarchaeology* 7: 221–9.

Haas, C.J., Zink, A., Molnar, E., Szeimies, U., Reischl, U., Marcsik, A., Ardagna, Y., Dutour, O., Pálfi, G. and Nerlich, A.G. 2000. Molecular evidence for different stages of tuberculosis in ancient bone samples from Hungary. *Am. J. Phys. Anthrop.* 113: 2933–3304.

Hackett, C. 1963. On the origin of the human treponematoses. *Bull. WHO* 29: 7–41.

Hackett, C. 1967. The human treponematoses. In D.R. Brothwell and A.T. Sandison (eds), *Diseases in antiquity.* Springfield, Ill., Charles Thomas, pp. 152–70.

Hackett, C. 1974. Possible treponemal changes in a Tasmanian skull. *Man* 9: 436–43.

Hackett, C. 1976a. Microscopic focal destruction (tunnels) in exhumed human bone. *Med. Sci. and the Law.* 21(4): 243–635.

Hackett, C. 1976b. *Diagnostic criteria of syphilis, yaws and treponarid (treponematoses) and of some other diseases in dry bones.* Sitzungsberichte der Heidelberger Akademie der Wissenschaften Mathematisch-naturwissenschaftliche Klasse, Abhandlung 4. Berlin, Springer-Verlag.

Hackett, C. 1981. Development of caries sicca in a dry calvaria. *Virchows Arch. (Pathol. Anat.)* 391: 53–79.

Hacking, P., Allen, T. and Rogers, J. 1994. Rheumatoid arthritis in a Medieval skeleton. *Int. J. Osteoarchaeology* 4: 251–5.

Halffman, C.A., Scott, G.R. and Pedersen, P.O. 1992. Palatine torus in the Greenlandic Norse. *Am. J. Phys. Anthrop.* 88: 145–61.

Hallbäck, D.A. 1976. A medieval (?) bone with a copper plate support indicating an open surgical treatment. *Ossa* 3/4: 63–82.

Ham, A.W. and Harris, W.R. 1956. Repair and transplantation of bone. In G.H. Bourne (ed.), *The biochemistry and physiology of bone*. New York, Academic Press.

Hamilton, G. 1998. Let them eat dirt. *New Scientist* 18 July: 26–31.

Hamperl, H. 1967. The osteological consequences of scalping. In D. Brothwell and A. Sandison (eds), *Diseases in antiquity*. Springfield, Ill., Charles C. Thomas, pp. 630–4.

Haneveld, G.T. and Perizonius, W.R.K. 1980. *Trepanning practice in the Netherlands*. Proceedings of the 3rd Paleopathology Association European Meeting, Caen, France.

Hanzlick, R. 1997. Death registration: history, methods and legal issues. *J. For. Sci.* 42(2): 265–9.

Hardy, A. 1994. Death is the cure of all diseases: using the General Register Office Cause of Death Statistics for 1837–1920. *Soc. Hist. Med.* 7(3): 472–92.

Harris, H.A. 1931. Lines of arrested growth in the long bones in childhood: the correlation of histological and radiographic appearances in clinical and experimental conditions. *Br. J. Radiol.* 18: 622–40.

Hart, G.D. 1980. Ancient diseases of the blood. In M.W. Wintrobe (ed.), *Blood pure and eloquent*. New York, pp. 33–56.

Hassan, F.A. 1973. On the mechanics of population growth during the Neolithic. *Curr. Anthrop.* 14(5): 535–42.

Hassan, M.M., Atkins, P.J. and Dunn, C.E. 2003. The spatial patterning of risk from arsenic poisoning: a Bangladesh case study. *J. Environmental Science and Health* 38: 1–24.

Hawkes, S.C. and Wells, C. 1975. Crime and punishment in an Anglo-Saxon cemetery. *Antiquity* 49: 118–22.

Hawkey, D. 1998. Disability, compassion and the skeletal record: using musculoskeletal stress markers (MSM) to construct an osteobiography from early New Mexico. *Int. J. Osteoarchaeology* 8: 326–40.

Hawkey, D. and Merbs, C.F. 1995. Activity-induced musculoskeletal stress markers (MSM) and subsistence strategy changes among ancient Hudson Bay Eskimos. *Int. J. Osteoarchaeology.* 5: 324–38.

Haynes, S., Searle, J.B., Bretman, A. and Dobney, K.M. 2002. Bone preservation and ancient DNA: the application of screening methods for predicting DNA survival. *J. Archaeological Science* 29: 585–92.

Henderson, C. 2003. Rethinking musculoskeletal stress markers. Poster presented at the Annual British Association of Biological Anthropology and Osteoarchaeology Conference, University of Southampton.

Henderson, J. 1987. Factors determining the state of preservation of human remains. In A. Boddington, A.N. Garland and R.C. Janaway (eds), *Death, decay and reconstruction: approaches to archaeology and forensic science*. Manchester, Manchester University Press, pp. 43–54.

Henneberg, M. and Henneberg, R.J. 1994. Treponematosis in an ancient Greek colony of Metaponto, Southern Italy, 580–250 BC. In O. Dutour, G. Pálfi, J. Bérato and J.-P. Brun (eds), *L'origine de la syphilis en Europe: avant ou après 1493?* Toulon, Centre Archéologique du Var, Éditions Errance, pp. 92–8.

Heoprich, P. 1989. Non-syphilitic treponematoses. In P. Hoeprich and M. Jordan (eds), *Infectious diseases*. 4th edn, Philadelphia, J.B. Lippincott, pp. 1021–34.

Her Majesty's Stationery Office 1985. *Manual of nutrition*. London, HMSO.

Herring, D.A., Saunders, S.R. and Katzenberg, M.A. 1998. Investigating the weaning process in past populations. *Am. J. Phys. Anthrop.* 105: 425–39.

Hershkovitz, I., Rothschild, B.M., Wish-Baratz, S. and Rothschild, C. 1994. Natural variation and differential diagnosis of skeletal changes in bejel (endemic syphilis). In O. Dutour, G. Pálfi, J. Bérato and J.-P. Brun (eds), *L'origine de la syphilis en Europe: avant ou après 1493?* Toulon, Centre Archéologique du Var, Éditions Errance, pp. 81–7.

Hershkovitz, I., Rothschild, B.M., Latimer, B.M., Dutour, O., Leonetti, G., Greenwald, C., Rothschild, C. and Jellema, L. 1997. Recognition of sickle cell anemia in skeletal remains of children. *Am. J. Phys. Anthrop.* 104: 213–26.

Hershkovitz, I., Greenwald, C., Rothschild, B.M., Latimer, B., Dutour, O., Jellema, L.M. and Wish-Baratz, S. 1999. Hyperostosis frontalis interna: an anthropological perspective. *Am. J. Phys. Anthrop.* 109: 303–25.

Hershkovitz, I., Greenwald, C.M., Latimer, B.M, Jellema, L.M., Wish-Baratz, S., Eshed, V., Dutour, O. and Rothschild, B.M. 2002. Serpens endocrania symmetrica (SES): a new term and possible clue for identifying intrathoracic disease in skeletal populations. *Am. J. Phys. Anthrop.* 118: 201–16.

Hess, A.F. 1929. *Rickets including osteomalacia and tetany.* Philadelphia, Lea and Febiger.

Hillson, S. 1986. *Teeth.* Cambridge, Cambridge University Press.

Hillson, S. 1992. Impression replica methods for studying hypoplasia and perikymata in human tooth crown surfaces from archaeological sites. *Int. J. Osteoarchaeology* 2: 65–78.

Hillson, S. 1996. *Dental anthropology.* Cambridge, Cambridge University Press.

Hillson, S. 1997. Relationship of enamel hypoplasia to the pattern of tooth crown growth: a discussion. *Am. J. Phys. Anthrop.* 104: 89–103.

Hillson, S. 2000. Dental pathology. In M.A. Katzenberg and S.R. Saunders (eds), *Biological anthropology of the human skeleton.* New York, Wiley-Liss, pp. 249–86.

Hillson, S. 2001. Recording dental caries in archaeological human remains. *Int. J. Osteoarchaeology* 11: 249–89.

Hillson, S. and Jones, S. 1989. Instruments for measuring surface profiles: an application in the study of ancient human tooth crown surfaces. *J. Archaeological Science* 16: 95–105.

Hillson, S., Grigson, C. and Bond, S. 1998. Dental defects of congenital syphilis. *Am. J. Phys. Anthrop.* 107: 25–40.

Hinton, R.J. 1981. Form and patterning of anterior tooth wear among Aboriginal human groups. *Am. J. Phys. Anthrop.* 54: 555–64.

Hodell, D.A., Quinn, R.L., Brenner, M. and Kamenov, G. 2004. Spatial variation of strontium isotopes (87Sr/86Sr) in the Maya region: a tool for tracking ancient human migration. *J. Archaeological Science* 31: 585–601.

Hodges, D.C. 1989. *Agricultural intensification and prehistoric health in the valley of Oaxaca, Mexico: prehistory and human ecology of the Valley of the Oaxaca.* Memoirs of the Museum of Anthropology, ed. K.V. Flannery, Volume 9, Number 22. Ann Arbor, University of Michigan.

Hodges, D.C. 1991. Temporomandibular joint osteoarthritis in a British skeletal population. *Am. J. Phys. Anthrop.* 85: 367–77.

Holcomb, R.C. 1940. The antiquity of congenital syphilis. *Bull. Hist. Med.* 10(2): 148–77.

Hollander, E. 1913. *Die Medizin in der Klassischen Malerie.* Stuttgart.

Hollingsworth, T.H. 1969. *Historical demography.* Ithaca, NY, Cornell Press.

Holmes, B. 1999. Grains of gold. *New Scientist* 14 August: 12.

Hooton, E.A. 1930. *The Indians of Pecos Pueblo: a study of their skeletal remains.* New Haven, Yale University Press.

Hopkins, D. 1980. News from the field. *Paleopathology Association Newsletter* 31: 6.

Horden, P. 2000. The Millennium Bug: health and medicine around the year 1000. *Soc. Hist. Med.* 13(2): 201–19.

Horne, P. 1995. Aspergillosis and dracunculiasis in mummies from the tomb of Parennefer. *Paleopathology Association Newsletter* 92: 10–12.

Howe, G.M. 1997. *People, environment, disease and death.* Cardiff, University of Wales Press.

Hrdlička, A. 1941. *Diseases of and artifacts on skull and bones from Kodiak Island.* Smithsonian Miscellaneous Collections 101(4). Washington, Smithsonian Institution.

Huber, B.R. and Anderson, R. 1995. Bonesetters and curers in a Mexican community: conceptual models, status and gender. *Med. Anthrop.* 17: 23–38.

Hudson, E.H. 1958. The treponematoses – or treponematosis. *Br. J. Venereal Dis.* 34: 22–3.

Hudson, E.H. 1963. Treponematosis and pilgrimage. *Am. J. Med. Sci.* 246: 645–56.

Hudson, E.H. 1965. Treponematosis and man's social evolution. *Am. Anthrop.* 67: 885–901.

Hudson, E.H. 1968. Christopher Columbus and the history of syphilis. *Acta Tropica* 25: 1–16.

Huffman, M.A. 1997. Current evidence for self-medication in primates: a multidisciplinary perspective. *Yearbook of Phys. Anthrop.* 40: 171–200.

Hughes, C., Heylings, D.J.A. and Power, C. 1996. Transverse (Harris) lines in Irish archaeological remains. *Am. J. Phys. Anthrop.* 101: 115–31.

Huijbers, P.M.J.F., Hendriks, J.L.M., Gerver, W.J.M., De Jong, P.J. and de Meer, K. 1996. Nutritional status and mortality of highland children in Nepal: impact of sociocultural factors. *Am. J. Phys. Anthrop.* 101: 137–44.

Hulse, E.V. 1972. Leprosy and ancient Egypt. *Lancet* 2: 1024.

Hulse, E.V. 1976. The nature of biblical leprosy and the use of alternative terms in modern translations of the Bible. *Med. Hist.* 20(2): 203.

Hummert, J.R. and Van Gerven, D.P. 1985. Observations on the formation and persistence of radiopaque transverse lines. *Am. J. Phys. Anthrop.* 66: 297–306.

Humphrey, J.H. and Hutchinson, D.L. 2001. Macroscopic characteristics of hacking trauma. *J. For. Sci.* 46(2): 228–33.

Humphrey, L. 2000. Growth studies of past populations: an overview and an example. In M. Cox and S. Mays (eds), *Human osteology in archaeology and forensic science.* London, Greenwich Medical Media, pp. 23–38.

Hunt, E.E., Jr and Hatch, J.W. 1981. The estimation of age at death and ages of formation of transverse lines from measurements of human long bones. *Am. J. Phys. Anthrop.* 54: 461–9.

Huss-Ashmore, R., Goodman, A.H. and Armelagos, G.J. 1982. Nutritional inference from paleopathology. In M.B. Schiffer (ed.), *Advances in archaeological method and theory* Volume 5. London, Academic Press, pp. 395–476.

Hutchinson, D.L. 1996. Brief encounters: Tatham Mound and the evidence for Spanish and Native American confrontation. *Int. J. Osteoarchaeology* 6: 51–65.

Hutchinson, D.L., Denise, C.B., Daniel, H.J. and Kalmus, G.W. 1997. A reevaluation of the cold water etiology of external auditory exostoses. *Am. J. Phys. Anthrop.* 103: 417–22.

Ikehara-Quebral, R. and Toomay Douglas, M. 1997. Cultural alteration of human teeth in the Mariana Islands. *Am. J. Phys. Anthrop.* 104: 381–91.

Ilani, S., Rosenfeld, A. and Dvorachek, M. 1999. Mineralogy and chemistry of a Roman remedy from Judea, Israel. *J. Archaeological Science* 26: 1323–6.

Inhorn, M.C. and Brown, P.J. 1990. The anthropology of infectious disease. *Ann. Rev. Anthrop.* 19: 89–117.

Inhorn, M.C. and Brown, P.J. 1997. The anthropology of infectious disease. In M.C. Inhorn and P.J. Brown (eds), *The anthropology of infectious disease: international health perspectives.* Canada, Gordon and Breach, pp. 31–67.

Iscan, M.Y. 1989 (ed.). *Age markers in the human skeleton.* Springfield, Ill., Charles C. Thomas.

Ives, R. and Brickley, M.B. 2004. A procedural guide to metacarpal radiogrammetry in archaeology. *Int. J. Osteoarchaeology* 14: 7–17.

Iyere, B.B. 1990. Leprosy deformities: experience in Molai leprosy hospital, Maiduguri, Nigeria.

Leprosy Review 61: 171–9.

Jackes, M.K. 1983. Osteological evidence for smallpox: a possible case from seventeenth century Ontario. *Am. J. Phys. Anthrop.* 60: 75–81.

Jackes, M.K. 2000. Building the bases for paleodemographic analysis. In M.A. Katzenberg and S.R. Saunders (eds), *Biological anthropology of the human skeleton.* New York, Wiley-Liss, pp. 417–66.

Jackson, D.W., Wiltse, L.L. and Cirincione, R.J. 1976. Spondylolysis in the female gymnast. *Clinical Orthopaedics* 117: 68–73.

Jacobi, K.P. and Danforth, M.E. 2002. Analysis of interobserver scoring patterns in porotic hyperostosis and cribra orbitalia. *Int. J. Osteoarchaeology* 12: 248–58.

Jaffe, H.L. 1958. *Tumors and tumorous conditions of bones and joints.* Philadelphia, Lea and Febiger.

Jaffe, H.L. 1972. *Metabolic, degenerative and inflammatory disease of bones and joints.* Philadelphia, Lea and Febiger.

James, R. and Nasmyth-Jones, R. 1992. The occurrence of cervical fractures in victims of judicial hanging. *For. Sci. Int.* 54: 81–91.

Janaway, R.C., Wilson, A.S., Caffell, A.C. and Roberts, C.A. 2001. Human skeletal collections: the responsibilities of project managers, physical anthropologists, conservators and the need for standardized condition assessments. In E. Williams (ed.), *Human remains: conservation, retrieval and analysis.* Proceedings of a conference held in Williamsburg, VA, 7–11 November 1999. British Archaeological Reports International Series 934. Oxford, Archaeopress, pp. 199–208.

Jankauskas, R. 2003. The incidence of diffuse idiopathic skeletal hyperostosis and social status correlations in Lithuanian skeletal materials. *Int. J. Osteoarchaeology* 13: 289–93.

Jans, M.M.E., Nielsen-Marsh, C.M., Smith, C.I., Collins, M.J. and Kars, H. 2004. Characterisation of microbial attack on archaeological bone. *J. Archaeological Science* 31: 87–95.

Janssen, H.A.M. and Maat, G.J.R. 1999. *Canons buried in the 'Stiftskapel' of the Saint Servaas Basilica at Maastricht AD 1070–1521.* A paleopathological study. Leiden, Barge's Anthropologica Number 5.

Janssens, P. 1970. *Palaeopathology.* London, John Baker.

Janssens, P. 1987. A copper plate on the upper arm in a burial at the church in Vrasene (Belgium). *J. Paleopathology* 1(1): 15–18.

Jarcho, S. 1966. The development and present condition of human paleopathology in the United States. In S. Jarcho (ed.), *Paleopathology.* New Haven, Yale University Press, pp. 3–42.

Jenner, E. 1801. *The origin of the vaccine inoculation.* Soho, D.N. Shury.

Johnston, F.E. 1963. Some observations on the roles of achondroplastic dwarfs through history. *Clin. Pediat.* 2: 703–8.

Jones, A.K.G. 1985. Trichurid ova in archaeological deposits: their value as indicators of ancient faeces. In N.J. Feiller, D.D. Gilbertson and N.G.A. Ralph (eds), *Palaeobiological investigations: research design, methods and data analysis.* British Archaeological Reports International Series 266. Oxford, BAR, pp. 105–19.

Jones, H.N., Priest, J.D., Hayes, W.C., Tichenor, C.C. and Nagel, D.A. 1977. Humeral hypertrophy in response to exercise. *J. Bone and Joint Surgery* 59A: 204–8.

Jones, J.H. 1993. *Bad blood: the Tuskagee syphilis experiment.* Toronto, The Free Press, A Division of Maxwell Macmillan.

Jones, M.W. 1990. A study of trauma in an Amish community. *J. Trauma* 30(7): 899–902.

Jónsdóttir, B., Ortner, D.J. and Frohlich, B. 2003. Probable destructive meningioma in an archaeological adult male skull from Alaska. *Am. J. Phys. Anthrop.* 122: 232–9.

Jónsson, B., Gardsell, P., Johnell, O., Redlund-Johnell, I. and Sernbo, I. 1992. Differences in fracture pattern between an urban and a rural population: a comparative population-based study in southern Sweden. *Osteoporosis Int.* 2: 269–73.

Jónsson, B., Gardsell, P., Johnell, O., Sernbo, I. and Gullberg, B. 1993. Life-style and different fracture prevalence: a cross sectional comparative population-based study. *Calcified Tiss. Int.* 52: 425–33.

Jopling, W.H. 1982. Clinical aspects of leprosy. *Tubercle* 63: 295–305.

Jopling, W.H. 1991. Leprosy stigma. *Leprosy Review* 62: 1–12.

Jopling, W.H. and McDougall, A.C. 1988. *Handbook of leprosy*. Oxford, Heinemann Medical Books.

Joseph, G.A. and Sundar Rao, P.S.S. 1999. Impact of leprosy on the quality of life. *Bull. WHO* 77(6): 515–17.

Judd, M. 2000. Trauma and interpersonal violence in ancient Nubia during the Kerma period (ca. 2500–1500 BC). Ph.D. thesis, University of Alberta, Edmonton, Canada.

Judd, M. 2002a. Comparison of long bone trauma recording methods. *J. Archaeological Science* 29: 1255–65.

Judd, M. 2002b. Ancient injury recidivism: an example from the Kerma period of ancient Nubia. *Int. J. Osteoarchaeology* 12: 86–106.

Judd, M. 2004. Trauma in the city of Kerma: ancient versus modern injury patterns. *Int. J. Osteoarchaeology* 14: 34–51.

Judd, M. and Roberts, C.A. 1998. Fracture patterns at the Medieval leper hospital in Chichester. *Am. J. Phys. Anthrop.* 105: 43–55.

Judd, M. and Roberts, C.A. 1999. Fracture trauma in a Medieval British farming village. *Am. J. Phys. Anthrop.* 109: 229–43.

Julkunen, H., Heinonen, O.P., Pyörälä, K. 1971. Hyperostosis of the spine in an adult population. *Ann. Rheum. Dis.* 30: 605–12.

Jurmain, R.D. 1980. The pattern of involvement of appendicular degenerative joint disease. *Am. J. Phys. Anthrop.* 53: 143–50.

Jurmain, R.D. 1990. Paleoepidemiology of a Central Californian prehistoric population from CA-ALA. I Degenerative joint disease. *Am. J. Phys. Anthrop.* 83: 83–94.

Jurmain, R.D. 1991. Paleoepidemiology of trauma in a prehistoric Central Californian population. In D. Ortner and A. Aufderheide (eds), *Human paleopathology: current syntheses and future options*. Washington, Smithsonian Institution Press, pp. 241–8.

Jurmain, R.D. 1997. Skeletal evidence of trauma in African apes, with special reference to the Gombe chimpanzees. *Primates* 38(1): 1–14.

Jurmain, R.D. 1999. *Stories from the skeleton: behavioral reconstruction in human osteology*. Amsterdam, Gordon and Breach Publishers.

Jurmain, R.D. 2001. Paleoepidemiological patterns of trauma in a prehistoric population from Central California. *Am. J. Phys. Anthrop.* 115: 13–23.

Jurmain, R.D. and Bellifemine, V.I. 1997. Patterns of cranial trauma in a prehistoric population from Central California. *Int. J. Osteoarchaeology* 7: 43–50.

Jurmain, R.D. and Kilgore, L. 1995. Skeletal evidence of osteoarthritis: a palaeopathological perspective. *Ann. Rheum. Dis.* 54: 443–50.

Jurmain, R.D., Nelson, H., Kilgore, L. and Trevathan, W. 1997. *Introduction to physical anthropology*. 7th edn, Belmont, California, Wadsworth Publishing Company.

Jurmain, R.D., Kilgore, L., Trevathan, W. and Nelson, H. 2003. *Introduction to physical anthropology*. 9th edn, Belmont, California, Wadsworth Publishing Company.

Kambe, T., Yonemitsu, K., Kibayashi, K. and Tsunenari, S. 1991. Application of a computer assisted image analyser to the assessment of area and number of sites of dental attrition and its use in age estimates. *For. Sci. Int.* 50: 97–109.

Kaplan, B.A. 1988. Migration and disease. In C.G.N. Maisie-Taylor and G.W. Lasker (eds), *Biological aspects of human migration*. Cambridge, Cambridge University Press, pp. 216–45.

Kapur, V., Whittam, T.S. and Musser, J.M. 1994. Is *Mycobacterium tuberculosis* 15,000 years old? *J. Infectious Diseases* 170: 1348–9.

Karn, K.W., Shockett, H.D., Moffitt, W.C. and Gray, J.L. 1984. Topographic classification of deformities of the alveolar process. *J. Periodontology* 55: 336–40.

Karsh, R.S. and McCarthy, J.D. 1960. Archaeology and arthritis. *Intern. Med.* 105: 640–4.

Katzenberg, M.A. 2000. Stable isotope analysis: a tool for studying past diet, demography, and life history. In M.A. Katzenberg and S.R. Saunders (eds), *Biological anthropology of the human skeleton*. New York, Wiley-Liss, pp. 305–27.

Katzenberg, M.A. and Lovell, N.C. 1999. Stable isotope variation in pathological bone. *Int. J. Osteoarchaeology* 9: 316–24.

Katzenberg, M.A., Kelley, M.A. and Pfeiffer, S. 1982. Hereditary multiple exostoses in an individual from a southern Ontario Iroquoian population. *Ossa* 8: 109–14.

Katzenberg, M.A., Schwarcz, H.P., Knyf, M. and Melbye, F.J. 1995. Stable isotope evidence for maize horticulture and paleodiet in southern Ontario, Canada. *Am. Antiq.* 60: 335–50.

Katzenberg, M.A., Herring, D.A. and Saunders, S.R. 1996. Weaning and infant mortality: evaluating the skeletal evidence. *Yearbook of Phys. Anthrop.* 39: 177–99.

Kaufman, M.H., Whitaker, D. and McTavish, J. 1997. Differential diagnosis of holes in the calvarium: application of modern clinical data to palaeopathology. *J. Archaeological Science* 24: 193–218.

Keene, D. 1983. Medieval urban environment in documentary records. *Archives* 16: 137–44.

Keers, R.Y. 1981. Laënnec: a medical history. *Thorax* 36(2): 91–4.

Kelley, M.A. and Eisenberg, L.E. 1987. Blastomycosis and tuberculosis in early American Indians: a biocultural view. *Midcontinental J. Archaeology* 12(1): 89–116.

Kelley, M. and Micozzi, M. 1984. Rib lesions in chronic pulmonary tuberculosis. *Am. J. Phys. Anthrop.* 65: 381–7.

Kelley, M., Murphy, S., Levesque, D. and Sledzik, P. 1994. Respiratory disease among Protohistoric and Early Historic Plains Indians. In D.W. Owsley and R.L. Jantz (eds), *Skeletal biology in the Great Plains: migration, warfare, health, and subsistence*. Washington, Smithsonian Institution Press, pp. 123–30.

Kemink, J.L., Niparko, J.K. and Telian, S.A. 1993. Mastoiditis. In K. Kiple (ed.), *The Cambridge world history of human disease*. Cambridge, Cambridge University Press, pp. 865–71.

Kennedy, G.E. 1986. The relationship between auditory exostoses and cold water: a latitudinal analysis. *Am. J. Phys. Anthrop.* 71: 401–15.

Kennedy, K.A.R. 1989. Skeletal markers of occupational stress. In M.Y. Iscan and K.A.R. Kennedy (eds), *Reconstruction of life from the skeleton*. New York, Alan Liss, pp. 129–60.

Kennedy, K.A.R. 1998. Markers of occupational stress: conspectus and prognosis of research. *Int. J. Osteoarchaeology* 8: 305–10.

Kent, S. 1987. The influence of sedentism and aggregation on porotic hyperostosis: a case study. *Man, New Series* 21: 605–36.

Kettel, B. 1996. Women, health and the environment. *Social Science and Medicine* 42(10): 1367.

Kilgore, L. 1989. A possible case of rheumatoid arthritis from Sudanese Nubia. *Am. J. Phys. Anthrop.* 79: 177–83.

Kilgore, L., Jurmain, R.D. and VanGerven, D. 1997. Palaeoepidemiological patterns of trauma in a medieval Nubian skeletal population. *Int. J. Osteoarchaeology* 7: 1103–14.

King, M., Speck, P. and Thomas, A. 1999. The effect of spiritual beliefs on outcome from illness. *Soc. Sci. Med.* 48: 1291–9.

King, S. 1992. Violence and death during the fall of the Roman Empire. Interpretations of a late 4th century/early 5th century charnel house deposit from Arras. Unpublished M.Sc. dissertation, University of Bradford.

King, S. 1994. The human skeletal remains from Glasgow Cathedral Excavations 1992–3. Unpublished skeletal report.

Klepinger, L.L. 1979. Paleopathological evidence for the evolution of rheumatoid arthritis. *Am. J. Phys. Anthrop.* 50: 119–22.

Klepinger, L.L. 1992. Innovative approaches to the study of past human health and subsistence strategies. In S.R. Saunders and M.A. Katzenberg (eds), *Skeletal biology of past peoples: research methods*. New York, John Wiley and Sons Ltd, pp. 121–30.

Klepinger, L.L., Kuhn, J.K. and Thomas, J., Jr 1977. Prehistoric dental calculus gives evidence for coca in early coastal Ecuador. *Nature* 269: 506–7.

Knight, B. 1981. History of wound treatment. *Nursing Times* 77(43): 5–8.

Knight, B. 1991. *Forensic pathology.* London, Edward Arnold.

Knüsel, C.J. 2001. Activity-related skeletal change. In V. Fiorato, A. Boylston and C. Knüsel (eds), *Blood red roses: the archaeology of a mass grave from the Battle of Towton AD 1461.* Oxford, Oxbow Books, pp. 103–18.

Knüsel, C.J., Kemp, R.L. and Budd, P. 1995. Evidence for remedial treatment of a severe knee injury from the Fishergate Gilbertine Monastery in the City of York. *J. Archaeological Science* 22: 369–84.

Knüsel, C.J., Roberts, C.A. and Boylston, A. 1996. Brief communication: when Adam delved . . . an activity-related lesion in three human skeletal populations. *Am. J. Phys. Anthrop.* 100: 427–34.

Knüsel, C.J., Göggel, S. and Lucy, D. 1997. Comparative degenerative joint disease of the vertebral column in the Medieval monastic cemetery of the Gilbertine Priory of St Andrew, Fishergate, England. *Am. J. Phys. Anthrop.* 103: 481–95.

Kohn, L.A., Leigh, S.R. and Cheverud, J. 1995. Asymmetric vault modification in Hopi crania. *Am. J. Physical Anthrop.* 98: 173–95.

Kolaridou, A. 1991. Harris lines as an indicator of stress in the post-Medieval population of Tours, France. Unpublished MA dissertation, University of Bradford, Department of Archaeological Sciences.

Kolman, C.J., Centurion-Lara, A., Lukehart, S.A., Owsley, D.W. and Tuross, N. 1999. Identification of *Treponema pallidum subspecies pallidum* in a 200-year-old skeletal specimen. *J. of Infectious Diseases* 180: 2060–3.

Kowal, W.A., Krahn, P.M. and Beattie, O. 1989. Lead levels in human tissues from the Franklin Forensic Project. *Int. J. of Environmental and Analytical Chem.* 35: 119–26.

Krieger, N., Rowley, D.L., Herman, A.A., Avery, B. and Phillips, M.T. 1995. Racism, sexism, and social class: implications for studies of health, disease, and well-being. *Am. J. Preventative Med. Supp.* 9: 82–122.

Krogman, W.M. and Iscan, M.Y. 1986 (eds). *The human skeleton in forensic medicine.* Springfield, Ill., Charles Thomas.

Kumar, S.S., Nasidze, I., Walimbe, S.R. and Stoneking, M. 2000. Brief communication: discouraging prospects for ancient DNA from India. *Am. J. Phys. Anthrop.* 113: 129–33.

Kustár, A. 1999. Facial reconstruction of an artificially distorted skull of the 4th to the 5th century from the site of Mözs. *Int. J. Osteoarchaeology* 9: 325–32.

Lai, P. and Lovell, N.C. 1992. Skeletal markers of occupational stress in the Fur Trade Period: a case study from a Hudson's Bay Company Fur Trade post. *Int. J. Osteoarchaeology* 2: 221–34.

Lallo, J., Armelagos, G.J. and Rose, J.C. 1978. Paleoepidemiology of infectious disease in Dickson Mounds population. *Med. Coll. Va. Quarterly* 14(1): 17–23.

Lambert, J.B., Xue, L. and Buikstra, J.E. 1989. Physical removal of contaminated inorganic material from buried bone. *J. Archaeological Science* 16: 427–36.

Lambert, P.M. 2002. Rib lesions in a prehistoric Puebloan sample from southwestern Colorado. *Am. J. Phys. Anthrop.* 117: 281–92.

Lancaster, H.O. 1990. *Expectations of life: a study on the demography, statistics and history of world mortality.* London, Springer-Verlag.

Larsen, C.S. 1984. Health and disease in prehistoric Georgia: the transition to agriculture. In M.N. Cohen and G.J. Armelagos (eds), *Paleopathology at the origins of agriculture.* London, Academic Press, pp. 367–92.

Larsen, C.S. 1985. Dental modifications and tool use in the Western Great Basin. *Am. J. Phys. Anthrop.* 67: 393–402.

Larsen, C.S. 1994. In the wake of Columbus: native population biology in postcontact Americas. *Yearbook of Phys. Anthrop.* 37: 109–54.

Larsen, C.S. 1995. Biological changes in human populations with agriculture. *Ann. Rev. of Anthrop.* 24: 185–213.

Larsen, C.S. 1997. *Bioarchaeology: interpreting behavior from the human skeleton.* Cambridge, Cambridge University Press.

Larsen, C.S. 1998. Gender, health, and activity in foragers and farmers in the American southeast: implications for social organisation in the Georgia Bight. In A.L. Grauer and P. Stuart-Macadam (eds), *Sex and gender in paleopathological perspective.* Cambridge, Cambridge University Press, pp. 165–87.

Larsen, C.S. and Milner, G. 1994 (eds). *In the wake of contact: biological responses to conquest.* New York, Wiley-Liss.

Larson, T.V. and Koenig, J.Q. 1994. Wood smoke: emissions and noncancer respiratory effects. *Ann. Rev. of Pub. Health* 15: 133–56.

Lascaratos, J. and Assimakopoulos, D. 1999. From the roots of otology: diseases of the ear and their treatment in Byzantine times (AD 324–1453). *Am. J. Otol.* 20(3): 397–402.

Laurence, K.M. 1958. The natural history of hydrocephalus. *Lancet* 29: 1152–4.

Lazenby, R. and Pfeiffer, S. 1993. Effects of a 19th century below-knee amputation and prosthesis on femoral morphology. *Int. J. Osteoarchaeology* 3: 19–28.

Learmonth, A. 1988. *Disease ecology.* Oxford, Basil Blackwell.

Le Page, M. 2002. Gene battle goes south. *New Scientist* 21–28 December: 25.

Lebel, S. and Trinkaus, E. 2002. Middle Pleistocene human remains from the Bau de l'Aubesier. *J. Hum. Evol.* 43(5): 659–85.

Lebel, S., Trinkaus, E., Fawe, M., Fernandez, P., Guérin, C., Richter, D., Mercier, N., Valladas, G. and Wagner, G.A. 2001. Comparative morphology and palaeobiology of Middle Pleistocene human remains from the Bau l'Aubesier, Vaucluse, France. *Proc. Nat. Acad. Sci.* 98(20): 11097–102.

Leden, I., Persson, E. and Persson, O. 1988. Aspects of the history of rheumatoid arthritis in the light of recent osteo-archaeological finds. *Scandinavian J. Rheum.* 37: 341–52.

Ledger, M., Holtzhausen, L.M., Constant, D. and Morris, A.G. 2000. Biomechanical beam analysis of long bones from a late 18th century slave cemetery in Cape Town, South Africa. *Am. J. Phys. Anthrop.* 112: 207–16.

Leestma, J.E. and Kirkpatrick, J.B. 1988. *Forensic Neuropathology.* New York, Raven Press.

Leisen, J.C.C., Duncan, H. and Riddle, J.M. 1991. Rheumatoid erosive arthropathy as seen in macerated (dry) bone specimens. In D.J. Ortner and A. Aufderheide (eds), *Human paleopathology: current syntheses and future options.* Washington, Smithsonian Institution Press, pp. 211–15.

Leitman, T., Porco, T. and Blower, S. 1997. Leprosy and tuberculosis: the epidemiological consequences of cross-immunity. *Am. J. Pub. Health* 87(12): 1923–7.

Levers, R.G.H. and Darling, A.I. 1983. Continuing eruption of some adult human teeth of ancient populations. *Arch. Oral Biol.* 28(5): 401–8.

Levy, H.S. 1967. *Chinese foot binding: the history of a curious erotic custom.* New York, Bell Publishing.

Lewis, B.A. 1998. Prehistoric juvenile rheumatoid arthritis in a precontact Louisiana native population reconsidered. *Am. J. Phys. Anthrop.* 106: 229–48.

Lewis, M.E. 1995. Inflammatory bone changes in leprous skeletons from the Medieval hospital of St James and St Mary Magdalene, Chichester, England. *Int. J. Leprosy* 63(1): 77–85.

Lewis, M.E. 2000. Non-adult palaeopathology: current status and future potential. In M. Cox and S. Mays (eds), *Human osteology in archaeology and forensic science.* London, Greenwich Medical Media, pp. 39–57.

Lewis, M.E. 2002a. Impact of industrialisation: comparative study of child health in four sites from Medieval and Postmedieval England (AD 850–1859). *Am. J. Phys. Anthrop.* 119(3): 211–23.

Lewis, M.E. 2002b. Infant and childhood leprosy: past and present. In C.A. Roberts, M.E. Lewis and K. Manchester (eds), *The past and present of leprosy: archaeological, historical, palaeopathological and clinical approaches*. British Archaeological Reports International Series 1054. Oxford, Archaeopress, pp. 163–70.

Lewis, M.E. 2004. Endocranial lesions in non-adult skeletons: understanding their aetiology. *Int. J. Osteoarchaeology* 14: 82–97.

Lewis, M.E., Roberts, C.A. and Manchester, K. 1995. A comparative study of the prevalence of maxillary sinusitis in Medieval urban and rural populations in Northern England. *Am. J. Phys. Anthrop.* 98(4): 497–506.

Lieverse, A.R. 1999. Diet and the aetiology of dental calculus. *Int. J. Osteoarchaeology* 9: 219–32.

Lilley, J.M., Stroud, G., Brothwell, D.R. and Williamson, M.H. 1994. *The Jewish burial ground at Jewbury*. The archaeology of York. The medieval cemeteries 12/3. York, Council for British Archaeology for York Archaeological Trust.

Lillie, M.C. and Richards, M.P. 2000. Stable isotope analysis and dental evidence of diet at the Mesolithic–Neolithic transition in Ukraine. *J. Archaeological Science* 27: 965–72.

Lillie, M.C., Richards, M.P. and Jacob, K. 2003. Stable isotope analysis of 21 individuals from the Epipalaeolithic cemetery of Vasilyevka III, Dnieper Rapids region, Ukraine. *J. Archaeological Science* 30: 743–52.

Lind, J. 1753. *A treatise on scurvy*. Edinburgh.

Lisowski, F.P. 1967. Prehistoric and early historic trepanation. In D. Brothwell and A.T. Sandison (eds), *Diseases in antiquity*. Springfield, Ill., Charles Thomas, pp. 651–72.

Littleton, J. 1999. Paleopathology of skeletal fluorosis. *Am. J. Phys. Anthrop.* 109: 465–83.

López-Durán, L. 1995. *Traumatología y Ortopedia*. Madrid, Luzán 5.

Loth, S. and Iscan, M.Y. 1989. Morphological assessment of age in the adult: the thoracic region. In M.Y. Iscan (ed.), *Age markers in the human skeleton*. Springfield, Ill., Charles Thomas, pp. 105–35.

Louis, D.S. 1990. Ramazzini and occupational diseases. *J. Hand Surg.* 15: 663–4.

Lovejoy, C.O. and Heiple, K.G. 1981. The analysis of fractures in skeletal populations with an example from the Libben site, Ottawa County, Ohio. *Am. J. Phys. Anthrop.* 55: 529–41.

Lovejoy, C.O., Meindl, R.S., Pryzbeck, T.R. and Mensforth, R.P. 1985. Chronological metamorphosis of the auricular surface of the ilium: a new method for the determination of adult skeletal age. *Am. J. Phys. Anthrop.* 68: 15–28.

Loveland, C.J., Gregg, J.B. and Bass, W.M. 1984. Osteochondritis dissecans from the Great Plains of North America. *Plains Anthrop.* 105: 239–46.

Lovell, N.C. 1990. *Patterns of injury and illness in great apes: a skeletal analysis*. Washington, Smithsonian Institution Press.

Lovell, N.C. 1994. Spinal arthritis and physical stress at Bronze Age Harappa. *Am. J. Phys. Anthrop.* 93: 149–64.

Lovell, N.C. 1997. Trauma analysis in palaeopathology. *Yearbook of Phys. Anthrop.* 40: 139–70.

Lovell, N.C. 2000. Paleopathological description and diagnosis. In M.A. Katzenberg and S.R. Saunders (eds), *Biological anthropology of the human skeleton*. New York, John Wiley and Sons Inc., pp. 217–48.

Lovell, N.C. and Dublenko, A.A. 1999. Further aspects of the Fur Trade life depicted in the skeleton. *Int. J. Osteoarchaeology* 9: 248–56.

Lubell, D., Jackes, M., Schwarcz, H.P., Knyf, M. and Meiklejohn, C. 1994. The Mesolithic–Neolithic transition in Portugal: isotopic and dental evidence of diet. *J. Archaeological Science* 21: 201–16.

Lucier, C.V., VanStone, J.W. and Keats, D. 1971. Medical practices and human anatomical knowledge among the Noatak eskimos. *Ethnology* 19: 251–64.

Lucy, S. 2000. *The Anglo-Saxon way of death*. Stroud, Sutton Publishing.

Luk, K.D.K. 1999. Tuberculosis of the spine in the new millennium. *Eur. J. Spine* 8: 338–45.

Lukacs, J.R. 1989. Dental paleopathology: methods for reconstructing dietary patterns. In M.Y. Iscan and K.A.R. Kennedy (eds), *Reconstruction of life from the skeleton*. New York, Alan Liss, pp. 261–86.

Lukacs, J.R. 1992. Dental paleopathology and agricultural intensification in South Asia: new evidence from Bronze Age Harappa. *Am. J. Phys. Anthrop.* 87: 133–50.

Lukacs, J.R. 1995. The 'caries correction factor': a new method of calibrating dental caries rates to compensate for antemortem loss of teeth. *Int. J. Osteoarchaeology* 5: 151–6.

Lukacs, J.R. and Pastor, R.F. 1988. Activity-induced patterns of dental abrasion in prehistoric Pakistan. *Am. J. Phys. Anthrop.* 76: 377–98.

Lukacs, J.R. and Walimbe, S.R. 1998. Physiological stress in prehistoric India: new data on localized hypoplasia of primary canines linked to climate and subsistence change. *J. Archaeological Science* 25: 571–85.

Lundberg, C. 1980. Dental sinusitis. *Swedish Dental J.* 4: 63–7.

Lurie, M.B. 1955. A pathogenetic relationship between tuberculosis and leprosy: the common denominators in the tissue response to Mycobacteria. In *CIBA Foundation Symposium on Experimental Tuberculosis*. Boston, Little Brown and Co., pp. 340–3.

Ma, K-W. 2000. Hare-lip surgery in the history of traditional Chinese medicine. *Med. Hist.* 44: 489–512.

Maat, G.J.R. 1982. *Scurvy in Dutch whalers buried at Spitsbergen*. Proceedings of the 4th European Meeting of the Paleopathology Association, Middelberg/Antwerpen, pp. 82–93.

Maat, G.J.R. 2004. Scurvy in adults and youngsters: the Dutch experience; a review of the history and pathology of a disregarded disease. *Int. J. Osteoarchaeology* 14: 77–81.

Maat, G.J.R. and Baig, M. 1991. Scanning electron microscopy of fossilised sickle cells. *Int. J. Anthrop.* 5(3): 271–6.

Maat, G.J.R. and Uytterschaut, H.T. 1984. *Microscopic observations on scurvy in Dutch whalers buried at Spitsbergen*. Proceedings of the Paleopathology Association 6th European Meeting, Siena, Italy, pp. 211–16.

Macchiarelli, R. and Bondioli, L. 1994. Linear densitometry and digital image processing of proximal femur radiographs: implications for archaeological and forensic anthropology. *Am. J. Phys. Anthrop.* 93: 109–22.

Macchiarelli, R., Bondioli, L., Censi, L., Hernaez, M.K., Salvadei, L. and Sperduti, A. 1994. Intra- and interobserver concordance in scoring Harris lines: a test on bone sections and radiographs. *Am. J. Phys. Anthrop.* 95: 77–83.

McCurdy, S.A., Ferguson, T.J., Goldsmith, D.F., Parker, J.E. and Schenker, M.B. 1996. Respiratory health of Californian rice farmers. *Am. J. Resp. Critical Care Med.* 153: 1553–9.

McDade, T.W. and Adair, L.S. 2001. Defining the 'urban' in urbanization and health: a factor analysis approach. *Soc. Sci. Med.* 53: 55–70.

MacDonald, B. 1997. *The plague and I*. New York, Akadine Press.

McDougall, A.C. 2002. Leprosy worldwide: current status. In C.A. Roberts, M.E. Lewis and K. Manchester (eds), *The past and present of leprosy: archaeological, historical, palaeopathological and clinical approaches*. British Archaeological Reports International Series 1054. Oxford, Archaeopress, pp. 17–20.

McElroy, A. and Townsend, P.K. 1996. *Medical anthropology in ecological perspective*. 3rd edn, Boulder, Colo., Westview Press.

MacKenzie, D. 2002. Suicide bombs leave a trail of disease. *New Scientist* 27 July: 9.

McKeown, T. and Record, R.G. 1960. Study of population for five years after birth. In *CIBA Foundation Symposium on Congenital Malformations*. Boston, Little Brown and Co., pp. 2–16.

McKinley, J.I. 1996. Hambledon Hill, Dorset: human bone report. Salisbury, Wessex Archaeology. Unpublished.

MacKinney, L. 1957. Medieval surgery. *J. Int. Coll. Surgeons* 27: 393–404.

Madhok, R., Melton III, L.J., Atkinson, E.J., O'Fallon, W.M. and Lewallen, D.G. 1993. Urban vs rural increase in hip fracture incidence: age and sex of 901 cases 1980–89 in Olmsted County, USA. *Acta Orthop. Scand.* 64(5): 543–8.

Malthus, T.R. 1798. *An essay on the principle of population.* London, Printed for J. Johnson.

Manchester, K. 1978a. *Executions in West Yorkshire.* Scient Presentes 5. Leeds, Yorkshire Archaeological Society.

Manchester, K. 1978b. Palaeopathology of a Royalist garrison. *Ossa* 5: 25–33.

Manchester, K. 1980a. Hydrocephalus in an Anglo-Saxon child. *Arch. Cantiana* 96: 77–82.

Manchester, K. 1980b. Jugular vein occlusion in the Bronze Age. *Yorkshire Archaeological J.* 52: 167–9.

Manchester, K. 1982. Spondylolysis and spondylolisthesis in two Anglo-Saxon skeletons. *Paleopathology Assoc. Newsletter* 37: 9–12.

Manchester, K. 1983a. Secondary cancer in an Anglo-Saxon female. *J. Archaeological Science* 10: 475–82.

Manchester, K. 1983b. *The archaeology of disease.* Bradford, Bradford University Press.

Manchester, K. 1991. Tuberculosis and leprosy: evidence for interaction of disease. In D. Ortner and A. Aufderheide (eds), *Human paleopathology: current syntheses and future options.* Washington, Smithsonian Institution Press, pp. 23–35.

Manchester, K. 1994. Rhinomaxillary lesions in syphilis: differential diagnosis. In O. Dutour, G. Pálfi, J. Bérato and J.-P. Brun (eds), *L'origine de la syphilis en Europe: avant ou après 1493?* Toulon, Centre Archéologique du Var, Éditions Errance, pp. 79–80.

Manchester, K. 2002. Infective bone changes of leprosy. In C.A. Roberts, M.E. Lewis and K. Manchester (eds), *The past and present of leprosy: archaeological, historical, palaeopathological and clinical approaches.* British Archaeological Reports International Series 1054. Oxford, Archaeopress, pp. 69–72.

Manchester, K. and Elmhirst, O.E.C. 1980. Forensic aspects of an Anglo-Saxon injury. *Ossa* 7: 179–88.

Manchester, K. and Knüsel, C. 1994. A medieval sculpture of leprosy in the Cistercian Abbaye de Cadouin. *Med. Hist.* 38(2): 204–6.

Mann, R.W. and Owsley, D.W. 1989. Anatomy of uncorrected talipes equinovarus in a fifteenth century American Indian. *J. Am. Podiatric Med. Assoc.* 79(9): 436–40.

Mann, R.W., Sledzik, P.S., Owsley, D.W. and Droulette, M.R. 1990. Radiographic examination of Chinese foot binding. *J. Am. Podiatric Med. Assoc.* 80(8): 405–9.

Mann, R.W., Roberts, C.A, Thomas, M.D. and Davy, D.T. 1991. Pressure erosion of the femoral trochlea, patella baja, and altered patellar surfaces. *Am. J. Phys. Anthrop.* 85: 321–7.

Mansilla, J. and Pijoan, C.M. 1995. Brief communication: a case of congenital syphilis during the colonial period in Mexico City. *Am. J. Phys. Anthrop.* 97: 187–95.

Manzi, G., Sperduit, A. and Passarello, P. 1991. Behavior-induced auditory exostoses in Imperial Roman society: evidence from coeval urban and rural communities near Rome. *Am. J. Phys. Anthrop.* 85: 253–60.

Maples, W.R. 1989. The practical application of age-estimation techniques. In M.Y. Iscan (ed.), *Age markers in the human skeleton.* Springfield, Ill., Charles Thomas, pp. 319–24.

Marchetti, A., Pelligrini, S., Bevilacqua, G. and Fornaciari, G. 1996. K-ras mutation of the tumour of Ferrante I of Aragon, King of Naples. *Lancet* 347: 1272.

Marcombe, D. and Manchester, K. 1990. The Melton Mowbray 'leper head': an historical and medical investigation. *Med. Hist.* 34: 86–91.

Margerison, B. and Knüsel, C. 2002. Paleodemographic comparison of a catastrophic and an attritional death assemblage. *Am. J. Phys. Anthrop.* 119: 134–43.

Mariani-Costantini, R., Catalano, P., di Gennaro, F., di Tota, G. and Angeletti, L.R. 2000. New light on cranial surgery in ancient Rome. *Lancet* 355: 305–7.

Markoe, G. 2000. *The Phoenicians.* London, British Museum Press.

Marota, I., Fornaciari, G. and Rollo, F. 1998. Hepatitis E virus (HEV) RNA sequences in the DNA of Maria of Aragon (1503–68): paleopathological evidence or anthropological marker? *J. Paleopathology* 10(2): 53–8.

Martens, W.J.M. 1998. *Health and climate change.* London, Earthscan Publications Ltd.

Martin, D.L. 1991. Bone histology and paleopathology: methodological considerations. In D. Ortner and A. Aufderheide (eds), *Human paleopathology, current syntheses and future options.* Washington, Smithsonian Institution Press, pp. 55–9.

Martin, D.L. 1997. Violence against women in the La Plata River Valley (AD 1000–1300). In D.L. Martin and D.W. Frayer (eds), *Troubled times: violence and warfare in the past.* Amsterdam, Gordon and Breach, pp. 45–75.

Martin, D.L. and Frayer, D. 1998 (eds). *Troubled times: violence and warfare in the past.* Amsterdam, Gordon and Breach.

Martin, D.L., Goodman, A.H. and Armelagos, G.J. 1985. Skeletal pathologies as indicators of diet. In R.I. Gilbert and J.H. Mielke (eds), *Analysis of prehistoric diets.* London, Academic Press, pp. 227–79.

Martin, D.L., Magennis, A.L. and Rose, J.C. 1987. Cortical bone maintenance in a historic Afro-American cemetery sample from Cedar Grove, Arkansas. *Am. J. Phys. Anthrop.* 74: 255–64.

Mascie-Taylor, C.G.N. and Lasker, G.W. 1988. *Biological aspects of human migration.* Cambridge, Cambridge University Press.

Masnicová, S. and Beňuš, R. 2003. Developmental anomalies in skeletal remains from the Great Moravia and Middle Ages cemeteries at Devin (Slovakia). *Int. J. Osteoarchaeology* 13: 266–74.

Masset, C. 1989. Age estimation on the basis of of cranial sutures. In M.Y. Iscan (ed.), *Age markers in the human skeleton.* Springfield, Ill., Charles Thomas, pp. 71–103.

Massler, M., Schour, J. and Poncher, H. 1941. Development pattern of the child as reflected in the calcification pattern of the teeth. *Am. J. Dis. Child.* 62: 33–67.

Masters, P.M. 1984. Age determination of an Alaskan mummy by amino acid racemization. *Arctic Anthropology* 21: 64–7.

Mather, C.D., Sadana, R., Salomon, J.A. and Murray C.J.L. 2000. Health and life expectancy in 191 countries, 1999. *Lancet* 357: 1685–91.

May, R.L., Goodman, A.H. and Meindl, R.S. 1993. Response of bone and enamel formation to nutritional supplementation and morbidity among malnourished Guatemalan children. *Am. J. Phys. Anthrop.* 92: 37–51.

May, W.P. 1897. Rheumatoid arthritis (osteitis deformans) affecting bones 5500 years old. *Br. Med. J.* 2: 1631–2.

Mays, S. 1985. The relationship between Harris line formation and bone growth and development. *J. Archaeological Science* 12: 207–20.

Mays, S. 1993. Infanticide in Roman Britain. *Antiquity* 67: 883–8.

Mays, S. 1995. The relationship between Harris lines and other aspects of skeletal development in adults and juveniles. *J. Archaeological Science* 22: 511–20.

Mays, S. 1996a. Healed limb amputations in human osteoarchaeology and their causes: a case study from Ipswich. *Int. J. Osteoarchaeology* 6: 101–13.

Mays, S. 1996b. Age-dependent cortical bone loss in a Medieval population. *Int. J. Osteoarchaeology* 6: 144–54.

Mays, S. 1997. A perspective on human osteoarchaeology in Britain. *Int. J. Osteoarchaeology* 7: 600–4.

Mays, S. 1999. A biomechanical study of activity patterns in a Medieval human skeletal assemblage. *Int. J. Osteoarchaeology* 9: 68–73.

Mays, S. 2000. Age-dependent cortical bone loss in women from 18th and early 19th century London. *Am. J. Phys. Anthrop.* 112: 349–61.

Mays, S. 2001. Effects of age and occupation on cortical bone in a group of 18th–19th century British men. *Am. J. Phys. Anthrop.* 116: 34–44.

Mays, S. 2002. Asymmetry in metacarpal cortical bone in a collection of British post-Medieval human skeletons. *J. Archaeological Science* 29: 435–41.

Mays, S. and Cox, M. 2000. Sex determination in skeletal remains. In M. Cox and S. Mays (eds), *Human osteology in archaeology and forensic science*. London, Greenwich Medical Media, pp. 117–30.

Mays, S. and Faerman, M. 2001. Sex identification in some putative infanticide victims from Roman Britain using ancient DNA. *J. Archaeological Science* 28: 555–9.

Mays, S. and Taylor, G.M. 2002. Osteological and biomolecular study of two possible cases of hypertrophic osteoarthropathy from Mediaeval England. *Am. J. Phys. Anthrop.* 29: 1267–76.

Mays, S. and Taylor, G.M. 2003. A first prehistoric case of tuberculosis from Britain. *Int. J. Osteoarchaeology* 13: 189–96.

Mays, S., Strouhal, E., Vyhnánek, L., Nemecková, A. 1996. A case of metastatic carcinoma of Medieval date from Wharram Percy, England. *J. Paleopathology* 8(1): 33–42.

Mays, S., Lees, B. and Stevenson, J.C. 1998. Age-dependent bone loss in the femur in a Medieval population. *Int. J. Osteoarchaeology* 8: 97–106.

Mays, S., Taylor, G.M., Legge, A.J., Young, D.B. and Turner-Walker, G. 2001. Paleopathological and biomolecular study of tuberculosis in a medieval skeletal collection from England. *Am. J. Phys. Anthrop.* 114: 298–311.

Mays, S., Fysh, S. and Taylor, G.M. 2002. Investigation of the link between visceral surface rib lesions and tuberculosis in a Medieval skeletal series from England using ancient DNA. *Am. J. Phys. Anthrop.* 119: 27–36.

Mays, S., Crane-Kramer, G. and Bayliss, A. 2003. Two probable cases of treponemal disease of Medieval date from England. *Am. J. Phys. Anthrop.* 120: 133–43.

Meiklejohn, C., Schentag, C. and Venema, A. 1984. Socioeconomic change and patterns of pathology and variation in the Mesolithic and Neolithic of Western Europe: some suggestions. In M.N. Cohen and G.J. Armelagos (eds), *Paleopathology at the origins of agriculture*. London, Academic Press, pp. 75–100.

Meiklejohn, C., Agelerakis, A., Akkermans, P.A., Smith, P.E.L. and Solecki, R. 1992. Artificial cranial deformation in the proto-Neolithic and Neolithic Near East and its possible origin: evidence from four sites. *Paleorient* 18(2): 83–97.

Meindl, R.S. and Lovejoy, C.O. 1989. Age changes in the pelvis: implications for paleodemography. In M.Y. Iscan (ed.), *Age markers in the human skeleton*. Springfield, Ill., Charles Thomas, pp. 137–68.

Melikian, M. and Waldron, T. 2003. An examination of skulls from two British sites for possible evidence of scurvy. *Int. J. Osteoarchaeology* 13: 207–12.

Mensforth, R.P. and Latimer, B.M. 1989. Hamann–Todd Collection aging studies: osteoporosis fracture syndrome. *Am. J. Phys. Anthrop.* 80: 461–79.

Mensforth, R.P., Lovejoy, C.O., Lallo, H. and Armelagos, G.J. 1978. The role of constitutional factors, diet and infectious disease in the etiology of porotic hyperostosis and periosteal reactions in prehistoric infants and children. *Med. Anthropol.* 2: 1–59.

Merbs, C.F. 1983. *Patterns of activity induced pathology in a Canadian Inuit population*. Archaeological Survey of Canada Paper No. 119. Ottawa, National Museums of Canada.

Merbs, C.F. 1989a. Trauma. In M.Y. Iscan and K.A.R. Kennedy (eds), *Reconstruction of life from the skeleton*. New York, Alan Liss, pp. 161–89.

Merbs, C.F. 1989b. Spondylolysis: its nature and significance. *Int. J. Anthrop.* 4(3): 143–9.

Merbs, C.F. 1992. A New World of infectious disease. *Yearbook of Phys. Anthrop.* 35: 3–42.

Merbs, C.F. 1995. Incomplete spondylolysis and healing: a study of ancient Canadian Eskimo skeletons. *Spine* 20(21): 2328–34.

Merbs, C.F. 1996. Spondylolysis and spondylolisthesis: a cost of being an erect biped or clever adaptation? *Yearbook of Phys. Anthrop.* 39: 201–28.

Merbs, C.F. 2002a. Asymmetrical spondylolysis. *Am. J. Phys. Anthrop.* 119: 156–74.

Merbs, C.F. 2002b. Spondylolysis in Inuit skeletons from Arctic Canada. *Int. J. Osteoarchaeology* 12: 279–90.

Mercer, W. 1964. Then and now: history of skeletal tuberculosis. *J. R. Coll. Surg. Edin.* 9: 243–54.

Merrett, D. and Pfeiffer, S. 2000. Maxillary sinusitis as an indicator of respiratory health in past populations. *Am. J. Phys. Anthrop.* 111: 301–18.

Meyer, K.F. 1964. Evolution of occupational diseases acquired from animals. *Indust. Med. Surg.* 33: 286–95.

Meyers, W., Walsh, G.P., Brown, H.L., Binford, C.H., Imes, G.D., Hadfield, T.L., Schlagel, C.J., Fukunishi, Y., Gerone, P.J., Wolf, R.H., Gormus, B.J., Martin, L.N., Harboe, M., Imaeda, T. 1985. Leprosy in a Mangabey monkey – naturally acquired infection. *Int. J. Leprosy* 53(1): 1–15.

Micozzi, M.S. 1991. Taphonomy and the study of disease in antiquity: the case of cancer. In M. Micozzi (ed.), *Postmortem change in human and animal remains.* Springfield, Ill., Charles Thomas, pp. 91–103.

Miles, A.E.W. 1963. The dentition in the assessment of individual age in skeletal material. In D. Brothwell (ed.), *Dental anthropology.* Oxford, Pergamon Press, pp. 191–209.

Miles, A.E.W. 1989. *An early Christian chapel and burial ground on the Isle of Ensay, Outer Hebrides, Scotland with a study of the skeletal remains.* British Archaeological Reports British Series 212, Oxford, BAR.

Miles, A.E.W. 1994. Non-union of the epiphysis of the acromion in the skeletal remains of a Scottish population of ca. 1700. *Int. J. Osteoarcheology* 4: 149–63.

Miles, A.E.W. 2001. The Miles method of assessing age from tooth wear. *J. Archaeological Science* 28: 973–82.

Miller, E., Ragsdale, B.D. and Ortner, D.J. 1996. Accuracy in dry bone diagnosis: a comment on palaeopathological methods. *Int. J. Osteoarchaeology* 6: 221–9.

Milner, G.R. and Larsen, C.S. 1991. Teeth as artifacts of human behavior: intentional mutilation and accidental modification. In M. Kelley and C.S. Larsen (eds), *Advances in dental anthropology.* New York, Alan Liss, pp. 351–78.

Milner, G.R., Wood, J.W. and Boldsen, J.L. 2000. Palaeodemography. In M.A. Katzenberg and S.R. Saunders (eds), *Biological anthropology of the human skeleton.* New York, Wiley-Liss, pp. 467–97.

Mitchell, P. 2003. Pre-Columbian treponemal disease from 14th century AD Safed, Israel, and implications for the Medieval Eastern Mediterranean. *Am. J. Phys. Anthrop.* 121: 117–24.

Mittler, D.M. and Van Gerven, D.P. 1994. Developmental, diachronic and demographic analysis of cribra orbitalia in the medieval Christian populations of Kulubnarti. *Am. J. Phys. Anthrop.* 93: 287–97.

Mittler, D.M., Van Gerven, D.P., Sheridan, S.G. and Beck, R. 1992. The epidemiology of enamel hypoplasia, cribra orbitalia and non-adult mortality in an ancient Nubian population. In A.H. Goodman and L. Capasso (eds), *Recent contributions to the study of enamel developmental defects.* Journal of Paleopathology Monographic Publications 2, Teramo, Italy, Edigrafital, pp. 143–50.

Miura, H., Araki, Y., Haraguchi, K., Arai, Y. and Umenai, T. 1997. Socioeconomic factors and dental caries in developing countries: a cross-national study. *Soc. Sci. Med.* 44(2): 269–72.

Moggi-Cecchi, J., Pacciani, E. and Pinto-Cisternas, J. 1994. Enamel hypoplasia and age at weaning in 19th century Florence. *Am. J. Phys. Anthrop.* 93: 299–306.

Mogle, P. and Zias, J. 1995. Trephination as a possible treatment for scurvy in a Middle Bronze Age (ca. 2200 BC) skeleton. *Int. J. Osteoarchaeology* 5: 77–81.

Møller, P. and Møller-Christensen, V. 1952. A Mediaeval female skull showing evidence of metastases from a malignant growth. *Acta Path. Microbiol. Scand.* 30: 336–42.

Møller-Christensen, V. 1953. *Ten lepers from Naestved.* Copenhagen, Danish Science Press.

Møller-Christensen, V. 1958. *Bogen om Abelholt Kloster.* Copenhagen, Danish Science Press.

Møller-Christensen, V. 1961. *Bone changes in leprosy.* Copenhagen, Munksgaard.

Møller-Christensen, V. 1967. Evidence of leprosy in earlier peoples. In D.R. Brothwell and A.T. Sandison (eds), *Disease in antiquity*. Springfield, Ill., Charles Thomas, pp. 295–307.

Møller-Christensen, V. 1969a. *A rosary bead as tooth filling in a human mandibular canine tooth: a unique case from the Danish Middle Ages*. 21st International Congress on the History of Medicine, Siena, Italy.

Møller-Christensen, V. 1969b. The history of syphilis and leprosy: an osteo-archaeological approach. *Abbotempo* 1: 20–5.

Møller-Christensen, V. 1978. *Leprosy changes of the skull*. Odense, University Press.

Møller-Christensen, V. and Hughes, D.R. 1966. An early case of leprosy from Nubia. *Man, New Series* 1: 242–3.

Molleson, T. 1989. Seed preparation in the Mesolithic: the osteological evidence. *Antiquity* 63: 356–62.

Molleson, T. and Cox, M. 1993. *The Spitalfields Project, Volume 2: the anthropology: the middling sort*. Council for British Archaeology Research Report 86. York, Council for British Archaeology.

Molnár, E. and Marcsik, A. 2002. Paleopathological evaluation of Hungarian skeletal remains from the 7th–9th centuries AD. *Antropologia Portuguesa* 19: 85–99.

Molnar, S. 1971. Human tooth wear, tooth function and cultural variability. *Am. J. Phys. Anthrop.* 34: 175–90.

Molnar, S. 1972. Tooth wear and culture: a survey of tooth function among some prehistoric populations. *Curr. Anthrop.* 13(5): 511–26.

Molnar, S. and Molnar, I. 1985. Observations of dental diseases among prehistoric populations of Hungary. *Am. J. Phys. Anthrop.* 67: 51–63.

Molto, J.E. 1990. Differential diagnosis of rib lesions: a case study from Middle Woodland, Southern Ontario. *Am. J. Phys. Anthrop.* 83: 439–47.

Molto, J.E. 2002. Leprosy in Roman period skeletons from Kellis 2, Dakhleh, Egypt. In C.A. Roberts, M.E. Lewis and K. Manchester (eds), *The past and present of leprosy: archaeological, historical, palaeopathological and clinical approaches*. British Archaeological Reports International Series 1054. Oxford, Archaeopress, pp. 179–92.

Montgomery, J., Budd, P. and Evans, J. 2000. Reconstructing the lifetime movement of ancient people: a Neolithic case study from southern England. *Eur. J. Archaeology* 3(3): 407–22.

Montgomery, P.Q., Williams, H.O.L., Reading, N. and Stringer, C.B. 1994. An assessment of the temporal bone lesions of the Broken Hill cranium. *J. Archaeological Science* 21: 331–7.

Moodie, R.L. 1923a. *Paleopathology: An introduction to the study of ancient evidence of disease*. Urbana, Ill., University of Illinois Press.

Moodie, R.L. 1923b. *The antiquity of disease*. Chicago, Chicago University Press.

Moodie, R.L. 1927. Injuries to the head among the pre-Columbian Peruvians. *Ann. Medieval History* 9(3): 277–307.

Moore, W.J. and Corbett, E. 1971. Distribution of dental caries in ancient British populations: Anglo-Saxon period. *Caries Res.* 5: 151–68.

Moore, W.J. and Corbett, E. 1973. Distribution of dental caries in British populations: Iron Age, Romano-British and Medieval periods. *Caries Res.* 7: 139–53.

Moore, W.J. and Corbett, E. 1975. Distribution of dental caries in ancient British populations III: the 17th century. *Caries Res.* 9: 163–75.

Morant, G.M. 1931. Study of the recently excavated Spitalfields crania. *Biometrika* 23: 191–248.

Morse, D., Brothwell, D. and Ucko, P. 1964. Tuberculosis in ancient Egypt. *Am. Rev. Resp. Dis.* 90: 524–41.

Morse, D., Dailey, R.C. and Bunn, J. 1974. Prehistoric multiple myeloma. *Bull. New York Acad. Med.* 54: 447–58.

Morse, S.S. 1995. Factors in the emergence of infectious diseases. *Emerging Infectious Diseases* 1(1): 7–15.

Mosekilde, L. 1990. Consequences of the remodelling process for vertebral bone structure: an SEM study (uncoupling of loaded structures). *Bone and Mineral* 10: 13–35.

Motluk, A. 2002. Tough choices. *New Scientist* 16 February: 12–13.

Munizaga, J., Allison, M.J., Gerszten, E. and Klurfeld, D.M. 1975. Pneumoconiosis in Chilean miners of the 16th century. *Bull. New York Acad. Med.* 5(11): 1281–93.

Murphy, E.M. 1996. A possible case of hydrocephalus in a Medieval child from Doonbought Fort, Co. Antrim, Northern Ireland. *Int. J. Osteoarchaeology* 6: 435–42.

Murphy, E.M. 2000. Developmental defects and disability: the evidence from the Iron Age semi-nomadic peoples of Aymyrlyg, south Siberia. In J. Hubert (ed.), *Madness, disability and social exclusion: the archaeology and anthropology of 'difference'*. London, Routledge, pp. 60–80.

Murphy, E.M., Gokhman, I., Christov, Y. and Barkova, L. 2002. Prehistoric Old World scalping: new cases from the cemetery of Aymyrlyg. *Am. J. Archaeology* 106: 1–10.

Murphy, K. 1999. A prehistoric case of polydactyly from the Iron Age site of Simbusenga, Zambia. *Am. J. Phys. Anthrop.* 108: 311–19.

Murphy, M.F., Wainscoat, J. and Colvin, B.T. 2002. Haematological disease. In P. Kumar and M. Clark (eds), *Clinical medicine*. 5th edn, Edinburgh, W.B. Saunders, pp. 405–71.

Murphy, T. 1959. The changing pattern of dentine exposure in human tooth attrition. *Am. J. Phys. Anthrop.* 17: 167–78.

Nathan, H. 1962. Osteophytes of the vertebral column. *J. Bone Joint Surg.* 44A(2): 243–68.

Nelson, D.A., Feingold, M., Bolin, F. and Parfitt, A.M. 1991. Principal components analysis of regional bone density in black and white women: relationship to body size and composition. *Am. J. Phys. Anthrop.* 86: 507–14.

Neri, R. and Lancelloti, L. 2004. Fractures of the lower limbs and their skeletal adaptations: a 20th century example of pre-modern healing. *Int. J. Osteoarchaeology* 14: 60–6.

Nerlich, A.G., Zink, A., Szeimies, U. and Haagedorn, H.G. 2000. Ancient Egyptian prosthesis of the big toe. *Lancet* 356: 2176–9.

Neves, W.A., Barros, A.M. and Costa, M.A. 1999. Incidence and distribution of postcranial fractures in the prehistoric population of San Pedro de Atacama, Northern Chile. *Am. J. Phys. Anthrop.* 109: 253–8.

Novak, S. 2001. Battle-related trauma. In V. Fiorato, A. Boylston and C. Knüsel (eds), *Blood red roses: the archaeology of a mass grave from the Battle of Towton AD 1461*. Oxford, Oxbow Books, pp. 90–102.

Oakberg, K., Levy, T. and Smith, P. 2000. A method for skeletal arsenic analysis applied to the Chalcolithic copper smelting site of Shiqmim, Israel. *J. Archaeological Science* 27: 895–901.

Oakley, K.P., Brooke, W.M.A., Akester, A.R. and Brothwell, D.R. 1959. Contributions on trepanning or trephination in ancient and modern times. *Man* 59: 93–6.

O'Connor, T.P. 2000. *The archaeology of animal bones*. Stroud, Sutton Publishing.

Olsen, S. and Shipman, P. 1994. Cutmarks and perimortem treatment of skeletal remains on the Northern Plains. In D.W. Owsley and R.L. Jantz (eds), *Skeletal biology of the Great Plains: migration, warfare, health and subsistence*. Washington, Smithsonian Institution Press, pp. 377–87.

O'Reilly, L.M. and Daborn, C.J. 1995. The epidemiology of *Mycobacterium bovis* infections in animals and man: a review. *Tubercle and Lung Disease* (Supplement 1): 1–46.

Ortner, D.J. 1979. Disease and mortality in the early Bronze Age people of Bab Edh-Dhra, Jordan. *Am. J. Phys. Anthrop.* 51: 589–98.

Ortner, D.J. 1981. Bone tumors in archeological human skeletons (paleopathology of human bone tumors). In H.E. Kaiser (ed.), *Neoplasms: comparative pathology of growth in animals, plants and man*. Baltimore, Williams and Wilkins, pp. 733–8.

Ortner, D.J. 1984. Bone lesions in a probable case of scurvy from Metlatavik, Alaska. *MASCA J.* 3: 79–81.

Ortner, D.J. 1991. Theoretical and methodological issues in paleopathology. In D. Ortner and A. Aufderheide (eds), *Human paleopathology: current syntheses and future options*. Washington, Smithsonian Institution Press, pp. 5–11.

Ortner, D.J. 1994. Descriptive methods in palaeopathology. In D.W. Owsley and R.L. Jantz (eds), *Skeletal biology in the Great Plains: migration, warfare, health and subsistence*. Washington, Smithsonian Institution Press, pp. 73–80.

Ortner, D.J. 1998. Male–female immune reactivity and its implications for interpreting evidence in human skeletal palaeopathology. In A. Grauer and P. Stuart-Macadam (eds), *Sex and gender in paleopathological perspective*. Cambridge, Cambridge University Press, pp. 79–82.

Ortner, D.J. 2002. Observations on the pathogensis of skeletal disease in leprosy. In C.A. Roberts, M.E. Lewis and K. Manchester (eds), *The past and present of leprosy: archaeological, historical, palaeopathological and clinical approaches*. British Archaeological Reports International Series 1054. Oxford, Archaeopress, pp. 73–80.

Ortner, D.J. 2003. *Identification of pathological conditions in human skeletal remains*. 2nd edn, London, Academic Press.

Ortner, D.J. and Ericksen, M.F. 1997. Bone changes in the human skull probably resulting from scurvy in infancy and childhood. *Int. J. Osteoarchaeology* 7: 212–20.

Ortner, D.J. and Mays, S.A. 1998. Dry bone manifestations of rickets in infancy and childhood. *Int. J. Osteoarchaeology* 8(1): 45–55.

Ortner, D. and Putschar, W.J. 1981. *Identification of pathological conditions in human skeletal remains*. Washington, Smithsonian Institution Press.

Ortner, D.J. and Ribas, C. 1997. Bone changes in a human skull from the early Bronze site of Bab Edh-Dhra', Jordan, probably resulting from scalping. *J. Paleopathology* 9(3): 137–42.

Ortner, D.J. and Utermohle, C.J. 1981. Polyarticular inflammatory arthritis in a pre-Columbian skeleton from Kodiak Island, Alaska, USA. *Am. J. Phys. Anthrop.* 56: 23–31.

Ortner, D.J., Manchester, K. and Lee, F. 1991. Metastatic carcinoma in a leper skeleton from a medieval cemetery in Chichester, England. *Int. J. Osteoarchaeology* 1: 91–8.

Ortner, D.J., Kimmerle, E. and Diez, M. 1999. Probable evidence of scurvy in non-adults from archeological sites in Peru. *Am. J. Phys. Anthrop.* 108: 321–31.

Ortner, D.J., Butler, W., Cafarella, J. and Milligan, L. 2001. Evidence of probable scurvy in non-adults from archeological sites in North America. *Am. J. Phys. Anthrop.* 114: 343–51.

Owsley, D.W. 1994. Warfare in coalescent traditional populations of the Northern Plains. In D.W. Owsley and R.L. Jantz (eds), *Skeletal biology of the Great Plains: migration, warfare, health and subsistence*. Washington, Smithsonian Institution Press, pp. 333–43.

Owsley, D.W. and Mann, R.W. 1990. An American Indian skeleton with clubfoot from the Cabin burial site (A1184), Hemphill County, Texas. *Plains Anthropologist* 35(128): 93–101.

Oyebola, D.D.O. 1980. Yoruba traditional bonesetters: the practice of orthopaedics in a primitive setting in Nigeria. *J. Trauma* 20(4): 312–22.

Ozbay, B., Uzun, K., Arslan, H. and Zehir, I. 2001. Functional and radiological impairment in women highly exposed to indoor biomass fuels. *Respirology* 6(3): 255–8.

Özbek, M. 2001. Cranial deformation in a non-adult sample from Değirmentepe (Chalcolithic, Turkey). *Am. J. Phys. Anthrop.* 115: 238–44.

Pabst, M.A. and Hofer, F. 1998. Deposits of different origin in the lungs of the 5,300 year old Tyrolean Iceman. *Am. J. Phys. Anthrop.* 107: 1–12.

Paget, J. 1877. On a form of chronic inflammation of bones (osteitis deformans). *Transactions of the Medical-Chirurgical Society* 60: 37–64.

Pales, L. 1929. Maladie de Paget préhistorique. *Anthrop. Paris* 39: 263–70.

Pálfi, G. 1991. The first osteoarchaeological evidence of leprosy in Hungary. *Int. J. Osteoarchaeology* 1: 99–102.

Pálfi, G., Dutour, O., Borreani, M., Brun, J.-P. 1992. Pre-Columbian congenital syphilis from the

Late Antiquity in France. *Int. J. Osteoarchaeology* 2: 245–61.

Pálfi, G., Dutour, O., Deák, J. and Hutás, I. 1999. *Tuberculosis: past and present.* Budapest/Szeged, Golden Book Publishers and Tuberculosis Foundation.

Panhuysen, R.G.A.M., Conenen, V. and Bruintjes, T.D. 1997. Chronic maxillary sinusitis in Medieval Maastricht, the Netherlands. *Int. J. Osteoarchaeology* 7: 610–14.

Panter-Brick, C. 2002. Sexual division of labor: energetic and evolutionary scenarios. *Am. J. Hum. Biol.* 14: 627–40.

Panuel, M. 1994. Radiographic manifestations of congenital syphilis. In O. Dutour, G. Pálfi, J. Bérato and J.-P. Brun (eds), *L'origine de la syphilis en Europe: avant ou après 1493?* Toulon, Centre Archéologique du Var, Éditions Errance, pp. 36–40.

Papathanasiou, A. 2003. Stable isotope analysis in Neolithic Greece and possible implications on human health. *Int. J. Osteoarchaeology* 13: 314–24.

Park, K. 1993. Black death. In K. Kiple (ed.), *The Cambridge world history of human disease.* Cambridge, Cambridge University Press, pp. 612–16.

Parker, S., Roberts, C.A. and Manchester, K. 1986. A review of British trepanations with reports on two new cases. *Ossa* 12: 141–57.

Parkhill, J., Wren, B.W., Thomson, N.R., Titball, R.W., Holden, M.T.G. and 30 other authors 2001. Genome sequence of *Yersinia pestis,* the causative agent of plague. *Nature* 413: 523–7.

Pate, F.D. and Hutton, J.T. 1988. Use of soil chemistry data to address post-mortem diagenesis in bone mineral. *J. Archaeological Science* 15: 729–39.

Pathria, M. 1995. Physical injury: spine. In D. Resnick (ed.), *Diagnosis of bone and joint disorders.* 3rd edn, London, W.B. Saunders, pp. 2825–98.

Patrick, P. and Waldron, T. 2003. Congenital absence of the patella in an Anglo-Saxon skeleton. *Int. J. Osteoarchaeology* 13: 147–9.

Paton, D.F. 1984. *Notes on Fractures.* Edinburgh, Churchill Livingstone.

Patterson, K.D. 1993. Meningitis. In K. Kiple (ed.), *The Cambridge world history of human disease.* Cambridge, Cambridge University Press, pp. 875–80.

Patton, M.A. 1987. Genetic aspects of congenital malformations. *Bailliere's Clin. Obstet. Gynaecology* 1(3): 723–5.

Patz, J.A., Epstein, P.R., Burke, T.A. and Balbus, J.M. 1996. Global climate change and emerging infectious diseases. *J. Am. Med. Assoc.* 275(3): 217–23.

Payne, D. 2000. Death keeps Irish doctors guessing. *Brit. Med. J.* 321: 468.

Pearce, D. and Goldblatt, P. 2001 (eds). *United Kingdom Health Statistics.* 2001 edn, London, Her Majesty's Stationery Office.

Pearce, F. 1998. Population bombshell. *New Scientist* 11 July: 1–4.

Pearce, F. 1999. Counting down. *New Scientist* 2 October: 20–1.

Pearce, F. 2002. Mama mia. *New Scientist* 20 July: 38–41.

Pease, A.S. 1940. Some remarks on the diagnosis and treatment of tuberculosis in antiquity. *Isis* 31: 380–93.

Pennington, R. 2001. Hunter-gatherer demography. In C. Panter-Brick, R.H. Layton and P.A. Rowley-Conwy (eds), *Hunter-gatherers: an interdisciplinary perspective.* Cambridge, Cambridge University Press, pp. 170–204.

Perzigian, A.J., Tench, P.A. and Braun, D.J. 1984. Prehistoric health in the Ohio River Valley. In M.N. Cohen and G.J. Armelagos (eds), *Paleopathology at the origins of agriculture.* London, Academic Press, pp. 347–92.

Pfeiffer, S. 1991. Rib lesions and New World tuberculosis. *Int. J. Osteoarchaeology* 1: 191–8.

Pfeiffer, S. 2000. Paleohistology: health and disease. In M.A. Katzenberg and S.R. Saunders (eds), *Biological anthropology of the human skeleton.* New York, Wiley-Liss, pp. 287–302.

Pfeiffer, S. and Crowder, C. 2004. An ill child among mid-Holocene foragers of Southern Africa. *Am. J. Phys. Anthrop.* 123: 23–9.

Pfeiffer, S. and Lazenby, R. 1994. Low bone mass in past and present populations. In H.H. Draper (ed.), *Advances in Nutritional Research 9*. New York, Plenum Press, pp. 35–51.

Philpott, R. 1991. *Burial practices in Roman Britain: a survey of grave treatment and furnishing*. British Archaeological Reports British Series 219. Oxford, Tempus Reparatum.

Pietrusewsky, M. and Douglas, M.T. 2002. *Ban Chiang, a prehistoric village site in northeast Thailand 1: the human skeletal remains*. Philadelphia, University of Pennsylvania, University Museum Monograph 11.

Piggott, S. 1940. A trepanned skull of the Beaker Period from Dorset and the practice of trepanning in prehistoric Europe. *Proc. Prehist. Soc.* 6: 112–33.

Pindborg, J.J. 1970. *Pathology of the dental hard tissues*. Copenhagen, Munksgaard.

Pineda, C., Mansilla, J., Pijoán, C., Fernández, S. and Martínez-Lavín, M. 1998. Radiographs of an ancient mortuary bundle support theory for the New World origin of syphilis. *Am. J. Radiol.* 171: 321–4.

Piperno, D. 1988. *Phytolith analysis: an archaeological and geological perspective*. London, Academic Press.

Pitt, M. 1995. Rickets and osteomalacia. In D. Resnick (ed.), *Diagnosis of bone and joint disorders*. 3rd edn, London, W.B. Saunders, pp. 1885–92.

Polednak, A.P. 1989. *Racial and ethnic differences in disease*. Oxford, Oxford University Press.

Polet, C. and Katzenberg, M.A. 2003. Reconstruction of the diet in a monastic community from the coast of Belgium. *J. Archaeological Science* 30: 525–33.

Polet, C., Dutour, O., Orban, R., Jadin, I. and Louryan, S. 1996. A healed wound caused by a flint arrowhead in a Neolithic human innominate from the Trou Rosette (Furfooz, Belgium). *Int. J. Osteoarchaeology* 6: 414–20.

Pollard, T.M. and Hyatt, S.B. 1999 (eds). *Sex, gender and health*. Cambridge, Cambridge University Press.

Polson, C.J., Gee, D.J. and Knight, B. 1985. *Essentials of forensic medicine*. Oxford, Pergamon Press.

Porter, R. 1997. *The greatest benefit to mankind: a medical history of humanity from antiquity to the present*. London, HarperCollins.

Pounds, N.J.G. 1974. *An economic history of medieval Europe*. London, Longman Group.

Powell, M.L. 1985. The analysis of dental wear and caries for dietary reconstruction. In R.I. Gilbert and J.H. Mielke (eds), *Analysis of prehistoric diets*. London, Academic Press, pp. 307–38.

Powell, M.L. 1988. *Status and health in prehistory: a case study of the Moundville Chiefdom*. Washington, Smithsonian Institution Press.

Power, C. 1992. The spread of syphilis and a possible early case in Waterford. *Archaeology (Ireland)* 6(4): 20–1.

Power, C. and O'Sullivan, V.R. 1992. Rickets in 19th century Waterford. *Archaeology (Ireland)* 6(1): 27–8.

Powlesland, D. 1980. West Heslerton – focus for a landscape project. *Rescue News* 21: 12.

Price, J.L. 1975. The radiology of excavated Saxon and Medieval human remains from Winchester. *Clin. Radiol.* 26: 363–70.

Price, T.D. 1989 (ed.). *The chemistry of prehistoric human bone*. Cambridge, Cambridge University Press.

Price, T.D., Blitz, J., Burton, J. and Ezzo, J.A. 1992. Diagenesis in prehistoric bone: problems and solutions. *J. Archaeological Science*. 19: 513–29.

Price, T.D., Bentley, R.A., Lüning, J., Gronenborn, D. and Wahl, J. 2001. Prehistoric human migration in the Linearbandkeramik of Central Europe. *Antiquity* 75: 593–603.

Prichard, P.D. 1993. A suicide by self-decapitation. *J. For. Sci. Soc.* 38(4): 981–4.

Prince, R.L., Knuiman, M.W. and Gulland, L. 1993. Fracture prevalence in an Australian population. *Aust. J. Pub. Health* 17(2): 124–8.

Privat, K.L., O'Connell, T.C. and Richards, M.P. 2002. Stable isotope analysis of human and faunal remains from the Anglo-Saxon cemetery at Berinsfield, Oxfordshire: dietary and social implications. *J. Archaeological Science* 29: 779–90.

Propst, K.B., Danforth, M.E. and Jacobi, K. 1994. Replicability in scoring enamel hypoplasias: a preliminary report. *Paleopathology Assoc. Newsletter* 87: 11–12.

Pyatt, F.B. and Grattan, J.P. 2001. Some consequences of ancient mining activities on the health of ancient and modern human populations. *J. of Pub. Health Med.* 23(3): 235–6.

Quatrehomme, G. and Iscan, M.Y. 1997. Post-mortem skeletal lesions. *For. Sci. Int.* 89: 155–65.

Quinn, M. and Babb, P. 1999. Cancer trends in England and Wales 1950–99. *Health Statistics Quarterly* 8: 5–19.

Rahtz, P. 1960. Sewerby. *Medieval Archaeology* 4: 134–65.

Ráliš, Z.A. 1981. Epidemic of fractures during period of snow and ice. *Br. Med. J.* 282: 603–5.

Randerson, J. 2002. Tainted talons could leave you with a nasty taste in your mouth. *New Scientist* 27 July: 8.

Ranjit, J.H. and Verghose, A. 1980. Psychiatric disturbances among leprosy patients: an epidemiological study. *Int. J. Leprosy* 48(4): 431–4.

Raoult, D., Aboudharam, G., Crubézy, E., Larrouy, G., Ludes, B. and Drancourt, M. 2000. Molecular identification by 'suicide PCR' of *Yersinia pestis* as the agent of Medieval Black Death. *Proc. Nat. Acad. Sci.* 97(23): 12800–30.

Rappuoli, R. 2002. Why we must pay more. *New Scientist* 31 August: 25.

Rawcliffe, C. 1997. *Medicine and society in later Medieval England.* Stroud, Sutton Publishing.

Reader, R. 1974. New evidence for the antiquity of leprosy in early Britain. *J. Archaeological Science* 1: 205–7.

Reber, V.B. 1999. Blood, coughs and fever: tuberculosis and the working classes of Buenos Aires, Argentina 1885–1915. *Soc. Hist. Med.* 12(3): 73–100.

Reichs, K. 1986a. Forensic implications of skeletal pathology: sex. In K. Reichs (ed.), *Forensic osteology: advances in the identification of human remains.* Springfield, Ill., Charles Thomas, pp. 112–42.

Reichs, K. 1986b. Forensic implications of skeletal pathology: ancestry. In K. Reichs (ed.), *Forensic osteology: advances in the identification of human remains.* Springfield, Ill., Charles Thomas, pp. 196–217.

Reichs, K. 1989. Treponematosis: a possible case from the late prehistoric of North Carolina. *Am. J. Phys. Anthrop.* 79: 289–303.

Reid, A.H., Fanning, T.G., Hultin, J.V. and Taubenberger, J.K. 1999. Origin and evolution of the 1918 'Spanish' influenza virus hemaglutinin gene. *Proc. Nat. Acad. Sci. USA* 96: 1651–6.

Reinhard, K. 1988. Cultural ecology of prehistoric parasitism on the Colorado plateau as evidenced by coprology. *Am. J. Phys. Anthrop.* 82: 145–63.

Reinhard, K. 1990. Archeoparasitology in North America. *Am. J. Phys. Anthrop.* 82: 145–63.

Reinhard, K., Geib, P.R., Callahan, M.M. and Hevly, R.H. 1992. Discovery of colon contents in a skeletonised burial: soil sampling for dietary remains. *J. Archaeological Science* 19: 697–705.

Renfrew, C. and Bahn, P. 1991. *Archaeology: theories, methods and practice.* London, Thames and Hudson.

Resnick, D. 1995a (ed.). *Diagnosis of bone and joint disorders.* 3rd edn, London, W.B. Saunders.

Resnick, D. 1995b. Target area approach to articular disorders: a synopsis. In D. Resnick (ed.), *Diagnosis of bone and joint disorders.* 3rd edn, London, W.B. Saunders, pp. 1757–80.

Resnick, D. and Goergen, T.G. 1995. Physical injury: extraspinal sites. In D. Resnick (ed.), *Diagnosis of bone and joint disorders.* 3rd edn, London, W.B. Saunders, pp. 2693–824.

Resnick, D. and Greenaway, G. 1982. Distal femoral cortical defects, irregularities and excavations. *Radiology* 143: 345–54.

Resnick, D. and Niwayama, G. 1988. *Diagnosis of bone and joint disorders*. 2nd edn, Philadelphia, W.B. Saunders.

Resnick, D. and Niwayama, G. 1995a. Rheumatoid arthritis. In D. Resnick (ed.), *Diagnosis of bone and joint disorders*. 3rd edn, London, W.B. Saunders, pp. 866–970.

Resnick, D. and Niwayama, G. 1995b. Osteomyelitis, septic arthritis, and soft tissue infection: mechanisms and situations. In D. Resnick (ed.), *Diagnosis of bone and joint disorders*. 3rd edn, London, W.B. Saunders, pp. 2325–418.

Resnick, D. and Niwayama, G. 1995c. Enostosis, hyperostosis, and periostitis. In D. Resnick (ed.), *Diagnosis of bone and joint disorders*. 3rd edn, London, W.B. Saunders, pp. 4396–466.

Resnick, D. and Niwayama, G. 1995d. Osteomyelitis, septic arthritis and soft tissue infection: organisms. In D. Resnick (ed.), *Diagnosis of bone and joint disorders*. 3rd edn, London, W.B. Saunders, pp. 2448–558.

Resnick, D. and Niwayama, G. 1995e. Osteoporosis. In D. Resnick (ed.), *Diagnosis of bone and joint disorders*. 3rd edn, London, W.B. Saunders, pp. 1783–853.

Resnick, D. and Niwayama, G. 1995f. Paget's disease. In D. Resnick (ed.), *Diagnosis of bone and joint disorders*. 3rd edn, London, W.B. Saunders, pp. 1923–68.

Resnick, D., Goergen, T.G. and Niwayama, G. 1995. Physical injury: concepts and terminology. In D. Resnick (ed.), *Diagnosis of bone and joint disorders*. 3rd edn, London, W.B. Saunders, pp. 2561–692.

Ribot, I. and Roberts, C.A. 1996. A study of non-specific stress indicators and skeletal growth in two Mediaeval non-adult populations. *J. Archaeological Science* 23: 67–79.

Richards, G.D. 1985. Analysis of a microcephalic child from the Late Period (ca. AD1100–1700) of Central California. *Am. J. Phys. Anthrop.* 68: 343–57.

Richards, G.D. 1995. Brief communication: earliest cranial surgery in North America. *Am. J. Phys.Anthrop.* 98: 203–9.

Richards, G.D. and Anton, S.C. 1991. Craniofacial configuration and postcranial development of a hydrocephalic child (ca. 2500 BC–AD 500): with a review of cases and comment on diagnostic criteria. *Am. J. Phys. Anthrop.* 85: 185–200.

Richards, L.C. 1990. Tooth wear and temporomandibular joint change in Australian aboriginal populations. *Am. J. Phys. Anthrop.* 82: 377–84.

Richards, M.P., Mays, S. and Fuller, B.T. 2002. Stable carbon and nitrogen isotope values of bone and teeth reflect weaning age at the Medieval Wharram Percy site, Yorkshire, UK. *Am. J. Phys. Anthrop.* 118: 205–10.

Richards, P. 1977. *The Mediaeval leper and his northern heirs*. Cambridge, D.S. Brewer.

Riddle, J.M., Duncan, H., Pitchford, W.C., Ellis, B.I., Brennan, T.A. and Fisher, L.J. 1988. Anteroposterior radiographic view of the knee: an unreliable indicator of bone damage. *Clin. Rheumatol.* 7(4): 504–13.

Ridley, D.S. and Jopling, W.H. 1966. Classification of leprosy according to immunity: a five group system. *Int. J. Leprosy* 34: 255–73.

Riojas-Rodriguez, H., Romano-Riquer, S., Santos-Burgoa, C. and Smith, K.R. 2001. Household firewood use and the health of children and women of Indian communities in Chiapas, Mexico. *Int. J. Occupation and Environmental Health* 7(1): 44–53.

Ripamonti, U. 1988. Paleopathology in *A. africanus*: a suggested case of a three million year old prepubertal periodontitis. *Am. J. Phys. Anthrop.* 76: 197–210.

Ritchie, W.A. and Warren, S.L. 1932. The occurrence of multiple bony lesions suggesting myeloma in the skeleton of a pre-Columbian Indian. *Am. J. Roentgenol.* 28: 622–8.

Robb, J. 1997. Intentional tooth removal in Neolithic Italian women. *Antiquity* 71(273): 659–69.

Robb, J., Bigazzi, R., Lazzarini, L., Scarsini, C. and Sonego, F. 2001. A comparison of grave goods and skeletal indicators from Pontecagnano. *Am. J. Phys. Anthrop.* 115(3): 213–22.

Roberts, C.A. 1985. Case report 5: osteochondroma. *Paleopathology Assoc. Newsletter* 50: 7–8.

Roberts, C.A. 1986a. Leprosy and leprosaria in medieval Britain. *MASCA J.* 4(1): 15–21.

Roberts, C.A. 1986b. Leprogenic odontodysplasia. In E. Cruwys and R. Foley (eds), *Teeth and anthropology*. British Archaeological Reports International Series 291. Oxford, BAR, pp. 137–47.

Roberts, C.A. 1987 Case report 9: scurvy. *Paleopathology Assoc. Newsletter* 57: 14–15.

Roberts, C.A. 1988a. Trauma and treatment in British antiquity: an osteoarchaeological study of macroscopic and radiological features of long bone fractures from the Historic period with a comparative study of clinical radiographs, supplemented by contemporary documentary, iconographical and archaeological evidence. Ph.D. thesis, University of Bradford, Department of Archaeological Sciences.

Roberts, C.A. 1988b. A rare case of dwarfism from the Roman Period. *J. Paleopathology* 2(1): 9–21.

Roberts, C.A. 1989. Trauma and treatment in British antiquity: a radiographic study. In J. Tate and E. Slater (eds), *Proceedings of the Science and Archaeology Conference, Glasgow, September, 1987*. British Archaeological Reports British Series 196. Oxford, BAR, pp. 339–59.

Roberts, C.A. 1991. Trauma and treatment in the British Historic period: a design for multidisciplinary research. In D. Ortner and A. Aufderheide (eds), *Human paleopathology: current syntheses and future options*. Washington, Smithsonian Institution Press, pp. 225–40.

Roberts, C.A. 1994. Treponematosis in Gloucester, England: a theoretical and practical approach to the pre-Columbian theory. In O. Dutour, G. Pálfi, J. Bérato and J.-P. Brun (eds), *L'origine de la syphilis en Europe: avant ou après 1493?* Toulon, Centre Archéologique du Var, Éditions Errance, pp. 101–8.

Roberts, C.A. 1999. Rib lesions and tuberculosis: the current state of play. In G. Pálfi, O. Dutour, J. Deák and I. Hutás (eds), *Tuberculosis: past and present*. Budapest/Szeged, Golden Book Publishers and Tuberculosis Foundation, pp. 311–16.

Roberts, C.A. 2000a. Did they take sugar: the use of skeletal evidence in the study of disability in past populations. In J. Hubert (ed.), *Madness, disability and social exclusion: the archaeology and anthropology of difference*. London, Routledge, pp. 46–59.

Roberts, C.A. 2000b. Trauma in biocultural perspective: past, present and future work in Britain. In M. Cox and S. Mays (eds), *Human osteology in archaeology and forensic science*. London, Greenwich Medical Media, pp. 337–56.

Roberts, C.A. 2000c. Infectious disease in biocultural perspective: past, present and future work in Britain. In M. Cox and S. Mays (eds), *Human osteology in archaeology and forensic science*. London, Greenwich Medical Media, pp. 145–62.

Roberts, C.A. 2002. The antiquity of leprosy in Britain: the skeletal evidence. In C.A. Roberts, M.E. Lewis and K. Manchester (eds), *The past and present of leprosy: archaeological, historical, palaeopathological and clinical approaches*. British Archaeological Reports International Series 1054. Oxford, Archaeopress, pp. 213–21.

Roberts, C.A. and Buikstra, J.E. 2003. *The bioarchaeology of tuberculosis: a global view on a reemerging disease*. Gainesville, Fla, University Press of Florida.

Roberts, C.A. and Cox, M. 2003. *Health and disease in Britain: prehistory to the present day*. Stroud, Sutton Publishing.

Roberts, C.A. and Lewis, M.E. 2002. Ecology and infectious disease in Britain from prehistory to the present: the case of respiratory infections. In P. Bennike, E. Bodzsár and C. Susanne (eds), *Ecological aspects of past human settlements in Europe: European Anthropological Association Biennial Yearbook*. Budapest, pp. 179–92.

Roberts, C.A. and McKinley, J. 2003. Review of trepanations in British antiquity focusing on funerary context to explain their occurrence. In R. Arnott, S. Finger and C.U.M. Smith (eds), *Trepanation: history, discovery, theory*. Lisse, Swets and Zeitlinger, pp. 56–78.

Roberts, C.A. and Manchester, K. 1995. *The archaeology of disease*. 2nd edn, Stroud, Sutton Publishing.

Roberts, C.A. and Wakely, J. 1992. Microscopical findings associated with the diagnosis of osteoporosis in palaeopathology. *Int. J. Osteoarchaeology* 2: 23–30.

Roberts, C.A., Lucy, D. and Manchester, K. 1994. Inflammatory lesions of ribs: an analysis of the Terry Collection. *Am. J. Phys. Anthrop.* 95(2): 169–82.

Roberts, C.A., Lewis, M.E. and Boocock, P. 1998. Infectious disease, sex and gender: the complexity of it all. In A. Grauer and P. Stuart-Macadam (eds), *Sex and gender in paleopathological perspective.* Cambridge, Cambridge University Press, pp. 93–113.

Roberts, C.A., Lewis, M.E. and Manchester, K. 2002. *The past and present of leprosy: archaeological, historical, palaeopathological and clinical approaches.* British Archaeological Reports International Series 1054. Oxford, Archaeopress.

Roberts, C.A., Knüsel, C. and Race, L. 2004. A foot deformity from a Romano-British cemetery at Gloucester, England and the current evidence for *Talipes* in palaeopathology. *Int. J. Osteoarchaeology* 14(5): 389–403.

Roberts, D.F., Fujiki, N. and Torizuka, K. 1992. *Isolation, migration and health.* Cambridge, Cambridge University Press.

Roberts, R.S. 1971. The use of literary and documentary evidence in the history of medicine. In E. Clarke (ed.), *Modern methods in the history of medicine.* London, Athlone Press, pp. 36–57.

Robling, A.G. and Stout, S.D. 2000. Histomorphometry of human cortical bone: applications to age estimation. In M.A. Katzenberg and S.R. Saunders (eds), *Biological anthropology of the human skeleton.* New York, Wiley-Liss, pp. 187–213.

Roches, E., Blondiaux, J., Cotton, A., Chastanet, P. and Flipo, R-M. 2002. Microscopic evidence for Paget's Disease in two osteoarchaeological samples from early Northern France. *Int. J. Osteoarchaeology* 12: 229–34.

Rogers, J. 2000. The palaeopathology of joint disease. In M. Cox and S. Mays (eds), *Human osteology in archaeology and forensic science.* London, Greenwich Medical Media, pp. 163–82.

Rogers, J. and Waldron, T. 1995. *A field guide to joint disease in archaeology.* Chichester, John Wiley and Sons.

Rogers, J. and Waldron, T. 2001. DISH and the monastic way of life. *Int. J. Osteoarchaeology* 11: 357–65.

Rogers, J., Waldron, T., Dieppe, P. and Watt, I. 1987. Arthropathies in palaeopathology: the basis of classification according to most probable cause. *J. Archaeological Science* 14: 179–93.

Rogers, J., Watt, I. and Dieppe, P. 1990. Comparison of visual and radiographic defects of bony changes at the knee joint. *Br. Med. J.* 300: 367–8.

Rogers, L. 1949. Meningeomas in Pharoah's people. *Br. J. Surg.* 36: 423–4.

Rollo, F., Luciani, S., Canpa, A. and Marota, I. 2000. Analysis of bacterial DNA in the skin and muscle of the Tyrolean Iceman offers new insight into the mummification process. *Am. J. Phys. Anthrop.* 111: 211–19.

Rollo, F., Ubaldi, M., Ermini, L. and Marota, I. 2002. Ötzi's last meals: DNA analysis of the intestinal content of the Neolithic glacier mummy from the Alps. *Proc. Nat. Acad. Sci.* 99(20): 12594–99.

Rose, B.S. 1975. Gout in the Maoris. *Seminars in Arthritis and Rheumatism* 5: 121–45.

Rose, J.C., Anton, S.C., Aufderheide, A.C., Eisenberg, L., Gregg, J.B., Neiburger, E.J. and Rothschild, B. 1991. *Skeletal database recommendations.* Detroit, Palaeopathology Association.

Rose, J.C., Green, T.J. and Green, V.D. 1996. NAGPRA is forever: osteology and the repatriation of skeletons. *Ann. Rev. Anthrop.* 25: 81–103.

Rosen, G. 1993. *A history of public health.* Baltimore, Md, Johns Hopkins University Press.

Rothschild, B.M. and Heathcote, G.M. 1993. Characterization of the skeletal manifestations of the treponemal disease yaws as a population phenomenon. *Clin. Infect. Dis.* 17: 198–203.

Rothschild, B.M. and Heathcote, G.M. 1995. Characterization of gout in a skeletal population sample: presumptive diagnosis in a Micronesian sample. *Am. J. Phys. Anthrop.* 98: 519–25.

Rothschild, B.M. and Rothschild, C. 1994. Distinguished: syphilis, yaws and bejel on the basis of differences in their respective osseous impact. In O. Dutour, G. Pálfi, J. Bérato and J.-P. Brun (eds), *L'origine de la syphilis en Europe: avant ou après 1493?* Toulon, Centre Archéologique du Var, Éditions Errance, pp. 68–71.

Rothschild, B.M. and Rothschild, C. 1995. Comparison of radiologic and gross examination for detection of cancer in defleshed skeletons. *Am. J. Phys. Anthrop.* 96: 357–63.

Rothschild, B.M. and Rothschild, C. 1998. Recognition of hypertrophic osteoarthropathy in skeletal remains. *J. Rheumatology* 25(11): 2221–7.

Rothschild, B.M., Woods, R.J. and Ortel, W. 1990. Rheumatoid arthritis 'in the buff': erosive arthritis in defleshed bones. *Am. J. Phys. Anthrop.* 82: 441–9.

Rothschild, B.M., Hershkovitz, I., Dutour, O., Latimer, B., Rothschild, C. and Jellema, L.M. 1997. Recognition of leukemia in skeletal remains: report and comparison of two cases. *Am. J. Phys. Anthrop.* 102: 481–96.

Rothschild, B.M., Hershkovitz, I. and Dutour, O. 1998. Clues potentially distinguishing lytic lesions of multiple myeloma from those of metastatic carcinoma. *Am. J. Phys. Anthrop.* 105: 241–50.

Rowling, J.T. 1961. Pathological changes in mummies. *Proc. R. Soc. Med.* 54: 409–15.

Ruff, C.B. 2000. Biomechanical analyses of archaeological skeletons. In M.A. Katzenberg and S.R. Saunders (eds), *Biological anthropology of the human skeleton.* New York, Wiley-Liss, pp. 71–102.

Ruff, C.B. and Jones, H.H. 1981. Bilateral asymmetry in cortical bone of the humerus and tibia. *Hum. Biol.* 53: 69–86.

Ruffer, M.A. 1910. Remarks on the histology and pathological anatomy of Egyptian mummies. *Cairo Scientific J.* 4: 1–5.

Ruffer, M.A. 1911. On arterial lesions found in Egyptian mummies. *J. Path. Bact.* 15: 453–62.

Ruffer, M.A. 1913. On pathological lesions found in Coptic bodies. *J. Path. Bact.* 18:149–62.

Ruffer, M.A. and Willmore, J.G. 1914. Note on a tumour of the pelvis dating from Roman times (AD 250) and found in Egypt. *J. Path. Bact.* 18: 480–4.

Ryan, A.S. 1997. Iron-deficiency anaemia in infant development: implications for growth, cognitive development, resistance to infection, and iron supplementation. *Yearbook Phys. Anthrop.* 40: 25–62.

Sager, P. 1969. *Spondylosis cervicalis: a pathological and osteoarchaeological study.* Copenhagen, Munksgaard.

Sahlin, Y. 1990. Occurrence of fractures in a defined population: a 1 year study. *Injury* 21: 158–60.

Sallares, R. and Gomzi, S. 2001. Biomolecular archaeology of malaria. *Ancient Biomolecules* 3: 195–212.

Salo, W.L., Aufderheide, A., Buikstra, J. and Holcomb, T.A. 1994. Identification of *Mycobacterium tuberculosis* DNA in a pre-Columbian mummy. *Proc. Nat. Acad. Sci. USA* 91: 2091–4.

Saluja, G., Fitzpatrick, K., Bruce, M. and Cross, J. 1986. Schmorl's Nodes (intravertebral herniations of intervertebral disc tissue) in two historic British populations. *J. Anat.* 145: 87–96.

Sandford, M.K. and Weaver, D. 2000. Trace element research in anthropology: new perspectives and challenges. In M.A. Katzenberg and S.R. Saunders (eds), *Biological anthropology of the human skeleton.* New York, Wiley-Liss, pp. 329–50.

Sandford, M.K., Van Gerven, D.P. and Meglen, R.R. 1983. Elemental hair analysis: new evidence on the etiology of cribra orbitalia in Sudanese Nubia. *Hum. Biol.* 55(4): 831–44.

Sandison, A.T. 1968. Pathological changes in the skeletons of earlier populations due to acquired disease and difficulties in their interpretation. In D.R. Brothwell (ed.), *Skeletal biology of earlier human populations.* New York, Pergamon Press, pp. 205–43.

Sandison, A.T. 1980a. Diseases in ancient Egypt. In A. Cockburn and E. Cockburn (eds), *Mummies, disease and ancient cultures.* Cambridge, Cambridge University Press, pp. 29–44.

Sandison, A.T. 1980b. Notes on some skeletal changes in pre-European contact Australian Aborigines. *J. Hum. Evol.* 9: 45–7.

Sandison, A.T. 1981. Diseases in the ancient world. In P.P. Anthony and R.N.M. Macsween (eds), *Recent advances in histopathology*. Edinburgh, Churchill Livingstone, pp. 1–18.

Santini, A., Land, M. and Raab, G.M. 1990. The accuracy of simple ordinal scoring of tooth attrition in age assessment. *For. Sci. Int.* 48: 175–84.

Santos, A.L. 2000. A skeletal picture of tuberculosis: macroscopic, radiological, biomolecular, and historical evidence from the Coimbra Identified Skeletal Collection. Ph.D. Thesis, Department of Anthropology, University of Coimbra, Portugal.

Santos, A.L. and Roberts, C.A. 2001. A picture of tuberculosis in young Portuguese people in the early 20th century: a multidisciplinary study of the skeletal and historical evidence. *Am. J. Phys. Anthrop.* 115: 38–49.

Sarnat, B.G. and Schour, J. 1941. Enamel hypoplasia (chronic enamel aplasia) in relation to systemic disease: a chronologic, morphologic and etiologic classification. *J. Am. Dental Assoc.* 28: 1989–2000.

Sartoris, D. 1995. Developmental dysplasia of the hip. In D. Resnick (ed.), *Diagnosis of bone and joint disorders*. 3rd edn, London, W.B. Saunders, pp. 4067–94.

Sattienspiel, L. 1990. Modeling the spread of infectious disease in human populations. *Yearbook Phys. Anthrop.* 33: 245–76.

Sauer, N. 1992. Forensic anthropology and the concept of race: if races don't exist, why are forensic anthropologists so good at identifying them? *Soc. Sci. Med.* 34(2): 107–11.

Saunders, S.R. 1989. Non-metric skeletal variation. In M.Y. Iscan and K.A.R. Kennedy (eds), *Reconstruction of life from the skeleton*. New York, Alan Liss, pp. 95–108.

Saunders, S.R. 1992. Non-adult skeletons and growth-related studies. In S.R. Saunders and M.A. Katzenberg (eds), *Skeletal biology of past peoples: research methods*. New York, Wiley-Liss, pp. 1–20.

Saunders, S.R. 2000. Non-adult skeletons and growth-related studies. In M.A. Katzenberg and S.R. Saunders (eds), *Biological anthropology of the human skeleton*. New York, Wiley-Liss, pp. 135–61.

Saunders, S.R. and Herring, A. 1995 (eds). *Grave reflections: portraying the past through cemetery studies*. Toronto, Canadian Scholars Press Inc.

Saunders, S.R., De Vito, C. and Katzenberg, M.A. 1997. Dental caries in 19th century Upper Canada. *Am. J. Phys. Anthrop.* 104: 71–87.

Sbonias, K. 1999. Investigating the interface between regional survey, historical demography and palaeodemography. In J. Bintliff and K. Sbonias (eds), *Reconstructing past population trends in Mediterranean Europe*. Oxford, Oxbow Books, pp. 219–43.

Schamall, D., Teschler-Nicola, M., Kainberger, F., Tangl, S., Brandstätter, F., Patzak, B., Muhsil, J. and Plenk, H. Jr. 2003. Changes in trabecular bone structure in rickets and osteomalacia: the potential of a medico-historical collection. *Int. J. Osteoarchaeology* 13: 282–8.

Schell, L.M. 1997. Culture as stressor: a revised model of biocultural interaction. *Am. J. Phys. Anthrop.* 102: 67–77.

Schell, L.M. and Czerwinski, S.A. 1998. Environmental health, social inequality and biological differences. In S.S. Strickland and P.S. Shetty (eds), *Human biology and social inequality*. Cambridge, Cambridge University Press, pp. 114–31.

Scheuer, L. and Black, S. 2000a. Development and ageing of the juvenile skeleton. In M. Cox and S. Mays (eds), *Human osteology in archaeology and forensic science*. London, Greenwich Medical Media, pp. 9–21.

Scheuer, L. and Black, S. 2000b. *Developmental juvenile osteology*. Cambridge, Cambridge University Press.

Schmidt, D., Hummel, S. and Herrmann, B. 2003. Brief communication: multiplex X/Y-PCR improves sex identification in a DNA analysis. *Am. J. Phys. Anthrop.* 121: 337–41.

Schmitt, A., Murail, P., Cunha, E. and Rougé, D. 2002. Variability of the pattern of aging on the human skeleton: evidence from bone indicators and implications on age at death estimation. *J. For. Sci.* 47(6): 1203–9.

Schultz, B. 1985. *Art and anatomy in Renaissance Italy.* Ann Arbor, Mich., UMI Research Press.

Schultz, M. 1979. Diseases of the ear region in early and prehistoric populations. *J. Hum. Evol.* 8(6): 575–80.

Schultz, M. 1994. Comparative histopathology of syphilitic lesions in prehistoric and historic human bones. In O. Dutour, G. Pálfi, J. Bérato and J.-P. Brun (eds), *L'origine de la syphilis en Europe: avant ou après 1493?* Toulon, Centre Archéologique du Var, Éditions Errance, pp. 63–7.

Schultz, M. 2001. Paleohistology of bone: a new approach to the study of ancient diseases. *Yearbook of Phys. Anthrop.* 44: 106–47.

Schultz, M. and Roberts, C.A. 2002. Diagnosis of leprosy in skeletons from an English later Medieval hospital using histological analysis. In C.A. Roberts, M.E. Lewis and K. Manchester (eds), *The past and present of leprosy: archaeological, historical, palaeopathological and clinical approaches.* British Archaeological Reports International Series 1054. Oxford, Archaeopress, pp. 89–104.

Schutkowksi, H., Schultz, M. and Holzgraefe, M. 1996. Fatal wounds in a late Neolithic double inhumation: a probable case of meningitis following trauma. *Int. J. Osteoarchaeology* 6: 179–84.

Schwartz, J.H., Brauer, J. and Gordon-Larsen, P. 1995. Brief communication: Tigaran (Point Hope, Alaska) tooth drilling. *Am. J. Phys. Anthrop.* 97: 77–82.

Scott, E.C. 1979. Dental scoring technique. *Am. J. Phys. Anthrop.* 51: 213–18.

Scott, G.R. and Turner, C.G. 1997. *The anthropology of modern human teeth.* Cambridge, Cambridge University Press.

Scott-Clark, C. and Levy, A. 2003. Spectre orange. *Guardian: Weekend* 29 March: 20–7

Scrimshaw, S.C.M. 1984. Infanticide in human populations: societal and individual concerns. In G. Hausfater and S. Blaffer (eds), *Infanticide: comparative and evolutionary perspectives.* New York, Aldine Publishing Company, pp. 441–4.

Scrimshaw, N.S. 2000. Iron deficiency. In A.H. Goodman, D.L. Dufour and G.H. Pelto (eds), *Nutritional anthropology: biocultural perspectives on food and nutrition.* London, Mayfield Publishing Company, pp. 252–8.

Sealy, J. 2000. Body tissue chemistry and palaeodiet. In D.R. Brothwell and A.M. Pollard (eds), *Handbook of archaeological sciences.* Chichester, John Wiley and Sons Ltd, pp. 269–79.

Sealy, J., Armstrong, R. and Schrire, C. 1995. Beyond lifetime averages: tracing life histories through isotopic analysis of different calcified tissues from archaeological human skeletons. *World Archaeology* 69: 290–300.

Šefčáková, A., Strouhal, E., Nemecková, A., Thurzo, M. and Stassíková-Stukovská, D. 2001. Case of metastatic carcinoma from end of the 8th-early 9th century Slovakia. *Am. J. Phys. Anthrop.* 116: 216–29.

Selye, H. 1950. *Stress.* Montreal, Medical Publishers.

Sevitt, S. 1981. *Bone repair and fracture healing in man.* Edinburgh, Churchill Livingstone.

Shaheen, M.A.E., Badr, A.A., Al-Khudairy, N., Khan, F.A. and Sabet, N. 1990. Patterns of accidental fractures and dislocations in Saudi Arabia. *Injury* 21: 347–50.

Shaw, J.L. and Sakellarides, H. 1967. Radial nerve paralysis associated with fractures of the humerus: a review of 45 cases. *J. Bone Joint Surg.* 49A(5): 899–902.

Shaw, M., Orford, S., Brimblecombe, N. and Dorling, D. 2000. Widening inequality between 160 regions of 15 European countries in the early 1990s. *Soc. Sci. Med.* 50: 1047–58.

Shipley, M., Black, C.M., Compston, J. and O'Gradaigh, D. 2002. Rheumatology and bone disease. In P. Kumar and M. Clark (eds), *Clinical medicine.* Edinburgh, W.B. Saunders, pp. 511–86.

Short, C.L. 1974. The antiquity of rheumatoid arthritis. *Arthritis and Rheumatism* 17(3): 193–205.

Sibbison, J.B. 1990. More about fluoride. *Lancet* 336: 737.

Sigerist, H.E. 1951. *A history of medicine Volume 1: primitive and archaic medicine.* New York, Oxford University Press.

Sjøvold, T., Swedborg, I. and Diener, I. 1974. A pregnant woman from the Middle Ages with exostosis multiplex. *Ossa* 1: 3–22.

Skinsnes, O.K. 1980. Leprosy in archaeologically recovered bamboo book in China. *Int. J. Leprosy* 48: 333.

Skinsnes, O.K. and Chang, P.H.C. 1985. Understanding of leprosy in ancient China. *Int. J. Leprosy* 53(2): 289–307.

Sledzik, P. and Barbian, L. 1997. Healing following cranial trauma. Paper presented at the Annual Meeting of the Paleopathology Association, 1–2 April, St Louis, Missouri.

Sledzik, P. and Bellantoni, N. 1994. Brief communication: bioarcheological and biocultural evidence for the New England vampire folk belief. *Am. J. Phys. Anthrop.* 94: 269–74.

Smith, B.E. 1995. *The emergence of agriculture.* New York, Scientific American Library.

Smith, B.H. 1984. Patterns of molar wear in hunter-gatherers and agriculturists. *Am. J. Phys. Anthrop.* 63: 39–56.

Smith, M.O. 2003. Beyond palisades: the nature and frequency of late Prehistoric deliberate violent trauma in the Chickamauga Reservoir of East Tennessee. *Am. J. Phys. Anthrop.* 121: 303–18.

Smith, P. and Kahila, G. 1992. Identification of infanticide in archaeological sites: a case study from the late Roman–early Byzantine periods at Ashkelon, Israel. *J. Archaeological Science* 19: 667–75.

Smrčka, V., Kuželka, V. and Melková, J. 2003. Meningioma probable reason for trephination. *Int. J. Osteoarchaeology* 13: 325–30.

Snow, C.E. 1943. Two prehistoric Indian dwarf skeletons from Moundville. *Alabama Museum of Natural History Museum Papers* 21: 1–90.

Soares, D. and Desar, N. 1995. Hand wounds in leprosy patients. *Leprosy Rev.* 66: 235–8.

Sofaer Deverenski, J.R. 2000. Sex differences in activity-related osseous change in the spine and the gendered division of labor at Ensay and Wharram Percy, UK. *Am. J. Phys. Anthrop.* 111: 333–54.

Sorg, M.H., Andrews, R.P. and Iscan, M.Y. 1989. Radiographic ageing in the adult. In M.Y. Iscan (ed.), *Age markers in the human skeleton.* Springfield , Ill., Charles C. Thomas, pp. 169–93.

Soulié, R. 1980. Un cas de métastases craniennes de carcinome datant du Bronze ancien; typologie des lésions: observations paléopathologiques analogues en Europe Centrale et Occidentale. In *Proceedings of the 3rd European Paleopathology Association Meeting, Caen, France, 1980*, Paris, Paleopathology Association, pp. 239–53.

Spigelman, M. and Donoghue, H.D. 2002. The study of ancient DNA answers a palaeopathological question. In C.A. Roberts, M.E. Lewis and K. Manchester (eds), *The past and present of leprosy: archaeological, historical, palaeopathological and clinical approaches.* British Archaeological Reports International Series 1054. Oxford, Archaeopress, pp. 293–6.

Spindler, K. 1994. *The man in the ice.* London, Weidenfeld and Nicolson.

Sreevatasan, H. 1993. Leprosy and arthropods. *Indian J. Leprosy* 65(2): 189–200.

Srinivasan, H. and Dharmendra. 1978. Deformities in leprosy (general considerations). In Dharmendra (ed.), *Leprosy.* Bombay, Kothari Medical Publishing House, pp. 197–204.

Standen, V.G. and Arriaza, B. 2000. Trauma in the preceramic coastal populations of Northern Chile: violence or occupational hazards. *Am. J. Phys. Anthrop.* 112: 239–49.

Standen, V.G., Arriaza, B.T. and Santoro, C.M. 1997. External auditory exostosis in prehistoric Chilean populations: a test of the cold water hypothesis. *Am. J. Phys. Anthrop.* 103: 119–29.

Stead, I.M., Bourke, J.E. and Brothwell, D. 1986. *Lindow man: the body in the bog.* London, Guild Publishing.

Stead, W.W. 2000. What's in a name: confusion of *Mycobacterium tuberculosis* and *Mycobacterium bovis* in ancient DNA analysis. *Paleopathology Assoc. Newsletter* 110: 13–16.

Steckel, R.H. 1995. Stature and the standard of living. *J. Economic Literature* 33: 1903–40.

Steckel, R.H. and Rose, J.C. 2002 (eds). *The backbone of history: health and nutrition in the Western Hemisphere.* Cambridge, Cambridge University Press.

Steckel, R.H., Sciulli, P.W. and Rose, J.C. 2002. A health index from skeletal remains. In R.H. Steckel and J.C. Rose (eds), *The backbone of history: health and nutrition in the Western Hemisphere.* Cambridge, Cambridge University Press, pp. 61–93.

Steele, J. 2000. Skeletal indicators of handedness. In M. Cox and S. Mays (eds), *Human osteology in archaeology and forensic science.* London, Greenwich Medical Media, pp. 307–23.

Steinbock, R.T. 1976. *Paleopathological diagnosis and interpretation.* Springfield, Ill., Charles Thomas.

Steinbock, R.T. 1993. Rickets and ostomalacia. In K. Kiple (ed.), *The Cambridge world history of human disease.* Cambridge, Cambridge University Press, pp. 978–80.

Stephan, R.M. 1966. Effects of different types of human foods on dental health in experimental animals. *J. Dent. Res.* 45: 1551–61.

Stevens, G.C. and Wakely, J. 1993. Diagnostic criteria for identification of seashell as a trephination implement. *Int. J. Osteoarchaeology* 3: 167–76.

Stewart, T.D. 1958. Stone age skull surgery: a general review with emphasis on the New World. *Smithsonian Inst. Ann. Rep.* 1957: 461–91.

Stewart, T.D. 1976. Non-union of fractures in antiquity, with descriptions of five cases from the New World involving the forearm. In S. Jarcho (ed.), *Essays on the history of medicine.* New York, New York Academy of Medicine, pp. 396–412.

Stewart, T.D. and Spoehr, A. 1967. Evidence on the palaeopathology of yaws. In D. Brothwell and A.T. Sandison (eds), *Diseases in antiquity.* Springfield, Ill., Charles Thomas, pp. 307–19.

Steyn, M. and Henneberg, M. 1995. Pre-Columbian presence of treponemal disease: a possible case from Iron Age southern Africa. *Curr. Anthrop.* 36(5): 869–73.

Stini, W.A. 1985. Growth rates and sexual dimorphism. In R.I. Gilbert and J.H. Mielke (eds), *Analysis of prehistoric diets.* London, Academic Press, pp. 191–226.

Stini, W.A. 1990 'Osteoporosis': etiologies, prevention and treatment. *Yearbook of Phys. Anthrop.* 33: 151–94.

Stini, W.A. 1995. Osteoporosis in biocultural perspective. *Ann. Rev. Anthrop.* 24: 397–421.

Stinson, S. 1985. Sex differences in environmental sensitivity during growth and development. *Yearbook of Phys. Anthrop.* 28: 123–47.

Stirland, A. 1986. A possible correlation between os acromiale in the burials from the *Mary Rose.* In *Proceedings of the 5th European Meeting of the Paleopathology Association, Siena, Italy, 1986,* pp. 327–34.

Stirland, A. 1991a. Pre-Columbian treponematosis in Medieval Britain. *Int. J. Osteoarchaeology* 1(1): 39–49.

Stirland, A. 1991b. Paget's disease (osteitis deformans): a classic case? *Int. J. Osteoarchaeology* 1: 173–7.

Stirland, A. 1994. Evidence for pre-Columbian treponematosis in Medieval Europe. In O. Dutour, G. Pálfi, J. Bérato and J.-P. Brun (eds), *L'origine de la syphilis en Europe: avant ou après 1493?* Toulon, Centre Archéologique du Var, Éditions Errance, pp. 109–15.

Stirland, A. 2000. *Raising the dead: the skeleton crew of Henry VIII's great ship, the Mary Rose.* Chichester, John Wiley.

Stirland, A. and Waldron, T. 1997. Evidence for activity-related markers in the vertebrae of the crew of the *Mary Rose. J. Archaeological Science* 24: 329–35.

Stodder, A.L.W. 1994. Bioarcheological investigations of protohistoric Pueblo health and demography. In C.S. Larsen and G.R. Milner (eds), *In the wake of contact: biological responses to contact.* New York, Wiley-Liss, pp. 97–107.

Stone, A.C. 2000. Ancient DNA from skeletal remains. In M.A. Katzenberg and S.R. Saunders (eds), *Biological anthropology of the human skeleton.* New York, Wiley-Liss, pp. 351–71.

Stone, A.C., Milner, G.R., Paabo, S. and Stoneking, M. 1996. Sex determination of ancient human skeletons using DNA. *Am. J. Phys. Anthrop.* 99: 231–8.

Stone, J.L. and Miles, M.L. 1990. Skull trepanation among the early Indians of Canada and the United States. *Neurosurgery* 26(6): 1015–20.

Strassman, B.I. and Dunbar, R.I.M. 1999. Human evolution and disease: putting the Stone Age in perspective. In S.C. Stearns (ed.), *Evolution in health and disease*. Oxford, Oxford University Press, pp. 91–101.

Stroud, G. and Kemp, R. 1993. *Cemeteries of St Andrew, Fishergate*. The archaeology of York. The medieval cemeteries 12/2. York, Council for British Archaeology for York Archaeological Trust.

Strouhal, E. 1976. Tumors in the remains of ancient Egyptians. *Am. J. Phys. Anthrop.* 45: 613–20.

Strouhal, E. 1994. Malignant tumors in the Old World. *Paleopathology Assoc. Newsletter* 85: 1–5.

Stuart-Macadam, P. 1985. Porotic hyperostosis: representative of a childhood condition. *Am. J. Phys. Anthrop.* 66: 391–8.

Stuart-Macadam, P. 1987. A radiographic study of porotic hyperostosis. *Am. J. Phys. Anthrop.* 74: 511–20.

Stuart-Macadam, P. 1989a. Porotic hyperostosis: relationship between orbital and vault lesions. *Am. J. Phys. Anthrop.* 80: 187–93.

Stuart-Macadam, P. 1989b. Nutritional deficiency disease: a survey of scurvy, rickets and iron deficiency anaemia. In M.Y. Iscan and K.A.R. Kennedy (eds), *Reconstruction of life from the skeleton*. New York, Alan Liss, pp. 201–22.

Stuart-Macadam, P. 1991. Anemia in Roman Britain: Poundbury Camp. In H. Bush and M. Zvelebil (eds), *Health in past societies: biocultural interpretations of human skeletal remains in archaeological contexts*. British Archaeological Reports International Series 567. Oxford, Tempus Reparatum, pp. 101–13.

Stuart-Macadam, P. 1992. Anemia in past human populations. In P. Stuart-Macadam and S.K. Kent (eds), *Diet, demography and disease: changing perspectives on anemia*. New York, Aldine De Gruyter, pp. 151–70.

Stuart-Macadam, P. 1998. Iron deficiency anemia: exploring the difference. In A. Grauer and P. Stuart-Macadam (eds), *Sex and gender in paleopathological perspective*. Cambridge, Cambridge University Press, pp. 45–63.

Stuart-Macadam, P. and Dettwyler, K.A. 1995 (eds). *Breastfeeding: biocultural perspectives*. New York, Aldine De Gruyter.

Sture, J. 2002. Biocultural perspectives on birth defects in late Medieval rural and urban populations in Northern England. Unpublished Ph.D. thesis, Department of Archaeology, University of Durham.

Sugiyama, L.S. 2004. Illness, injury, and disability among Shiwiar forager-horticulturists: implications of health-risk buffering for the evolution of human life history. *Am. J. Phys. Anthrop.* 123: 371–89.

Sumner, D.R., Morbeck, M. and Lobick, J.T. 1989. Apparent age-related bone loss among adult female Gombe chimpanzees. *Am. J. Phys. Anthrop.* 79: 225–34.

Sussman, R.W. 1973. Child transport, family size, and increase in human population during the Neolithic. *Curr. Anthrop.* 14(5): 285–9.

Suzuki, T. 1987. Paleopathological study on a case of osteosarcoma. *Am. J. Phys. Anthrop.* 74: 309–18.

Swabe, J. 1999. *Animals, disease and human society*. London, Routledge.

Swedlund, A.C. and Armelagos, G.J. 1990 (eds). *Disease in populations in transition: anthropological and epidemiological perspectives*. New York, Bergin and Garvey.

Swerdlow, A., Doll, R. and dos Santos Silva, I. 1997. Time trends in cancer incidence and mortality in England and Wales. In J. Charlton and M. Murphy (eds), *The health of adult Britain 1841–1994*. Volume 2. London, HMSO, pp. 30–59.

Tanner, J.M. 1978. *Foetus into man: physical growth from conception to maturity*. Cambridge, Mass., Harvard University Press.

Tayles, N. 1996. Anemia, genetic diseases, and malaria in prehistoric mainland Southeast Asia. *Am. J. Phys. Anthrop.* 101: 11–27.

Tayles, N. 1999. *The excavation of Khok Phanom Di: a prehistoric site in Central Thailand. Volume 5: The People.* London, Society of Antiquaries.

Tayles, N., Dommett, K. and Nelsen, K. 2000. Agriculture and dental caries: the case of rice in prehistoric Southeast Asia. *World Archaeology* 32(1): 68–83.

Taylor, G.M., Widdison, S., Brown, I.N. and Young, D. 2000. A Mediaeval case of lepromatous leprosy from 13th–14th century Orkney, Scotland. *J. Archaeological Science* 27: 1133–8.

Taylor, M., Rutland, P. and Molleson, T. 1997. A sensitive polymerase chain reaction method for the detection of *Plasmodium species* in ancient human remains. *Ancient Biomolecules* 1: 192–203.

Taylor, S.E. 1995 (ed.). *Health psychology.* 3rd edn, New York, McGraw-Hill Inc.

Teaford, M.F. 1991. Dental microwear: what can it tell us about diet and dental function? In M. Kelley and C.S. Larsen (eds), *Advances in dental anthropology.* New York, Alan Liss, pp. 341–56.

Teaford, M.F. and Lytle, J.D. 1996. Brief communication: diet-induced changes in rates of human tooth microwear: a case study involving stone-ground maize. *Am. J. Phys. Anthrop.* 100: 143–7.

Thoen, C.O. and Steele, J.H. 1995 (eds). *Mycobacterium bovis infection in animals and humans.* Ames, Iowa State University Press.

Thomas, F.D., Kassab, J.Y. and Jones, B.M. 1995. Fluoridation in Anglesey 1993: a clinical study of dental caries in 5-year-old children who had experienced sub-optimal fluoridation. *Br. Dent. J.* 178: 55–9.

Thompson, D.D. and Cowen, K.S. 1984. Age at death and bone biology of the Barrow mummies. *Arctic Anthrop.* 21: 83–8.

Tillier, A.-M., Arensburg, B., Duday, H. and Vandermeersch, B. 2001. Brief communication: an early case of hydrocephalus: the Middle Paleolithic Qafzeh child (Israel). *Am. J. Phys. Anthrop.* 114: 166–70.

Tkocz, I. and Bierring, F. 1984. A medieval case of metastasizing carcinoma with multiple osteosclerotic bone lesions. *Am. J. Phys. Anthrop.* 65: 373–80.

Torres-Rouff, C. 2003. Oral implications of labret use: a case from pre-Columbian Chile. *Int. J. Osteoarchaeology* 13: 247–51.

Trembly, D. 1995. On the antiquity of leprosy in Western Micronesia. *Int. J. Osteoarchaeology* 5: 377–84.

Trevor, J.C. 1950. Notes on the human remains of Romano-British date from Norton, Yorkshire. In P. Corder (ed.), *Roman Pottery at Norton, East Yorkshire.* Roman Malton and District Report 7, Leeds, Roman Antiquities Committee of the Yorkshire Achaeological Society, pp. 39–40.

Trinkhaus, E. 1983. *Shanidar Neanderthals.* London, Academic Press.

Trinkhaus, E. 1985. Pathology and posture of the La Chapelle-Aux-Saints Neandertal. *Am. J. Phys. Anthrop.* 67: 19–41.

Trotter, M. 1970. Estimation of stature from intact long limb bones. In T.D. Stewart (ed.), *Personal identification in mass disasters.* Washington, National Museum of Natural History, Smithsonian Institution, pp. 71–83.

Truman, R.W., Kumaresan, J.A., McDonough, C.M., Job, C.K. and Hastings, R.C. 1991. Seasonal and spatial trends in the detectability of leprosy in wild armadillos. *Epidemiology and Infection* 106: 549–60.

Tucker, B.K., Hutchinson, D.L., Gilliland, M.F.G., Charles, T.M., Daniel, H.J. and Wolfe, L.D. 2001. Microscopic characteristics of hacking trauma. *J. For. Sci.* 46(2): 234–40.

Turkel, S.J. 1989. Congenital abnormalities in skeletal populations. In M.Y. Iscan and K.A.R. Kennedy (eds), *Reconstruction of life from the skeleton.* New York, Alan Liss, pp. 109–27.

Turner, C. 1993. Cannibalism in Chaco Canyon: the charnel pit excavated in 1926 at Small House Ruin by Frank H.H. Roberts Jr. *Am. J. Phys. Anthrop.* 91: 421–39.

Turner, G. and Anderson, T. 2003. Marked occupational dental abrasion from Medieval Kent. *Int. J. Osteoarchaeology* 13: 168–72.

Turner, T. 2002. Changes in biological anthropology: results of the 1998 American Association of Physical Anthropologists membership survey. *Am. J. Phys. Anthrop.* 118: 111–16.

Tyrrell, A. 2000. Skeletal non-metric traits and the assessment of inter- and intra-population diversity: past problems and future potential. In M. Cox and S. Mays (eds), *Human osteology in archaeology and forensic science.* London, Greenwich Medical Media, pp. 289–306.

Tyson, R.A. 1997 (ed). *Human paleopathology and related subjects: an international bibliography.* San Diego, Museum of Man.

Ubaldi, M., Luciani, S., Marota, I., Fornaciari, G., Cano, R.J. and Rollow, F. 1998. Sequence analysis of bacterial DNA in the colon of an Andean mummy. *Am. J. Phys. Anthrop.* 107: 285–95.

Ubelaker, D. 1979. Skeletal evidence for kneeling in prehistoric Ecuador. *Am. J. Phys. Anthrop.* 51: 679–85.

Ubelaker, D. 1989. *Human skeletal remains: excavation, analysis and interpretation.* Washington, Taraxacum Press.

Ubelaker, D. 1992. Hyoid fracture and strangulation. *J. For. Sci.* 37(5): 1216–22.

Ubelaker, D. and Adams, B.J. 1995. Differentiation of perimortem and post-mortem trauma using taphonomic indicators. *J. For. Sci.* 40(3): 509–12.

Ucko, P. 1969. Ethnoarchaeological interpretations of funerary remains. *World Archaeology* 1: 262–90.

Umbelino, C., Cunha, E. and Silva, A.M. 1996. A possible case of poliomyelitis in a Portuguese skeleton dated from the 15th century. In A. Pérez-Pérez (ed.), *Salud, Enfermedad Y Muserte en el Pasado Consucuencìas biológicas del esters y la patología.* Fundación Uriach 1838, pp. 229–35.

Urteaga, O. and Pack, G.T. 1966. On the antiquity of melanoma. *Cancer* 19: 607–10.

Valentin, F. and d'Errico, F. 1995. Brief communication: skeletal evidence of operations on cadavers from Sens (Yonne, France) at the end of the 15th century. *Am. J. Phys. Anthrop.* 98: 375–90.

Van Beek, G.C. 1983. *Dental morphology: an illustrated guide.* Bristol, P.S.G. Wright.

Vaughan, V.C. and MacKay, R.J. 1975. *Textbook of paediatrics.* Philadelphia, W.B. Saunders.

Verano, J.W., Anderson, L.S. and Franco, R. 2000. Foot amputation by the Moche of ancient Peru: osteological evidence and archaeological context. *Int. J. Osteoarchaeology* 10: 177–88.

Vernon-Roberts, B. and Pirie, C.J. 1973. Healing trabecular microfractures in the bodies of lumbar vertebrae. *Ann. Rheum. Dis.* 32: 406–12.

Villa, P., Bouville, C., Courtin, J., Helmer, D., Mahieu, E., Shipman, P., Belluomini, P. and Branca, M. 1986. Cannibalism in the Neolithic. *Science* 233: 431–6.

Vincent, V. and Gutierrez Perez, M.C. 1999. The agent of tuberculosis. In G. Pálfi, O. Dutour, J. Deák and I. Hutás (eds), *Tuberculosis: past and present.* Budapest/Szeged, Golden Book Publishers and Tuberculosis Foundation, pp. 139–43.

Vogel, F. 1970. ABO blood groups and disease. *Am. J. Hum. Gen.* 22: 464–75.

Vrebos, J. 1986. Cleft lip surgery in Anglo-Saxon Britain: The Leech Book (circa AD 920). *Plast. Reconstr. Surg.* 77: 850–3.

Vreeland, J.M. and Cockburn, A. 1980. Mummies of Peru. In A. Cockburn and E. Cockburn (eds), *Mummies, disease and ancient cultures.* Cambridge, Cambridge University Press, pp. 135–74.

Vuorinen, H.S., Tapper, U. and Mussalo-Rauhama, H. 1990. Trace and heavy metals in infants, analysis of long bones from Ficana, Italy, 8th–6th century BC. *J. Archaeological Science* 17: 237–54.

Wacher, J. 2000. *A portrait of Roman Britain.* London, Routledge.

Wakely, J. and Young, I. 1995. A Medieval wrist injury fracture of the hook of the hamate bone. *J. Paleopathology* 7(1): 51–6.

Wakely, J., Manchester, K. and Roberts, C. 1991. Scanning electron microscopy of rib lesions. *Int. J. Osteoarchaeology* 1: 185–9.

Wakely, J., Anderson, T. and Carter, A. 1995. A multidisciplinarian case study of prostatic (?) carcinoma from Mediaeval Canterbury. *J. Archaeological Science* 22: 469–77.

Wakely, J., Strouhal, E., Vyhnánek, L. and Nemeckova, A. 1998. Case of a malignant tumour from Abingdon, Oxfordshire. *J. Archaeological Science* 25: 949–55.

Waldron, T. 1985. DISH at Merton Priory: evidence for a 'new' occupational disease. *Br. Med. J.* 291: 1762–3.

Waldron, T. 1987a. The relative survival of the human skeleton: implications for palaeopathology. In A Boddington, A.N. Garland and R.C. Janaway (eds), *Death, decay and reconstruction: approaches to archaeology and forensic science.* Manchester, Manchester University Press, pp. 55–64.

Waldron, T. 1987b. Lytic lesions in a skull: a problem in diagnosis. *J. Paleopathology* 1(1): 5–14.

Waldron, T. 1989. The effects of urbanisation on human health. In D. Serjeantson and T. Waldron (eds), *Diet and crafts in towns: the evidence of animal remains from the Roman to the post-Medieval periods.* British Archaeological Reports British Series 199. Oxford, BAR, pp. 55–73.

Waldron, T. 1993a. The distribution of osteoarthritis of the hands in a skeletal population. *Int. J. Osteoarchaeology* 3: 213–18.

Waldron, T. 1993b. The health of the adults. In T. Molleson and M. Cox (eds), *The Spitalfields Project, Volume 2: the anthropology: the middling sort.* Council for British Archaeology Research Report 86. York, Council for British Archaeology, pp. 67–89.

Waldron, T. 1994. *Counting the dead: the epidemiology of skeletal populations.* New York, Wiley.

Waldron, T. 1995. Changes in the distribution of osteoarthritis over historical time. *Int. J. Osteoarchaeology* 5: 385–9.

Waldron, T. 1996. What was the prevalence of malignant disease in the past? *Int. J. Osteoarchaeology* 6: 463–70.

Waldron, T. 1997a. Osteoarthritis of the hip in past populations. *Int. J. Osteoarchaeology* 7: 186–9.

Waldron, T. 1997b. A nineteenth century case of carcinoma of the prostate, with a note on the early history of the disease. *Int. J. Osteoarchaeology* 7: 241–7.

Waldron, T. 1998. An unusual cluster of meningiomas? *Int. J. Osteoarchaeology* 8: 213–17.

Waldron, T. 2000. The study of the human remains from Nubia: the contribution of Grafton Elliot Smith and his colleagues to palaeopathology. *Med. Hist.* 44: 363–88.

Waldron, T. and Cox, M. 1989. Occupational arthropathy: evidence from the past. *Br. J. Industrial Med.* 46: 420–2.

Waldron, T. and Rogers, J. 1991. Inter-observer variation in coding osteoarthritis in human skeletal remains. *Int. J. Osteoarchaeology* 1: 49–56.

Waldron, T. and Rogers, J. 1994. Rheumatoid arthritis in an English post-Medieval skeleton. *Int. J. Osteoarchaeology* 4: 165–7.

Walker, E.G. 1983. Evidence for prehistoric cardiovascular disease of syphilitic origin on the Northern Plains. *Am. J. Phys. Anthrop.* 60: 499–503.

Walker, P.L. 1986. Porotic hyperostosis in a marine-dependent Californian Indian population. *Am. J. Phys. Anthrop.* 69: 345–54.

Walker, P.L. 1989. Cranial injuries as evidence of violence in prehistoric Southern California. *Am. J. Phys. Anthrop.* 80: 313–23.

Walker, P.L. 1995. Problems of preservation and sexism in sexing: some lessons from historical collections for palaeodemographers. In S. Saunders and A. Herring (eds), *Grave reflections: portraying the past through cemetery studies.* Toronto, Canadian Scholars Press, pp. 31–47.

Walker, P.L. 1997. Wife beating, boxing and broken noses: skeletal evidence for the cultural patterning of violence. In D.L. Martin and D.W. Frayer (eds), *Troubled times: violence and warfare in the past.* Amsterdam, Gordon and Breach, pp. 145–79.

Walker, P.L. and Cook, D. 1998. Brief communication: gender and sex: *vive la différence. Am. J. Phys. Anthrop.* 106: 255–9.

Walker, P.L. and Hollimon, S.E. 1989. Changes in osteoarthritis with the development of a maritime economy among southern Californian Indians. *Int. J. Anthrop.* 4(3): 171–83.

Walker, P.L., Dean, G. and Shapiro, P. 1991. Estimating age from tooth wear in archaeological populations. In M. Kelley and C.S. Larsen (eds), *Advances in dental anthropology.* New York, Wiley Liss, pp. 169–78.

Walker, P.L., Cook, D.C. and Lambert, P.M. 1997. Skeletal evidence for child abuse: a physical anthropological perspective. *J. For. Sci.* 42(2): 196–207.

Walker, R., Parsche, F., Bierbrier, M. and McKerrow, J.H. 1987. Tissue identification and histologic study of six lung specimens from Egyptian mummies. *Am. J. Phys. Anthrop.* 72: 43–8.

Wapler, U., Crubézy, E. and Schultz, M. 2004. Is cribra orbitalia synonymous with anemia? Analysis and interpretation of cranial pathology in Sudan. *Am. J. Phys. Anthrop.* 123: 333–9.

Warren, H.V., Delavault, R.E. and Cross, O.H. 1967. Possible correlations between geology and some disease patterns. *Ann. New York Acad. Sci.* 136(22): 657–710.

Weaver, D. 1998. Osteoporosis in the bioarchaeology of women. In A. Grauer and P. Stuart-Macadam (eds), *Sex and gender in paleopathological perspective.* Cambridge, Cambridge University Press, pp. 27–44.

Webb, S. 1988. Two possible cases of trephination from Australia. *Am. J. Phys. Anthrop.* 75: 541–8.

Website 1. http://www.who.int/lep/stat2002/global02.htm (accessed 1 June 2005).

Website 2. http://www.global.sbs.ohio-state.edu (accessed 7 June 2005).

Weiner, A.S. 1970. Blood groups and disease. *Am. J. Human Genetics* 22: 476–83.

Weinstein, R.S., Simmons, D.J. and Lovejoy, C.O. 1981. Ancient bone disease in a Peruvian mummy revealed by quantitative skeletal histomorphometry. *Am. J. Phys. Anthrop.* 54: 321–6.

Weiss, D.L. and Møller-Christensen, V. 1971a. An unusual case of tuberculosis in a mediaeval leper. *Danish Med. Bull.* 18: 11–14.

Weiss, D.L. and Møller-Christensen, V. 1971b. Leprosy, echinococcosis and amulets: a study of a Mediaeval Danish inhumation. *Med. Hist.* 15(3): 260–7.

Weiss, E. 2003a. Effects of rowing on humeral strength. *Am. J. Phys. Anthrop.* 121: 293–302.

Weiss, E. 2003b. Understanding muscle markers: aggregation and construct validity. *Am. J. Phys. Anthrop.* 121: 230–40.

Weiss, K.M. 1993. *Genetic variation and human disease: principles and evolutionary approaches.* Cambridge, Cambridge University Press.

Welch, M. 1992. *Anglo-Saxon England.* London, Batsford/English Heritage.

Wells, C. 1962. Three cases of aural pathology of Anglo-Saxon date. *J. Laryng. Otol.* 76: 931–3.

Wells, C. 1963. Ancient Egyptian pathology. *J. Laryng. Otol.* 77(3): 261–5.

Wells, C. 1964a. *Bones, bodies and disease.* London, Thames and Hudson.

Wells, C. 1964b. The study of ancient disease. *Surgo* 32(1): 3–7.

Wells, C. 1964c. Chronic sinusitis with alveolar fistulae of Mediaeval date. *J. Laryng. Otol.* 78(3): 320–2.

Wells, C. 1964d. Two medieval cases of malignant disease. *Br. Med. J.* 1064: 1611–12.

Wells, C. 1965. Osteogenesis imperfecta from an Anglo-Saxon burial ground at Burgh Castle, Suffolk. *Med. Hist.* 9: 88–9.

Wells, C. 1967. Pseudopathology. In D. Brothwell and A.T. Sandison (eds), *Diseases in antiquity.* Springfield, Ill., Charles Thomas, pp. 5–19.

Wells, C. 1974a. Osteochondritis dissecans in ancient British skeletal material. *Med. Hist.* 18(4): 365–9.

Wells, C. 1974b. The results of 'bone setting' in Anglo-Saxon times. *Med. Biol. Ill.* 24: 215–20.

Wells, C. 1976a. Fractures of the heel bones in early and prehistoric times. *The Practitioner* 217: 294–8.

Wells, C. 1976b. Romano-British pathology. *Antiquity* 50: 53–5.

Wells, C. 1977. Disease of the maxillary sinus in antiquity. *Med. Biol. Ill.* 27: 173–8.

Wells, C. 1978. A medieval burial of a pregnant woman. *The Practitioner* 221: 442–4.

Wells, C. 1982. The human remains. In A. McWhirr, L. Viner and C. Wells (eds), *Romano-British cemeteries at Cirencester*. Cirencester, Excavations Committee, pp. 135–202.

Wells, C. and Woodhouse, N. 1975. Paget's disease in an Anglo-Saxon. *Med. Hist.* 19(4): 396–400.

Wenham, S. 1987. Anatomical interpretations of Anglo-Saxon weapon injuries. In *Weapons and warfare in Anglo-Saxon England*. Oxford University Committee for Archaeology Monograph 21, pp. 123–39.

White, C.D. 1996. Sutural effects of fronto-occipital cranial modification. *Am. J. Phys. Anthrop.* 100: 397–410.

White, C.D. and Armelagos, G.J. 1997. Osteopenia and stable isotope ratios in bone collagen of Nubian female mummies. *Am. J. Phys. Anthrop.* 103: 185–99.

White, C.D., Healy, P.F. and Schwarcz, H.P. 1993. Intensive agriculture, social status, and Maya diet at Pacbitun, Belize. *J. Anthrop. Res.* 49: 347–75.

White, C.D., Spence, M.W., Stuart-Williams, H.L.Q. and Schwarcz, H.P. 1998. Oxygen isotopes and the identification of geographical origins: the Valley of Oaxaca versus the Valley of Mexico. *J. Archaeological Science* 25: 643–55.

White, T.D. 1992. *Prehistoric cannibalism at Mancos. 5MTUMR-2346*. Princeton, Princeton University Press.

White, T.D., DeGusta, D., Richards, G.D. and Baker, S.D. 1997. Brief communication: prehistoric dentistry in the American Southwest: a drilled canine from Sky Aerie, Colorado. *Am. J. Phys. Anthrop.* 103: 409–14.

White, W. 1988. *The cemetery of St Nicholas Shambles*. London, Museum of London and the London and Middlesex Archaeological Society.

Whittaker, D.K. 1993. Oral health. In T. Molleson and M. Cox (eds), *The Spitalfields Project, Volume 2: the anthropology: the middling sort*. Council for British Archaeology Research Report 86. York, Council for British Archaeology, pp. 49–65.

Whittaker, D.K. 2000. Ageing from the dentition. In M. Cox and S. Mays (eds), *Human osteology in archaeology and forensic science*. London, Greenwich Medical Media, pp. 83–99.

Whittaker, D.K., Molleson, T., Daniel, A.T., Williams, J.T., Rose, P. and Resteghini, R. 1985. Quantitative assessment of tooth wear, alveolar crest height and continuing eruption in a Romano-British population. *Arch. Oral Biol.* 30(6): 493–501.

Wienker, C.W. and Wood, J.F. 1987. Osteological individuality indicative of migrant citrus laboring. *J. For. Sci.* 33(2): 562–7.

Wiggins, R., Boylston, A. and Roberts, C.A. 1993. Report on the human skeletal remains from Blackfriars, Gloucester (19/91). Unpublished.

Wilbur, A.K., Buikstra, J.E. and Stojanowski, C. 2002. Mycobacterial disease in North America: an epidemiological test of Chaussinand's cross-immunity hypothesis. In C.A. Roberts, M.E. Lewis and K. Manchester (eds), *The past and present of leprosy: archaeological, historical, palaeopathological and clinical approaches*. British Archaeological Reports International Series 1054. Oxford, Archaeopress, pp. 247–58.

Wiley, A.S. and Pike, I.L. 1998. An alternative method for assessing early mortality in contemporary populations. *Am. J. Phys. Anthrop.* 107: 315–30.

Wilkinson, C. and Neave, R. 2003. The reconstruction of a face showing a healed wound. *J. Archaeological Science* 30: 1343–8.

Wilkinson, L. 1993. Brucellosis. In K. Kiple (ed.), *The Cambridge world history of human disease*. Cambridge, Cambridge University Press, pp. 625–8.

Wilkinson, R.G. 1997. Violence against women: raiding and abduction in prehistoric Michigan. In D.L. Martin and D.W. Frayer (eds), *Troubled times: violence and warfare in the past*. Amsterdam, Gordon and Breach, pp. 21–43.

Willey, P. and Scott, D.D. 1996. 'The bullets buzzed like bees': gunshot wounds in skeletons from the Battle of the Little Bighorn. *Int. J. Osteoarchaeology* 6: 15–27.

Williamson, M.A., Johnston, C.A., Symes, S.A. and Schultz, J.J. 2003. Interpersonal violence between 18th century native Americans and Europeans in Ohio. *Am. J. Phys. Anthrop.* 122: 113–22.

Willis, R.A. 1973. *The spread of tumors in the human body.* London, Butterworth.

Wilson, C.S. 1985. Staples and calories in Southeast Asia: the bulk of consumption. In D.J. Cattle and K.H. Schwerin (eds), *Food energy in tropical ecosystems.* New York, Gordon and Breach Publishers, pp. 65–82.

Wilson, M.E. 1995. Travel and the emergence of infectious diseases. *Emerging Infectious Diseases* 1(2): 39–46.

Wiseman, R. 1696. *Eight chirurgical treatises.* London, Tooke and Meredith.

Wolinsky, E. 1992. Mycobacterial diseases other than tuberculosis. *Clin. Infect, Dis.* 15: 1–12.

Wood, J.W., Milner, G.R., Harpending, H.C. and Weiss, K.M. 1992. The osteological paradox: problems of inferring prehistoric health from skeletal samples. *Curr. Anthrop.* 33(4): 343–70.

Woods, R. and Woodward, J. 1984. Mortality, poverty and the environment. In R. Woods and J. Woodward (eds), *Urban disease and mortality in 19th century England.* London, Batsford, pp. 19–36.

Woodward, M. and Walker, A.R.P. 1994. Sugar consumption and dental caries: evidence from 90 countries. *Br. Dent. J.* 176(8): 297–302.

Woolf, A.D. and St John Dixon, A. 1988. *Osteoporosis: a clinical guide.* London, Martin Dunitz.

World Health Organization 1997. *World health report.* Geneva, World Health Organization

World Health Organization 2000. *Weekly Epidemiological Record* 75: 226–32, 361–8.

Wright, L.E. and Schwarcz, H.P. 1998. Stable carbon and oxygen isotopes in human tooth enamel: identifying breastfeeding and weaning in prehistory. *Am. J. Phys. Anthrop.* 106: 1–18.

Wyatt, H.V. 1993. Poliomyelitis. In K. Kiple (ed.), *The Cambridge world history of human disease.* Cambridge, Cambridge University Press, pp. 942–50.

Zias, J. 2002. New evidence for the history of leprosy in the Ancient Near East: an overview. In C.A. Roberts, M.E. Lewis and K. Manchester (eds), *The past and present of leprosy: archaeological, historical, palaeopathological and clinical approaches.* British Archaeological Reports International Series 1054. Oxford, Archaeopress, pp. 259–68.

Zias, J. and Mitchell, P. 1996. Psoriatic arthritis in a fifth-century Judaean monastery. *Am. J. Phys. Anthrop.* 101: 491–502.

Zias, J. and Mumcuoglu, K. 1991. Pre-pottery Neolithic B headlice from Nahal Hemar Cave. *Atiquot (Jerusalem)* 20: 167–8.

Zias, J. and Numeroff, K. 1987. Operative dentistry in the 2nd century BC. *J. Am. Dental Assoc.* 114: 665–6.

Zias, J. and Pomeranz, S. 1992. Serial craniectomies for intracranial infection 5.5 millenia ago. *Int. J. Osteoarchaeology* 2: 183–6.

Zias, J. and Sekeles, E. 1985. The crucified man from Giv'at Ha-Mivtar. *Israel Exploration Soc.* 35: 22–7.

Zimmerman, M.R. 2000. The study of preserved human tissues. In D.R. Brothwell and A.M. Pollard (eds), *Handbook of archaeological sciences.* Chichester, John Wiley and Sons Ltd, 249–57.

Zimmerman, M.R. and Aufderheide, A.C. 1984. The frozen family of Utqiagvik: the autopsy findings. *Arctic Anthrop.* 21: 53–64.

Zimmerman, M.R., Yeatman, G.W. and Sprinz, H. 1971. Examination of an Aleutian mummy. *Bull. New York Acad. Med.* 47(1): 80–103.

Zink, A.R., Sola, C., Reschel, U., Grabner, W., Rastogi, N., Wolf, H. and Nerlich, A. 2003. Characterization of *Mycobacterium tuberculosis* complex DNAs by spoligotyping. *J. Clin. Microbiology* 41(1): 359–67.

Index

Page numbers in *italics* denote an illustration. Page numbers in **bold** denote a main reference to the subject.

Printed in the USA
CPSIA information can be obtained
at www.ICGtesting.com
LVHW081115081223
765863LV00007B/573